Empty Nose Syndrome

Empty Nose Syndrome
Evidence Based Proposals for Inferior Turbinate Management

Eugene Barton Kern

*George M. and Edna B. Endicott Professor of Medicine Emeritus,
Mayo Foundation for Medical Education and Research,
Rochester, Minnesota, United States*

*Professor, Rhinology and Facial Plastic Surgery Emeritus,
Mayo Clinic School of Medicine
Clinical Professor, Department of Otorhinolaryngology
Head and Neck Surgery, State University of New York (SUNY),
Buffalo, New York, United States*

*Director and Vice President, Gromo Foundation for Medical
Education and Research, Buffalo, New York, United States*

Oren Friedman

*Director, Facial Plastic Surgery,
Associate Professor,
Otorhinolaryngology Head & Neck Surgery,
University of Pennsylvania School of Medicine,
Philadelphia, Pennsylvania, United States*

ELSEVIER

Empty Nose Syndrome   ISBN: 978-0-443-10715-3

Publisher: Sarah Barth
Acquisitions Editor: Jessica L. McCool
Editorial Project Manager: Tracy I. Tufaga
Project Manager: Swapna Srinivasan
Cover Designer: Miles Hitchen

3251 Riverport Lane
St. Louis, Missouri 63043

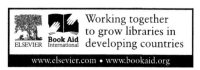

Working together to grow libraries in developing countries

www.elsevier.com • www.bookaid.org

For my darling wife Ruthie, our children, and grandchildren. Yours, mine, ours… evermore. EBK
To my family, whose love and encouragement empower me…everything I do, I do for you. OF

In large measure, this book is also dedicated to our patients, trusting that we will care for them with knowledge, integrity, and compassion for their well-being and happiness. Thus, it is our dedication.

Contents

Foreword...xi
Preface xiii
Acknowledgments... xvii

CHAPTER 1 Introduction and overview 1
   1 Introduction and overview 1
   2 Empty nose syndrome (ENS) in print media, TV; with ubiquity
      on the World Wide Web.. 7
   3 Nasal physiology: olfaction, breathing ("perfect nasal
      resistance"), internal nasal valve area, defensive
      immunoglobulins, cytokines plus T and B lymphocytes 21

CHAPTER 2 The scope of the empty nose syndrome (ENS).........33
   1 Definition: what is empty nose syndrome (ENS)?.....................33
   2 Symptoms of the empty nose syndrome (ENS).........................39
   3 Empty nose syndrome or atrophic rhinitis? A definition
      of terms..40
      3.1 Primary atrophic rhinitis 47
      3.2 Secondary atrophic rhinitis 49
      3.3 Differential diagnosis of nasal atrophy............................ 50
   4 Diagnosis of ENS..54
   5 Iatrogenic wonderland-etiology of ENS 56

**CHAPTER 3 Pathophysiology of the empty nose
           syndrome (ENS)** 57

CHAPTER 4 Treatment options for ENS 63
   1 Introduction 63
      1.1 Medical... 63
      1.2 Surgical.. 65
      1.3 Preventing ENS 67

CHAPTER 5 The turbinates—an overview................................69
   1 Historical perspective..69
   2 Turbinate anatomy...87
      2.1 Anatomy of the *middle turbinate* 87
      2.2 Anatomy of the *inferior turbinate*.................................. 88
   3 Physical examination 93
   4 Rhinologic evaluation with assessment tests and biopsy............95

CHAPTER 6   Brief history of evidence-based medicine—David Sackett, MD...97

CHAPTER 7   The turbinates—management..............................107
    1 Middle turbinate management 107
    2 Inferior turbinate management...117
        2.1 Classification: inferior turbinate enlargement ("hypertrophy")..117
        2.2 Turbinate reduction: surgical and nonsurgical procedures... 117

CHAPTER 8   How do you find the "Best Reduction Method" for inferior turbinate enlargement ("hypertrophy") reduction?...135
    1 A Context with Discussion of some specific critical confounding questions 135
        1.1 Randomized controlled trials searching for the "Best Reduction Method" from the literature.................136
        1.2 Future studies—designing the "Best Study" for finding the "Best Reduction Method".....................................137
        1.3 Thoughts for designing a "Best Study" for finding the "Best Reduction Method" for treating patients with inferior turbinate enlargement ("hypertrophy")...............138
        1.4 When are randomized controlled trials NOT needed?......139
        1.5 Asking answerable questions: empiricism versus rationalism..140
        1.6 Are controlled trials (RCTs) really needed? Can they actually be accomplished in a surgical setting?...............142
        1.7 Evidence first, but what to do when RCT data are limited, incomplete, inconclusive, conflicting, or starkly nonexistent? 144
        1.8 What are the influences of "placebo effects" in research and practice outcomes? 145
        1.9 What are the ethics of using placebos in *medicine*?.........147
       1.10 What are the ethics of using placebos in *surgery*?...........147
       1.11 *"Sham"* surgery, is there an ethical place for research surgical trials or is it forbidden? 149
       1.12 What are the limitations, if any, to the doctrine of randomized controlled trials?.................................. 151
       1.13 Is there an ethical approach to surgical and invasive procedures within randomized controlled trials?............. 153

1.14 What are the obligations and accountability to
     our patients regarding surgical *innovations*?................... 154
1.15 What are the CONSORT requirements and what's their
     importance for researchers and journals?....................... 155
1.16 What is propensity score matching all about?................ 157
1.17 What about using clinical practice guidelines and
     associated conflicts of interest?................................... 158
1.18 What about practice replacement, reversal,
     and the nature of medical progress? 165

CHAPTER 9   Children and inferior turbinate reduction 169

**CHAPTER 10   Medical journals: judging the quality of the editors,
               the peer reviewers, plus the issue
               of plagiarism** 175

CHAPTER 11   Review, finishing touches, and closure 181
     1 Managing the empty nose syndrome patient—summary........... 185
         1.1 Empty nose syndrome exists 185
         1.2 Pertinent nasal physiology 185
         1.3 Symptoms of ENS.. 186
         1.4 History and symptoms 188
         1.5 Nasal endoscopy 189
         1.6 Imaging... 189
         1.7 Testing in ENS 189
         1.8 Etiology of ENS 193
         1.9 Pathophysiology of ENS.. 194
         1.10 Preventing ENS 199
         1.11 Medical treatment of ENS 200
         1.12 Surgical treatment of ENS 204
     2 Evidence-based medicine—David Sackett, MD...................... 212
     3 Consolidated standards of reporting trials........................... 212
     4 Replacement or reversal of a medical practice....................... 213
     5 Managing middle turbinate enlargement.............................. 214
     6 Managing inferior turbinate enlargement ("hypertrophy") 215
         6.1 Evidence-based proposals.. 215
     7 Regarding children 218

8 Summary, future directions, and closing thoughts 219

    8.1 Summary... 219

    8.2 Medical management.. 221

    8.3 Surgical management 222

    8.4 Future directions.. 222

    8.5 Closing thoughts.. 227

Appendix 233

References... 239

Index 263

Foreword

When, in the middle and late 19th century, specialization in medicine started, rhinology gradually developed as a separate specialty and became part of the Triological Oto-Rhino-Laryngology. In the early years of the new specialty, various surgical procedures and new instruments were developed; among them were the surgical reduction and resection of the inferior and the middle turbinate. It soon turned out, however, that resecting parts of the turbinates had to be performed conservatively and with care as these structures play an essential role in nasal function. Even partial resection of those physiological important structures may lead to permanent complaints. Eugene B. Kern, Professor of Rhinology at the Mayo Clinics, was one of the first to stress the need to be careful and conservative in reducing the nasal turbinates. A too wide nasal cavity produces various permanent complaints, symptoms that were coined by him the "Empty Nose Syndrome." His lectures and writings about this syndrome have been of historical importance and have led to the awareness among otorhinolaryngologists to treat the nasal turbinates with care.

Egbert Huizing, MD, PhD
Professor Emeritus of The University
Medical Centre Utrecht, The Netherlands
Chair Department of Oto-Rhino-Laryngology, 1980-1998
Laren, The Netherlands
October 2022

Preface

Our goal with this text is to create an awareness of the *empty nose syndrome (ENS)* among physicians, surgeons, and patients.

After subject exploration, new understandings were realized allowing us to advocate treatment recommendations for patients with ENS, strategies for preventing ENS, and certain *evidenced-based proposals* for treating the turbinates, especially the inferior turbinates, so as to avoid ENS.

First, we validate our patients' experiences by broadcasting loudly that the *ENS* exists. Yes, it is a true clinical entity that frequently occurs subsequent to "excessive," *iatrogenic*, and "trauma" to turbinate tissue. The true incidence of ENS after therapeutic turbinate "trauma" is unknown, although with our experience, it is not as "rare" as some assume.

In 2020, on the ***American Rhinologic Society*** website, the following quotation appeared specifically speculating; suggesting that there are ***thousands of patients*** with the ***ENS***.

> *"The exact incidence of ENS is currently unknown. There are still **thousands** of patients experiencing ENS." (Bold italics added)*

Second, for us, the primary purpose for inferior turbinate surgery is to reduce nasal airway obstruction (improve breathing), all the while *preserving* nasal function and *preventing* the scourge of the ENS. To this end, we offer reflections regarding *evidence-based management* of breathing difficulty secondary to pathology of the inferior turbinate in both *adults* and *children*. Realize, from the literature and our own (anecdotal) experience, of performing "conservative" turbinate surgery that adding an *adequate* inferior turbinate out-fracture (lateralization), the ***nasal airway can be*** effectively *enlarged and maintained* (durable) for a "prolonged" period (time).[212,246–250,252,254]

Third, we condense and concentrate much of the known knowledge into this single "comprehensive" resource, so practitioners may review diagnosis, etiology, and treatment (medical and surgical) of this *underappreciated* syndrome (ENS) along with the risks associated with aggressive turbinate excision, especially when nasal physiology is often seemingly slighted so we offer a brief summary of the "latest" principle "purposes" of the human nose.

Ideally, all our clinical decisions should be based on evidence-based medicine (EBM), a subject that we review in this book, recognizing the supremacy of the randomized controlled trial (RCT); however, when data from a RCT are limited, incomplete, inconclusive, conflicting, or starkly nonexistent, there is no choice but to rely upon clinical reasoning, the rationalism of "clinical judgment," yet awareness of a possible flawed conclusion must always be kept in mind.[280]

The all-inclusive concept of EBM underscores the difference between ***decisions based on hard scientific evidence*** from well-designed and competent RCTs as ***opposed to decisions based on expert opinion.***

Recall that in 2013, Prasad et al., from the National Institute of Health (NIH), asserted that, "the reversal of established medical practice is common and occurs across all classes of medical practice." In fact, these investigators documented that 146 (40.2 %) of certain formerly "validated" established medical practices (they reviewed 2044 original articles) were reversed (discontinued); vexing is the unexpected realization that practices previously believed "rational" and "logical" were ultimately *proven to be flawed, useless or harmful.*[274]

As physicians and surgeons, all clinicians, we are duty-bound *"to do the best we can"* for our patients within the boundaries of prevailing knowledge, understanding that "good" medicine utilizes the current "best information available," allowing for "educated guesses," which is obviously subject to alteration, as medical dogmas and practices are subject to continuous change, corrections with amendments, adjustments, and improvements since that's the actual course of medical progress, the ever minting of a new and current *"approximate temporary truth."*[326]

As adroitly pointed out by Sergio Cocchei (2017) in his paper, *"Error, contradiction and reversal in science and medicine,"* the concept of *"approximate temporary truth"* was introduced by, the esteemed philosopher of science, Professor Sir Karl Raimund Popper (1902−1994). Professor Popper reflected on the temporal quality of "truth" since biomedical research and clinical practice have witnessed, as Prasad et al. (2013) has exposed, numerous examples of reversals and rejections of once dearly and "rationally" held beliefs.[274,326]

By definition, surgery is the medical practice of managing diseases, deformities, and injuries by actually "cutting" into a part of the body while, on the other hand, electrocautery, chemocautery, lasers, radiofrequency, coblation, or ultrasound is not surgery in the traditional "strict sense" of "cold knife" cutting, but nonetheless they are currently covered beneath the umbrella of "surgery," although we prefer to label them "nonsurgical" procedures.

We think that with a physiologic understanding, practitioners pursuing inferior turbinate reduction have an unambiguous obligation to preserve the pseudostratified epithelial mucociliary transport system, minimizing submucosal (lamina propria, stroma) neurovascular damage; thereby avoiding adverse physiologic penalties, with resultant sequelae, all the while improving nasal breathing function.

Consequently, in our opinion, "cold knife" techniques have the edge for now, *avoiding thermal trauma* as submucosal vascular choking fibrosis deprives the overlying epithelium with the necessary nutrition to maintain normal mucociliary transport; depriving the moisture necessary for charging the inspired air with heat and humidity; permitting optimal exchange of O_2-CO_2 at the alveolar level.

The final arbitrator, "Father Time," must "weigh in" before issuing a "final" adjudication (concrete guidelines) regarding turbinate surgery.

For "today" only, treatment options for the inferior turbinate are limited since guidelines from quality RCTs are presently *nonexistent for children, so* we offer our own *"approximate temporary truth."* For now, we suggest that submucosal resection (microdebrider-submucosal) and inferior turbinoplasty (*without* bony resection unless conchal enlargement) *with* out-fracture (lateralization) as the most rational current conservative surgical alternative, after failed medical therapy; suggested by Argenbright et al.[333] (2015) *for children*; reinforced by Passali et al.'s (1999, 2003) prospective randomized trial *in adults* ($N = 382$) with data collected before intervention and at *four years and six years* after intervention.[212,218]

For adults, with *evidence-based treatment proposals* in mind, it was Larrabee and Kacker[267] who reviewed five studies that they rated as level 1 evidence, prospective and randomized trials. These include the following notable *evidence-based treatment* contributions including: "cold knife" submucosal resection of inferior turbinate tissue (turbinoplasty), radiofrequency treatment, microdebrider-assisted turbinoplasty, and ultrasound turbinate reduction.[26,27,212,232,237]

The *evidence-based treatment proposal* for "surgical" management of the inferior turbinate(s) favored by Larrabee and Kacker[267] was the laudable paper presented by Passali et al. (1999, 2003) who reported on the randomized outcomes for all their *adult* patients ($N = 382$) having nasal airway obstruction, secondary to inferior turbinate enlargement ("hypertrophy") who were refractory ("failed") to medical management and treated with various procedures including: electrocautery, cryotherapy, laser cautery, submucosal resection *without* lateral displacement-out-fracture, submucosal resection *with* lateral displacement, and turbinectomy. They performed objective testing including rhinomanometry and acoustic rhinometry plus measuring mucociliary transport times and determining levels of secretory immunoglobulin A.[212,218]

And in the words of Passali et al.:

"These data indicate that submucosal resection with lateral displacement of the inferior turbinate results in the greatest increases in airflow and nasal respiratory function with the lowest risk of long-term complications." [212]

"After 6 years, only submucosal resection resulted in optimal long-term normalization of nasal patency and in restoration of mucociliary clearance and local secretory IgA production to a physiological level with few postoperative complications ($p < .001$)." [212]

As a consequence of these findings, Larrabee and Kacker[267] recommended Passali et al.'s *inferior turbinate submucosal resection (turbinoplasty) combined with out-fracture (lateral displacement)* as the *first-choice* technique for treating inferior turbinate enlargement ("hypertrophy").[212,218] This *inferior turbinate submucosal resection (turbinoplasty)* may be accomplished by either a "cold knife" or with a microdebrider.

We submit to you, our perspectives for your consideration, recognizing that our collective rhinologic knowledge was earned by the tangible experience of caring for countless thousands of rhinology patients and specifically treating more than 300 souls suffering with the *ENS*.

The Authors 2023

Acknowledgments

A very special appreciation goes to Monika Stenkvist Asplund, M.D., Ph.D. Associate Professor Emerita, Department of Otorhinolaryngology Head and Neck Surgery, Uppsala University, Uppsala, Sweden, who, with her extraordinary observational powers, as a visiting surgeon and scientist to the Mayo Clinic in 1994, was the first to say, "Dr. Kern, that nose looks empty." With that moniker, a syndrome begot a name.

The authors also acknowledge two indispensable colleagues, Joyce R. Mc Fadden, MLS, AHIP, Librarian and Julie A. Swenson, Interlibrary Loan Coordinator of the Mayo Clinic Libraries and Historical Unit, Rochester, Minnesota, who skillfully and with great alacrity, orchestrated the collection of over 300 original papers and books—some in French, others in Dutch and German—from the Mayo collection and by interlibrary loan; a most grateful thank you to you both; we could not have effectively accomplished this work without you.

It was the steady guiding hands of Tracy Tufaga, Editorial Project Manager, Swapna Srinivasan and Kiruthika Govindaraju Project Managers at Elsevier who "stewarded" us properly through the minefields of permissions, copyrights, and other assorted challenges before attaining the dream, a beautiful finished polished product, the "book." So, it is with great appreciation for all you quietly and competently did and do; we humbly offer one major magnificent thank you.

Additionally, this work was immeasurably enhanced by the knowledgeable assistance of Michael A. Hohberger, who provided effective editorial advice.

Moreover, we owe a great debt of gratitude to our teachers, colleagues, and students who collectively imbued in us the rank of absolute integrity, assertive curiosity, insistent skepticism, the virtue of conscientiousness, and a sublime compassion for the human condition and all that entails.

We are exceptionally appreciative that this work was partially funded by an educational grant from: The Gromo Foundation for Medical Education and Research, Buffalo, New York.
The Authors 2023

Data Sources

Materials for this book were identified by PubMed database, Medline, Google, Wikipedia, YouTube, and the lay press merging the literature searches up to and including January 1, 2023.

Review Methods

References were evaluated and chosen if they directly addressed aspects of nasal physiology, the *empty nose syndrome* (ENS) or indirectly discussed sequalae (side effects) of nasal procedures producing symptoms consistent with ENS including both surgical turbinate resections (complete, partial, and turbinoplasty procedures) and nonsurgical turbinate reduction adjunctive procedures (n-sTRAP) producing symptoms consistent with the protean symptoms seen in ENS. We searched for pertinent papers based on the guidance for conducting methodological reviews.[1] This type of review represents a distinct "literature synthesis method," and its methodology remains relatively underdeveloped. The eligibility criteria were limited to books and papers published, translated or referenced in the English language, although some papers were translated from the original language of publication.

It is possible that we may have unintentionally introduced a selection bias and regrettably, some important papers may have been inadvertently omitted. For this we, the authors, apologize.

Introduction and overview

1. Introduction and overview

Debate concluded, the *empty nose syndrome (ENS)* exists. ENS was initially recognized and formally presented to the profession by the Mayo Clinic team in 1994. With over a quarter of a century experience of treating hundreds of patients devastated by ENS, we reexamined the existing thinking concerning the etiology, differential diagnosis, diagnosis, treatment, and ultimately preventing this crippling disorder.

We found more than 60 specific citations exclusively for the *ENS* on the PubMed database. With our own, more than 300 ENS patients and conceivably countless others in the United States of America, feasibly approaching thousands globally including reports in the medical literature and on the World Wide Web from Africa, Canada, Chile, China, France, Germany, Israel, Italy, Korea, Malaysia, the Middle East, the Netherlands, Portugal, Russia, Spain, and Turkey posing the question, is ENS really a *rare* condition?

In 2020, on the **American Rhinologic Society** website, the following quotation appeared specifically speculating, suggesting that there are thousands of patients with the *ENS*.

> *"The exact incidence of ENS is currently unknown. There are still thousands of patients experiencing ENS."*

Moreover, the Internet is awash with numerous patient posts regarding their ENS symptoms along with support websites for the "postnasal surgery dysfunction community" including: https//www.change.org/emptynose, https://www.usasinus.org/empty-nose-syndrome and https://www.nasalcripple.com.

In this chapter, we offer an introduction and overview of the subject, ENS, highlighting subjects we will consider in detail with corresponding citations from the literature (broad bibliography of 376 references), besides providing complete commentary regarding the fundamental features of ENS along with a review of pertinent nasal physiology, a comprehensive differential diagnosis and an analysis of the various medical, surgical, and psychological treatment options for these desperately distraught patients, some of whom, have *committed suicide* because of their horrific torment.

Empty Nose Syndrome. https://doi.org/10.1016/B978-0-443-10715-3.00001-9

ENS is frequently initiated by an iatrogenic traumatic violation of the physiologic integrity of the nasal mucosa and submucosal structures of the turbinates inducing a *secondary atrophic rhinitis*. The nasal mucosa, "the organ of the nose," comparable to all human organ systems, has limits to its functional capacity before failure ensues; therefore, recommendations for both inferior and middle turbinate management to evade and prevent the calamity of ENS are considered and presented.

For example, apropos the middle turbinate, we champion saving it for both its physiological function and as a crucial anatomical landmark unless reduced or destroyed by polypoid disease concomitant to chronic rhinosinusitis, then removal of variable amounts of polypoid tissue is required along with the inadvertent and unintended concomitant turbinate tissue resection. Most unfortunately, since there is no hard scientific evidence, no evidence-based medicine (EBM) imperative of a randomized controlled trial (RCT), we awkwardly and regrettably must rely on the potentially biased and placebo effect prone possibilities of expert opinion.

Regarding the inferior turbinate, with today's "approximate temporary truth,"* the inferior turbinate should also be totally preserved at best; out-fracture (lateralization) is one of the non-surgical Turbinate Reduction Adjunctive Procedures (n-sTRAPs), as an attractive atraumatic alternative with some evidence if performed "adequately" can be very effective in maintaining a fixed lateral position contrary to and divergent from some citations in the literature.

*The term, **"approximate temporary truth,"** is from Professor Sir Karl Raimund Popper (1902—1994), the Austrian-British philosopher of science, from his 1959 book "The Logic of Scientific Discovery" Basic Books, Inc. New York translated from the German "Logik der Forschung" by the author with assistance of Dr. Julius Freed and Lan Freed. His assertions regarding science are extremely revealing: "Science is not a system of certain, or well-established statements; nor is it a system which steadily advances towards a state of finality. Our science is not knowledge (epistēmē): it can never claim to have attained truth, or even a substitute for it, such as probability. Yet science has more than mere biological survival value. It is not only a useful instrument. Although it can attain neither truth nor probability, do striving for knowledge and the search for truth are still the strongest motives of scientific discovery. We do not know: we can only guess." (Italics **not** added) Those lines are quoted directly and exactly from "The Logic of Scientific Discovery" page 278.

Specifically, surgery is: the medical practice of managing diseases, deformities, and injuries by actually "cutting" into a part of the body, while, on the other hand, electrocautery, chemocautery, lasers, radiofrequency, coblation, or ultrasound are not surgery in the traditional sense of cold knife "cutting," but nonetheless they are currently considered "surgery" by some authors, we choose to call these practices the **n**on-surgical **t**urbinate **r**eduction **a**djunctive **p**rocedures (n-sTRAPs).

If a more assertive surgical intervention to improve nasal breathing is required, then focus intervention exclusively at the inferior turbinate head (the posterior portion of the critical internal nasal valve area) as a very *limited submucosal micro-debrider turbinoplasty* that can be complemented with an inferior turbinate out-fracture (lateralization). With an affirming nod to **evidence based medicine (EBM)**, this strategy is supported by two papers, with level one evidence of a randomized controlled trial (RCT), from the literature.

Most assuredly, ***aggressive surgery*** to the lateral wall of the nose, including the middle and inferior turbinates, is indicated and *justified for inverting papilloma, juvenile angiofibroma, and a number of malignant disorders*, which may unfortunately also result in symptoms of the *ENS*.

Total inferior turbinectomy for inferior turbinate enlargement ("hypertrophy") has been **condemned** by a number of surgeons and baptized a **nasal crime** by two European academic authors with whom we are totally in agreement. We state unequivocally that **total inferior turbinectomy** for inferior turbinate enlargement ("hypertrophy") is a **nasal crime, especially in children without the benefit of a well-designed RCT or without future follow-up into the years of adulthood.**

Total inferior turbinectomy was trumpeted and supported by some surgeons on the "other side" of the divide who claimed they **never** observed the long-lasting signs and symptoms of persistent nasal airway obstruction, crusting, postoperative pain, and emotional issues including depression and anxiety seen in the multitude of *ENS* patients after total or near total (subtotal) inferior turbinectomy for inferior turbinate enlargement ("hypertrophy").

It is clear that the optimal turbinate management lies in **prevention** to avoid the catastrophic calamity of ENS. Unfortunately, it is unknown, at the present moment, as to the precise amount of nasal mucosa and submucosa that must be preserved during intranasal turbinate procedures to prevent ENS. Therefore, we should *always minimize* turbinate manipulation with attendant mucosal and submucosal damage whenever possible, especially radical excision of the turbinate(s) unless absolutely mandatory dictated by specific pathology as noted above.

The ideas behind EBM comes from the "father" of EBM, David Sackett, MD. EBM is primarily about discovery of the "best medical evidence," for crafting clinical choices, judgments, and rational therapeutic decisions in the best interest of the patient. The entire concept of EBM is the distinction between decisions based on **hard scientific evidence** from well-designed and competent RCTs as opposed to decisions **based on expert opinion**.

Unvalidated therapies need scrutiny with attempts at verification with proof before being embraced and approved as sensible and successful or discarded as useless or harmful. Proof is obtained through well-conceived and well-done RCTs, which avoid bias and are absolutely indispensable for intelligently comparing competing medical practices.

The time-honored bedrock of principled moral care of patients requires that **unvalidated care must not** be undertaken unless in a structured evidence-based RCT. The ideal double-blind placebo-controlled trial **cannot easily** be applied to surgical comparisons, but the optimal design of RCTs for surgery must be attempted nonetheless.

We believe that in well-done RCTs, ***blinding is possible*** for surgical and procedural studies when the operator remains "silent" as to his/her specific involvement with subjective and objective outcome studies performed by blinded evaluators-coded study.

With the emergence of EBM and its reliance on RCTs, it was soon recognized that the results of the RCTs were not generalizable, meaning that these RCTs results were not widely transferable from the broad trial study population to a specific unique individual surgical patient; therefore, surgeons lost their enthusiasm for the soul of EBM, the RCT.

As recently as 2015, it was determined that RCTs in the ENT literature are under 4% because they are difficult, regularly expensive, and at times ethically challenging to perform, and observational studies are utilized more frequently with a retrospective investigation to make connections concerning treatment effectiveness, which then can be followed by confirmatory studies.

CONSORT stands for, **CON**solidated **S**tandards **O**f **R**eporting **T**rials, which is a uniform method of reporting RCTs that markedly improve trial methodological construction thereby avoiding publishing flawed studies. CONSORT was developed to promote consistency, clarity, accuracy, and transparency of reporting of RCTs. Unfortunately, it was found as recently as 2015 that the reporting quality of ENT journals was considered ***"suboptimal"*** and could be improved especially by using the CONSORT requirements.

Propensity score matching (PSM), propensity score systems can be used in observational studies to decrease a confounding variable; an indication of bias. When performed with proper methodology using PSM, it is possible to obtain results that "approximate" a "randomized prospective study."

Clinical practice guidelines (CPGs) require authoritative judgments from various individuals, thereby potentially introducing bias and a possible conflict of interest (COI). When and if the data from RCTs are limited, incomplete, inconclusive, conflicting, or starkly nonexistent then contemporary CPGs and or advisories are often relied upon for an honest expert opinion as to how to proceed caring for a unique individual patient.

There are twofold reasons that medical therapies decline in approval and are no longer used:

(1) ***Replacement*** occurs when a practice is displaced by one that is ***better***.
(2) ***Reversal (discontinued)*** occurs when a practice is ***withdrawn*** when it is realized that the practice was never really successful or it was discovered to be harmful, it is then reversed. The solution to a ***reversal*** is finding the answer by RCTs. Preferably, questionable medical practices are replaced by better ones, based on strong and substantial comparative trials (RCTs) where new practices overtake older ones inaugurating novel canons and new standards of care. In fact, it is well-known that once "time-honored" medical and surgical practices are repeatedly ***reversed*** (***discontinued***), which is the nature of medical progress. In 2013, several investigators, in a 10-year review of the literature, found

146 (40.2%) verified and validated medical practices that were ***reversed***, no doubt, at first, those practices seemed logical and exquisitely rational when in fact they were ultimately flawed.

Medical journals are extremely influential voices in setting standards for accepting and adjudicating submitted research to accurately and unbiasedly update the profession. The unwritten covenant with peer reviewers and their editors is that they all act in the best interest of the profession, ultimately, for the best interest of the patient. Recently, in 2019, a comprehensive search for tools for determining the quality of peer review reports was undertaken. Assessors of the peer review process asked:

1. Is peer review: a flawed process at the heart of science and journals?
2. Who reviews the reviewers?
3. Editorial peer reviewers' recommendations at a general medical journal: are they reliable and do editors care?
4. Rereviewing peer review.
5. Peer review for biomedical publications: we can improve the system.
6. Make peer review scientific.
7. Custodians of high-quality science: are editors and peer reviewers good enough?

Realizing the need for validated tools that define the quality of peer-reviewed research reports, investigators found 24 tools: 23 scales and one checklist, which could define the quality of peer review reports. It was noted there was no single tool that defined the word "quality". They concluded that the contemporary tools available for assessing peer review quality are of questionable validity.

"Several tools are available to assess the quality of peer review reports; however, the development and validation process is questionable and the concepts evaluated by these tools vary widely."

Some studies have found that the peer reviewer's competence, especially in biostatistics, and overall capability to uncover errors and detect reporting deficiencies is unacceptably wanting. Other studies showed that the need is urgent for improving the quality of peer review reporting and for finding instruments (tools) for evaluating and improving the quality of those reports.

The consequences of the reviewer's findings are obviously critical, requiring astute interpretative rigor, comprehension and understanding of the scientific work, and an operational understanding of statistical analysis, so the editorial decision is scientifically justified. The outside investigators plan to survey journal editors and authors alike by initiating and managing an international online survey regarding the quality of peer reviewer's reports for developing new evaluation tools that can be used for appraising interventions aimed at improving the peer review process especially in the analysis of RCTs.

The first International Peer Review Congress was held approximately about 30 years ago and is still on going as in 2017, David Moher presented a plenary talk at the eighth International Congress on Peer Review and Scientific Publication (below) entitled: ***"Custodians of High-Quality Science: Are Editors and Peer Reviewers Good Enough?"*** https://www.youtube.com/watch?v=RV2tknDtyDs&t=454s.

According to several investigators, there has been an increase in plagiarism, deception, and malfeasance with falsification of data and inappropriate statistics in some recently published medical journals. We must all be alert to possible crimes and misdemeanors in the name of medical research, *never naïve please.*

Regarding children, we think, surgeons operating on the turbinates of children have an *explicit moral and ethical obligation to the follow, report, and publish on the trajectory* of these *children* as they passage into adulthood. Considering turbinate surgery in children, some responsible colleagues concluded that:

"There is currently little evidence to support turbinate reduction surgery in children. The role of surgery, if any, has not been properly examined. Furthermore, the long-term effects on nasal airflow dynamics, nasal physiology, and long-term complications remain to be studied."

Today, if pediatric surgery is indicated, some type of *"conservative"* turbinoplasty is the plausible treatment of choice, for those children failing the mandatory three month trial of intense medical management. Microdebrider submucosal inferior turbinoplasty (most often *without* bone resection) but with additional out-fracture (lateralization) of an inferior turbinate makes the most sense at this juncture without guidance from any RCTs. Until well-executed RCTs are available, we along with others *caution* the profession *not to remove* turbinates in children, since meager, if any, evidence exists supporting any type of turbinate reduction surgery in this population. A position that we unequivocally and wholeheartedly support despite journal reports of total inferior turbinectomies in children.

Ultimately, when considering any "new" innovative procedure or "reevaluation" of a current procedure, we think that it is necessary to inaugurate a formal approach for developing an RCT for bias elimination and placebo control, by creating an authorized ***research*** protocol to answer the question following the CONSORT statement. This applies to all future treatment approaches to the middle and inferior turbinates, except for the study by Professor Desiderio Passali and associates (n = 328), with an inferior turbinate RCT, followed and reported after four and six years, respectively, the profession still lacks confirming RCTs with long-term follow-up (measured in years) for both adults and children to avoid the tragic calamity of the ***"ENS."*** This importantly noteworthy study by Passali et al. is cited and discussed in detail later in the text.

Medicine utilizes the "best information available" at the time, allowing for "educated guesses," with rejections of once dearly held beliefs, which, of course, is always subject to change. We physicians and surgeons should tolerate "uncertainty" acknowledging the reality that medical theories and practices are subject to dislocation, disruption, and unceasing modification and improvements because that's the nature of medical and scientific advancement.

Since, according to Professor Sir Karl Raimund Popper's concept of "approximate temporary truth," as noted above, we cannot know *truth* and can only guess; therefore, we can only *approximate* the truth. The approximation of truth that holds authority today is only *temporary* because it may be replaced tomorrow by an alternative and superior "approximate temporary truth." This concept of "approximate temporary truth" powers the engine of scientific progress from leeches, purges, and bloodletting to antibiotics, DNA, deoxyribonucleic acid, proton beam therapy, and gene-editing, clustered regularly interspaced short palindromic repeats, (CRISPR) "genetic engineering".

2. Empty nose syndrome (ENS) in print media, TV; with ubiquity on the World Wide Web

Just as in the Dostoyevsky novel, *Crime and Punishment*, an individual surgeon faces a moral crisis after performing a *total turbinectomy*, subsequently realizing the tangible adverse consequences to the patient and eventually recoiling with disgust at the deed and experiences a titanic internal struggle with the horror and guilt for performing such an abhorrent surgical act.

We ask, can a profession collectively come face to face, with such a moral crisis, about performing a total inferior turbinectomy? What about "lesser" inferior turbinate procedures?

Long ago and not so far away at the University of Nebraska, in 1985, G. F. Moore and colleagues published, in the journal *The Laryngoscope*, their observations after an extended patient follow-up of 3−5 years, following total inferior turbinate resection, they ended their journal abstract with the subsequent two analytical critical, compelling sentences. "In this study, patients who had previously undergone total inferior turbinectomy were evaluated with the use of an extensive questionnaire. It confirms that total inferior turbinectomy carries significant morbidity and should be ***condemned***."[2] (Bold italics added)

Going beyond condemnation, Egbert Huizing and John de Groot, from the Netherlands, writing on page 300 of their well-received *Functional Reconstructive Nasal Surgery*, second edition 2015, Thieme Publishers, roared denunciation again, as in their first edition, 2003, that, ***"Total turbinectomy must be considered a nasal crime"***.[3,4] (Bold italics added)

The discussion of the ENS is no longer limited to arcane debates at obscure medical meetings or an occasional report in the literature of the occult. The ENS is now in the public domain and has been for some time. For instance, the ENS is in print media, with both the *LA Times*, circulation 650,000 and the *New York Post*, circulation 500,000:

Zitner, Adam (Los Angeles Times, May 10, 2001). *Sniffing at Empty Nose Idea.*

"SUFFOCATING"
THE NIGHTMARE OF EMPTY NOSE SYNDROME

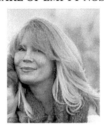

FIGURE 1.1

The patient stated that: "My nightmare condition makes me feel like I'm constantly suffocating". The story about *"Empty Nose Syndrome"* can be seen on YouTube: *A Condition Called **Empty Nose Syndrome** Left This Woman Struggling to Breathe.* https://youtu.be/QERIZS-XEC4 (71, 885 views as of October 1, 2022).

Cohen, Joyce (New York Post/Mirror.co.uk, July 15, 2018). *My nightmare condition makes me feel like I'm constantly suffocating.* Fig. 1.1.

An example of a computerized tomography (CT) scan in a patient exhibiting the common findings of the "ENS" can be seen in Fig. 1.2.

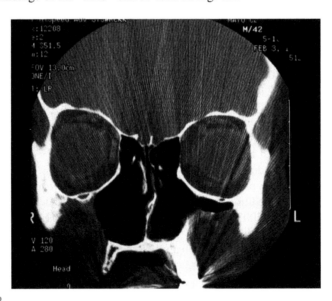

FIGURE 1.2

Coronal CT scan of a patient exhibiting the common findings seen in patients with the "***empty nose syndrome.***" There is a cavernous expansion of the intranasal airway with the absence of the lateral nasal walls and both inferior turbinates, which have been previously surgically resected (removed-not by a Mayo Clinic surgeon) after bilateral total inferior turbinectomies. The mucosa covering the right middle turbinate remnant is atrophic.
From: Moore EJ, Kern EB. Atrophic rhinitis: a review of 242 cases American Journal of Rhinology. 2001;15(6): 355–361. Note: we do not advocate total or subtotal turbinectomies for benign turbinate enlargement ("hyperplastic"). (By permission of Mayo Foundation for Medical Education and Research. All Rights Reserved).

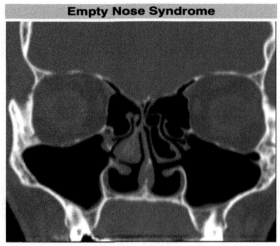

Empty Nose Syndrome

Altered nasal anatomy after bilateral subtotal inferior turbinectomy.

Empty nose syndrome

From Wikipedia, the free encyclopedia

FIGURE 1.3

From the free online encyclopedia https://en.wikipedia.org/wiki/Empty_nose_syndrome, an example of a CT scan of an **empty nose syndrome** patient with *"altered nasal anatomy after bilateral subtotal inferior turbinectomy."*

Additionally, ENS is now a prominent part of the Internet lexicon. A concise discussion of the "ENS" appears on the free online encyclopedia, https://www.Wikipedia.org along with an example of a CT scan of an ENS patient with *"altered nasal anatomy after bilateral subtotal inferior turbinectomy."* Fig. 1.3 from Wikipedia. Fig. 1.4 is the CT scan of a "normal" individual and a CT scan of an "ENS" patient seen in our practice.

If you commence a Google reference search for the ENS, you will be astonished and overwhelmed by more than 60 citations on Google and over 60 medical references on the PubMed database specifically with the term, ENS in the title of the medical paper, as of November 01, 2022. Table 1.1.

Furthermore, realize that the social media platform Facebook has an *Empty Nose Syndrome Forum,* while YouTube has over 40 videos with a tsunami of over 80,000 views including a segment devoted to the **empty nose syndrome** by the television hostess Megyn Kelly. (Bold italics added)

Megyn Kelly On the Today Show, NBC News. August 30, 2018.

A Condition Called Empty Nose Syndrome Left This Woman Struggling to Breathe. (Bold italics added)

https://youtu.be/QERIZS-XEC4.

(70,287 views as of August 2022)

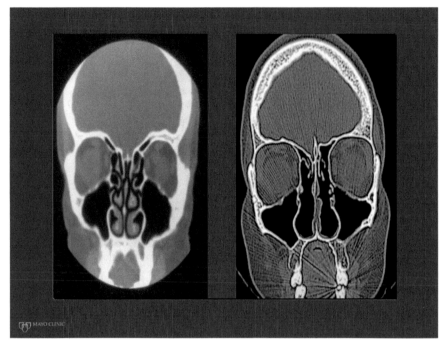

FIGURE 1.4

Coronal CT scan of a **"normal" individual** on the **left side**. Note the presence of a straight nasal septum, normal lateral nasal walls, and both middle and inferior turbinates along with well-aerated maxillary and ethmoid sinuses are present. On the **right side** is a coronal CT scan of an *"empty nose syndrome"* **patient** exhibiting the common findings seen in these patients. There is a cavernous expansion of the intranasal airway with the absence of both middle and inferior turbinates that have been previously surgically resected (removed-not by a Mayo Clinic surgeon) after a bilateral total middle and inferior turbinectomies. The ethmoid sinuses have been partially resected, and the majority of the lateral nasal wall is presently intact bilaterally. Note: we do not advocate total or subtotal turbinectomies for benign turbinate enlargement ("hyperplastic").

(Kern and Friedman. By permission of Mayo Foundation for Medical Education and Research. All Rights Reserved).

Oliphant J. Is the *empty nose* real? (Bold italics added) And if not, why are people killing themselves over it?

BuzzFeed.com April 14, 2016.

Brett Helling a *Suicide*. (Bold italics added)

Table 1.1 PubMed database references: *Empty nose syndrome* (ENS) in the title from 2001−November 1, 2022.

2022

1. Kanjanawasee D, Campbell RG, Rimmer J, Alvarado R, Kanjanaumporn J, Snidvongs K, Kalish L, Harvey RJ, Sacks R. *Empty nose syndrome* pathophysiology: a systematic review. Otolaryngol Head Neck Surg. 2022 Sep; 167(3):434−451. https://doi.org/10.1177/01945998211052919. Epub 2021 Oct 19. PMID: 34665687.
2. Huang CC, Wu PW, Lee CC, Chang PH, Huang CC, Lee TJ. Suicidal thoughts in patients with *empty nose syndrome*. Laryngoscope Investig Otolaryngol. 2022 Jan 19; 7(1):22−28. https://doi.org/10.1002/lio2.730. PMID: 35155779; PMCID: PMC8823180.
3. Lamb M, Bacon DR, Zeatoun A, Onourah P, Thorp BD, Abramowitz J, Ebert CS Jr, Kimple AJ, Senior BA. Mental health burden of *empty nose syndrome* compared to chronic rhinosinusitis and chronic rhinitis. Int Forum Allergy Rhinol. 2022 Mar 25. https://doi.org/10.1002/alr.22997. Epub ahead of print. PMID: 35333009.
4. Huang CC, Wu PW, Chuang CC, Lee CC, Lee YS, Chang PH, Fu CH, Huang CC, Lee TJ. Identifying obstructive sleep apnoea in patients with *empty nose syndrome*. Diagnostics (Basel). 2022 Jul 15; 12(7):1720. https://doi.org/10.3390/diagnostics12071720. PMID: 35885624; PMCID: PMC9323833.
5. Hosokawa Y, Miyawaki T, Omura K, Akutsu T, Kimura R, Ikezono T, Otori N. Surgical treatment for *empty nose syndrome* using autologous dermal fat: evaluation of symptomatic improvement. Ear Nose Throat J. 2022 Sep 29:1455613221130885. https://doi.org/10.1177/01455613221130885. Epub ahead of print. PMID: 36174975.
6. Chang MT, Bartho M, Kim D, Tsai EF, Yang A, Dholakia SS, Khanwalkar A, Rao VK, Thamboo A, Lechner M, Nayak JV. Inferior meatus augmentation procedure (IMAP) for treatment of *empty nose syndrome*. Laryngoscope. 2022 Jun; 132(6):1285−1288. https://doi.org/10.1002/lary.30001. Epub 2022 Jan 24. PMID: 35072280.
7. Huang CC, Wu PW, Lee YS, Huang CC, Chang PH, Fu CH, Lee TJ. Impact of sleep dysfunction on psychological burden in patients with *empty nose syndrome*. Int Forum Allergy Rhinol. 2022 Jun 5. https://doi.org/10.1002/alr.23040. Epub ahead of print. PMID: 35665478.
8. Piazza F. In reference to inferior meatus augmentation procedure (IMAP) for treatment of *empty nose syndrome*. Laryngoscope. 2022 Jun; 132(6):E21. https://doi.org/10.1002/lary.30118. Epub 2022 Apr 2. PMID: 35366012.
9. Lindemann J, Goldberg-Bockhorn E, Stupp F, Scheithauer M, Sieron HL, Hoffmann TK, Sommer F, Zimmermann L. Erstellung einer deutschen Version des *empty nose syndrome* 6 item questionnaire "(ENS6Q) [Adaption of the "Empty Nose 6 Item Questionnaire" (ENS6Q) into German language]. Laryngorhinootologie. 2022 May 18. German. https://doi.org/10.1055/a-1841-6542. Epub ahead of print. PMID: 35584746.
10. Chang MT, Nayak JV. In response to inferior meatus augmentation procedure (IMAP) for treatment of *empty nose syndrome*. Laryngoscope. 2022 Jun; 132(6):E22. https://doi.org/10.1002/lary.30119. Epub 2022 Apr 2. PMID: 35366011.
11. Maul X, Thamboo A. The clinical effect of psychosomatic interventions on *empty nose syndrome* secondary to turbinate-sparing techniques: A prospective self-controlled study. Int Forum Allergy Rhinol. 2021 May; 11(5):955−956. https://doi.org/10.1002/alr.22724. Epub 2020 Nov 5. PMID: 33151623.

Continued

Table 1.1 PubMed database references: *Empty nose syndrome* (ENS) in the title from 2001–November 1, 2022.—*cont'd*

2021

1. Law RH, Ahmed AM, Van Harn M, Craig JR. Middle turbinate resection is unlikely to cause *empty nose syndrome* in first year postoperatively. Am J Otolaryngol. 2021 Jan 26; 42(4):102,931. https://doi.org/10.1016/j.amjoto.2021.102931. Epub ahead of print. PMID: 33550027.

2. Wu CL, Fu CH, Lee TJ. Distinct histopathology characteristics in *empty nose syndrome*. Laryngoscope. 2021 Jan; 131(1):E14-E18. https://doi.org/10.1002/lary.28586. Epub 2020 Mar 3. PMID: 32125703.

3. Chang FY, Fu CH, Lee TJ. Outcomes of olfaction in patients with *empty nose syndrome* after submucosal implantation. Am J Otolaryngol. 2021 Feb 18; 42(4):102,989. https://doi.org/10.1016/j.amjoto.2021.102989. Epub ahead of print. PMID: 33676069.

4. Kim CH, Kim J, Song JA, Choi GS, Kwon JH. The degree of stress in patients with *empty nose syndrome*, compared with chronic rhinosinusitis and allergic rhinitis. Ear Nose Throat J. 2021 Feb; 100(2):NP87-NP92. https://doi.org/10.1177/0145561319858912. Epub 2019 Jul 4. PMID: 31272211.

5. Huang CC, Wu PW, Fu CH, Huang CC, Chang PH, Lee TJ. Impact of psychologic burden on surgical outcome in *empty nose syndrome*. Laryngoscope. 2021 Mar; 131(3):E694-E701. https://doi.org/10.1002/lary.28845. Epub 2020 Jul 21. PMID: 32692881.

6. Wu CL, Fu CH, Lee TJ. In response to distinct histopathology characteristics in *empty nose syndrome*. Laryngoscope. 2021 Apr; 131(4):E1039. https://doi.org/10.1002/lary.29183. Epub 2021 Jan 18. PMID: 33459370.

7. Salzano FA, Vaira LA, Maglitto F, Mesolella M, De Riu G. In reference to distinct histopathology characteristics in *empty nose syndrome*. Laryngoscope. 2021 Apr; 131(4):E1038. https://doi.org/10.1002/lary.29181. Epub 2021 Jan 18. PMID: 33459372.

8. Gordiienko IM, Gubar OS, Sulik R, Kunakh T, Zlatskiy I, Zlatska A. *Empty nose syndrome* pathogenesis and cell-based biotechnology products as a new option for treatment. World J Stem Cells. 2021 26; 13(9):1293–1306. https://doi.org/10.4252/wjsc.v13.i9.1293. PMID: 34630863; PMCID: PMC8474723.

9. La Rosa R, Passali D, Passali GC, Ciprandi G. A practical classification of the *empty nose syndrome*. J Biol Regul Homeost Agents. 2021 Jan–Feb; 35(1 Suppl. 2):51–54. https://doi.org/10.23812/21-1supp2-10. PMID: 33982539.

10. Chang CF. Using platelet-rich fibrin scaffolds with diced cartilage graft in the treatment of *empty nose syndrome*. Ear Nose Throat J. 2021 Sep 25:1455613211045567. https://doi.org/10.1177/01455613211045567. Epub ahead of print. PMID: 34569297.

11. Dholakia SS, Yang A, Kim D, Borchard NA, Chang MT, Khanwalkar A, Lechner M, Nayak JV. Long-term outcomes of inferior meatus augmentation procedure to treat *empty nose syndrome*. Laryngoscope. 2,021,131(11):E2736-E2741. https://doi.org/10.1002/lary.29593. Epub 2021 May 15. PMID: 33991117.

12. Fu CH, Chen HC, Huang CC, Chang PH, Lee TJ. Serum high-sensitivity C-reactive protein is associated with postoperative psychiatric status in patients with *empty nose syndrome*. Diagnostics (Basel). 2021 Dec 18; 11(12):2388. https://doi.org/10.3390/diagnostics11122388. PMID: 34943627; PMCID: PMC8700485.

Table 1.1 PubMed database references: *Empty nose syndrome* (ENS) in the title from 2001–November 1, 2022.—*cont'd*

13. Amanian A, Hari K, Habib AR, Dholakia SS, Nayak J, Thamboo A. The *empty nose syndrome* 6-item questionnaire (ENS6Q): a diagnostic tool to distinguish *empty nose syndrome* from primary nasal obstruction. Int Forum Allergy Rhinol. 2021 Jul; 11(7): 1113–1115. https://doi.org/10.1002/alr.22761. Epub 2021 Jan 18. PMID: 33460303.

14. Tian P, Hu J, Ma Y, Zhou C, Liu X, Dang H, Zou H. The clinical effect of psychosomatic interventions on *empty nose syndrome* secondary to turbinate-sparing techniques: a prospective self-controlled study. Int Forum Allergy Rhinol. 2021 Jun; 11(6):984–992. https://doi.org/10.1002/alr.22726. Epub 2020 Nov 5. PMID: 33151634.

15. Maul X, Thamboo A. The clinical effect of psychosomatic interventions on *empty nose syndrome* secondary to turbinate-sparing techniques: A prospective self-controlled study. Int Forum Allergy Rhinol. 2021 May; 11(5):955–956. https://doi.org/10.1002/alr.22724. Epub 2020 Nov 5. PMID: 33151623.

16. Malik J, Dholakia S, Spector BM, Yang A, Kim D, Borchard NA, Thamboo A, Zhao K, Nayak JV. Inferior meatus augmentation procedure (IMAP) normalizes nasal airflow patterns in *empty nose syndrome* patients via computational fluid dynamics (CFD) modeling. Int Forum Allergy Rhinol. 2021 May; 11(5):902–909. https://doi.org/10.1002/alr.22720. Epub 2020 Nov 29. PMID: 33249769; PMCID: PMC8062271.

17. Hassan CH, Malheiro E, Béquignon E, Coste A, Bartier S. Sublabial bioactive glass implantation for the management of primary atrophic rhinitis and *empty nose syndrome*: operative technique. Laryngoscope Investig Otolaryngol. 2021 Dec 8; 7(1):6–11. https://doi.org/10.1002/lio2.713. PMID: 35155777; PMCID: PMC8823167.

2020

1. Gill AS, Said M, Tollefson TT, Strong EB, Nayak JV, Steele TO. Patient-reported outcome measures and provocative testing in the workup of *empty nose syndrome*-advances in diagnosis: a systematic review. Am J Rhinol Allergy. 2020 Jan; 34(1):134–140. https://doi.org/10.1177/1945892419880642. Epub 2019 Oct 8. PMID: 31594386.

2. Tranchito E, Chhabra N. Rhinotillexomania manifesting as *empty nose syndrome*. Ann Otol Rhinol Laryngol. 2020 Jan; 129(1):87–90. https://doi.org/10.1177/0003489419870832. Epub 2019 Aug 16. PMID: 31416334.

3. Patel P, Most SP. Functionally crippled nose. Facial Plast Surg. 2020 Feb; 36(1):66–71. doi:10.55/s-0040-1701488. Epub 2020 Mar 19. PMID: 32191961. (Bold italics ours) Note: This paper is one of 3 exceptions but is included in this Table 1 since the authors stated: "A variety of surgical interventions can also result in a functionally crippled nose and diagnoses including nasal valve stenosis, septal perforations, and *empty nose syndrome* are discussed."

4. Le Bon SD, Horoi M, Le Bon O, Hassid S. Intranasal trigeminal training in *empty nose syndrome*: a pilot study on 14 patients. Clin Otolaryngol. 2020 Mar; 45(2):259–263. https://doi.org/10.1111/coa.13483. Epub 2019 Dec 11. PMID:31777150.

5. Thamboo A, Dholakia SS, Borchard NA, Patel VS, Tangbumrungtham N, Velasquez N, Huang Z, Zarabanda D, Nakayama T, Nayak JV. Inferior meatus augmentation procedure (IMAP) to treat *empty nose syndrome*: a pilot study. Otolaryngol Head Neck Surg. 2020 Mar; 162(3):382–385. https://doi.org/10.1177/0194599819900263. Epub 2020 Jan 14. PMID: 31935161.

Continued

Table 1.1 PubMed database references: *Empty nose syndrome* (ENS) in the title from 2001–November 1, 2022.—*cont'd*

6. Malik J, Thamboo A, Dholakia S, Borchard NA, McGhee S, Li C, Zhao K, Nayak JV. The cotton test redistributes nasal airflow in patients with *empty nose syndrome*. Int Forum Allergy Rhinol. 2020 Apr; 10(4):539–545. https://doi.org/10.1002/alr.22489. Epub 2020 Jan 17. PMID: 31951101; PMCID: PMC7182493.

7. Malik J, Dholakia S, Spector BM, Yang A, Kim D, Borchard NA, Thamboo A, Zhao K, Nayak JV. Inferior meatus augmentation procedure (IMAP) normalizes nasal airflow patterns in *empty nose syndrome* patients via computational fluid dynamics (CFD) modeling. Int Forum Allergy Rhinol. 2020 Nov 29. https://doi.org/10.1002/alr.22720. Epub ahead of print. PMID: 33249769.

8. Maul X, Thamboo A. The clinical effect of psychosomatic interventions on *empty nose syndrome* secondary to turbinate-sparing techniques: A prospective self- controlled study. Int Forum Allergy Rhinol. 2020 Nov 5. https://doi.org/10.1002/alr.22724. Epub ahead of print. PMID: 33151623.

9. Tian P, Hu J, Ma Y, Zhou C, Liu X, Dang H, Zou H. The clinical effect of psychosomatic interventions on *empty nose syndrome* secondary to turbinate-sparing techniques: a prospective self-controlled study. Int Forum Allergy Rhinol. 2020 Nov 5. https://doi.org/10.1002/alr.22726. Epub ahead of print. PMID: 33151634.

2019

1. Maza G, Li C, Krebs JP, Otto BA, Farag AA, Carrau RL, Zhao K. Computational fluid dynamics after endoscopic endonasal skull base surgery-possible *empty nose syndrome* in the context of middle turbinate resection. Int Forum Allergy Rhinol. 2019 Feb; 9(2):204–211. https://doi.org/10.1002/alr.22236. Epub 2018 Nov 29. PMID: 30488577; PMCID: PMC6358472.

2. Alnæs M, Andreassen BS. Osteomyelitis after radiofrequency turbinoplasty. Tidsskr nor Laegeforen. 2019 May 16; 139(9). Norwegian, English. https://doi.org/10.4045/tidsskr.18.0843. PMID: 31140260. Note: One patient developed *"empty nose syndrome"*

3. Borchard NA, Dholakia SS, Yan CH, Zarabanda D, Thamboo A, Nayak JV. Use of intranasal submucosal fillers as a transient implant to alter upper airway aerodynamics: implications for the assessment of *empty nose syndrome*. Int Forum Allergy Rhinol. 2019 Jun; 9(6):681–687. https://doi.org/10.1002/alr.22299. Epub 2019 Feb 4. PMID: 30715801.

4. Manji J, Patel VS, Nayak JV, Thamboo A. Environmental triggers associated with *empty nose syndrome* symptoms: a cross-sectional study. Ann Otol Rhinol Laryngol. 2019 Jul; 128(7):601–607. https://doi.org/10.1177/0003489419833714. Epub 2019 Feb 28. PMID: 30818962.

5. Gill AS, Said M, Tollefson TT, Steele TO. Update on *empty nose syndrome*: disease mechanisms, diagnostic tools, and treatment strategies. Curr Opin Otolaryngol Head Neck Surg. 2019 Aug; 27(4):237–242. https://doi.org/10.1097/MOO.0000000000000544. PMID: 31116142.

6. Fu CH, Wu CL, Huang CC, Chang PH, Chen YW, Lee TJ. Nasal nitric oxide in relation to psychiatric status of patients with *empty nose syndrome*. Nitric Oxide. 2019 Nov 1; 92:55–59. https://doi.org/10.1016/j.niox.2019.07.005. Epub 10. PMID: 31408674.

7. Talmadge J, Nayak JV, Yao W, Citardi MJ. Management of postsurgical *empty nose syndrome*. Facial Plast Surg Clin North Am. 2019 Nov; 27 (4):465–475. https://doi.org/10.1016/j.fsc.2019.07.005. PMID: 31587766.

8. Huang CC, Wu PW, Fu CH, Huang CC, Chang PH, Wu CL, Lee TJ. What drives depression in *empty nose syndrome*? a sinonasal outcome test-25 subdomain analysis. Rhinology. 2019 Dec 1; 57(6):469–476. https://doi.org/10.4193/Rhin19.085. PMID: 31502597.

Table 1.1 PubMed database references: *Empty nose syndrome* (ENS) in the title from 2001–November 1, 2022.—*cont'd*

2018

1. Li C, Farag AA, Maza G, McGhee S, Ciccone MA, Deshpande B, Pribitkin EA, Otto BA, Zhao K. Investigation of the abnormal nasal aerodynamics and trigeminal functions among *empty nose syndrome* patients. Int Forum Allergy Rhinol. 2018 Mar; 8(3): 444–452. https://doi.org/10.1002/alr.22045. Epub 2017 Nov 22. PMID: 29165896; PMCID: PMC6015742.

2. Lee TJ, Fu CH, Wu CL, Lee YC, Huang CC, Chang PH, Chen YW, Tseng HJ. Surgical outcome for *empty nose syndrome*: impact of implantation site. Laryngoscope. 2018 Mar; 128(3):554–559. https://doi.org/10.1002/lary.26769. Epub 2017 Jul 17. PMID: 28714537.

3. Tan NC, Goggin R, Psaltis AJ, Wormald PJ. Partial resection of the middle turbinate during endoscopic sinus surgery for chronic rhinosinusitis does not lead to an increased risk of *empty nose syndrome*: a cohort study of a tertiary practice. Int Forum Allergy Rhinol. 2018 Apr 6. https://doi.org/10.1002/alr.22127. Epub ahead of print. PMID: 29633570.

4. Dzhenkov DL, Stoyanov GS, Georgiev R, Sapundzhiev N. Histopathological findings in an unclassifiable case of *empty nose syndrome* with long-term follow-up. Cureus. 2018 May 20; 10(5):e2655. https://doi.org/10.7759/cureus.2655. PMID: 30042906; PMCID: PMC6054367.

5. Manji J, Nayak JV, Thamboo A. The functional and psychological burden of *empty nose syndrome*. Int Forum Allergy Rhinol. 2018 Jun; 8(6):707–712. https://doi.org/10.1002/alr.22097. Epub 2018 Feb 14. PMID: 29443458.

6. Kim DY, Hong HR, Choi EW, Yoon SW, Jang YJ. Efficacy and safety of autologous stromal vascular fraction in the treatment of *empty nose syndrome*. Clin Exp Otorhinolaryngol. 2018 Dec; 11(4):281–287. https://doi.org/10.21053/ceo.2017.01634. Epub 2018 May 16. PMID: 29764011; PMCID: PMC6222192.

2017

1. Velasquez N, Thamboo A, Habib AR, Huang Z, Nayak JV. The *empty nose syndrome* 6-item questionnaire (ENS6Q): a validated 6-item questionnaire as a diagnostic aid for *empty nose syndrome* patients. Int Forum Allergy Rhinol. 2017 Jan; 7(1):64–71. https://doi.org/10.1002/alr.21842. Epub 2016 Aug 24. PMID: 27557473.

2. Konstantinidis I, Tsakiropoulou E, Chatziavramidis A, Ikonomidis C, Markou K. Intranasal trigeminal function in patients with *empty nose syndrome*. Laryngoscope. 2017 Jun; 127(6):1263–1267. https://doi.org/10.1002/lary.26491. Epub 2017 Feb 22. PMID: 28224626.

3. Li C, Farag AA, Leach J, Deshpande B, Jacobowitz A, Kim K, Otto BA, Zhao K. Computational fluid dynamics and trigeminal sensory examinations of *empty nose syndrome* patients. Laryngoscope. 2017 Jun; 127(6):E176-E184. https://doi.org/10.1002/lary.26530. Epub 2017 Mar 9. PMID: 28278356; PMCID: PMC5445013.

4. Thamboo A, Velasquez N, Habib AR, Zarabanda D, Paknezhad H, Nayak JV. Defining surgical criteria for *empty nose syndrome*: Validation of the office-based cotton test and clinical interpretability of the validated *empty nose syndrome* 6-item questionnaire. Laryngoscope. 2017 Aug; 127(8):1746–1752. https://doi.org/10.1002/lary.26549. Epub 2017 Mar 27. PMID: 28349563.

Continued

Table 1.1 PubMed database references: *Empty nose syndrome* (ENS) in the title from 2001–November 1, 2022.—*cont'd*

5. Mangin D, Bequignon E, Zerah-Lancner F, Isabey D, Louis B, Adnot S, Papon JF, Coste A, Boyer L, Devars du Mayne M. Investigating hyperventilation syndrome in patients suffering from *empty nose syndrome*. Laryngoscope. 2017 Sep; 127(9):1983–88. https://doi.org/10.1002/lary.26599. Epub 2017 Apr 13. PMID: 28407251.
6. Balakin BV, Farbu E, Kosinski P. Aerodynamic evaluation of the *empty nose syndrome* by means of computational fluid dynamics. Comput Methods Biomech Biomed Engin. 2017 Nov; 20(14):1554–1561. https://doi.org/10.1080/10255842. 2017.1385779. Epub 2017 Oct 24. PMID: 29064287.
7. Ma ZX, Quan-Zeng, Jie-Liu, Hu GH. Assessment of postsurgical outcomes between different implants in patients with *empty nose syndrome*: a meta-analysis. J Int Med Res. 2017 Dec; 45(6):1939–1948. https://doi.org/10.1177/0300060517715167. Epub 2017 Nov 3. PMID: 29098901; PMCID: PMC5805217.

2016

1. Hong HR, Jang YJ. Correlation between remnant inferior turbinate volume and symptom severity of *empty nose syndrome*. Laryngoscope. 2016 Jun; 126(6): 1290–1295. https://doi.org/10.1002/lary.25830. Epub 2015 Dec 21. PMID: 26692010.
2. Lee TJ, Fu CH, Wu CL, Tam YY, Huang CC, Chang PH, Chen YW, Wu MH. Evaluation of depression and anxiety in *empty nose syndrome* after surgical treatment. Laryngoscope. 2016 Jun; 126(6):1284–1289. https://doi.org/10.1002/lary.25814. Epub2015 Dec 15. PMID: 26667794.
3. Shah K, Guarderas J, Krishnaswamy G. *Empty nose syndrome* and atrophic rhinitis. Ann Allergy Asthma Immunol. 2016 Sep; 117(3):217–220. https://doi.org/10.1016/j. anai.2016.07.006. PMID: 27613452.
4. Thamboo A, Velasquez N, Ayoub N, Nayak JV. Distinguishing computed tomography findings in patients with *empty nose syndrome*. Int Forum Allergy Rhinol. 2016 Oct; 6(10):1075–1082. https://doi.org/10.1002/alr.21774. Epub 2016 Jul 13. PMID: 27409044.

2015

1. Sozansky J, Houser SM. Pathophysiology of *empty nose syndrome*. Laryngoscope. 2015 Jan; 125(1):70–74. https://doi.org/10.1002/lary.24813. Epub 2014 Jun 30. PMID: 24978195.
2. Kuan EC, Suh JD, Wang MB. *Empty nose syndrome*. Curr Allergy Asthma Rep. 2015 Jan; 15(1):493. https://doi.org/10.1007/s11882-014-0493-x. PMID: 25430954.
3. Lemogne C, Consoli SM, Limosin F, Bonfils P. Treating *empty nose syndrome* as a somatic symptom disorder. Gen Hosp Psychiatry. 2015 May–Jun; 37(3):273.e9–10. https://doi.org/10.1016/j.genhosppsych.2015.02.005. Epub 2015 Feb 25. PMID: 25754986.
4. Leong SC. The clinical efficacy of surgical interventions for *empty nose syndrome*: a systematic review. Laryngoscope. 2015 Jul; 125(7):1557–1562. https://doi.org/10. 1002/lary.25170. Epub 2015 Feb 3. PMID: 25647010.
5. Chang AA, Watson D. Inferior turbinate augmentation with auricular cartilage for the treatment of *empty nose syndrome*. Ear Nose Throat J. 2015 Oct–Nov; 94(10–11): E14–E15. PMID: 26535824.

Table 1.1 PubMed database references: *Empty nose syndrome* (ENS) in the title from 2001–November 1, 2022.—*cont'd*

6. Velasquez N, Huang Z, Humphreys IM, Nayak JV. Inferior turbinate reconstruction using porcine small intestine submucosal xenograft demonstrates improved quality of life outcomes in patients with *empty nose syndrome*. Int Forum Allergy Rhinol. 2015 Nov; 5(11):1077–1081. https://doi.org/10.1002/alr.21633. Epub 2015 Sep 2. PMID: 26332403.

2014

1. Tam YY, Lee TJ, Wu CC, Chang PH, Chen YW, Fu CH, Huang CC. Clinical analysis of submucosal medpor implantation for *empty nose syndrome*. Rhinology. 2014 Mar; 52(1):35–40. https://doi.org/10.4193/Rhin13.086. PMID: 24618626.
2. Jiang C, Wong F, Chen K, Shi R. Assessment of surgical results in patients with *empty nose syndrome* using the 25-item sino-nasal outcome test evaluation. JAMA Otolaryngol Head Neck Surg. 2014 May; 140(5):453–458. https://doi.org/10.1001/jamaoto.2014.84. PMID: 24626391.

2013

1. Saafan ME. Acellular dermal (alloderm) grafts versus silastic sheets implants for management of *empty nose syndrome*. Eur Arch Otorhinolaryngol. 2013 Feb; 270(2): 527–533. doi:10.1007/s00405-012-1955-1. Epub 2012 Apr 19. PMID: 22526572.
2. Bastier PL, Bennani-Baiti AA, Stoll D, de Gabory L. β-Tricalcium phosphate implant to repair *empty nose syndrome*: preliminary results. Otolaryngol Head Neck Surg. 2013 Mar; 148(3):519–522. https://doi.org/10.1177/0194599812472436. Epub 2013 Jan 8. PMID: 23300225.
3. Jiang C, Shi R, Sun Y. Study of inferior turbinate reconstruction with Medpor for the treatment of *empty nose syndrome*. Laryngoscope. 2013 May; 123(5):1106–1111. https://doi.org/10.1002/lary.23908. Epub 2012 Dec 3. PMID: 23208803.
4. Jung JH, Baguindali MA, Park JT, Jang YJ. Costal cartilage is a superior implant material than conchal cartilage in the treatment of *empty nose syndrome*. Otolaryngol Head Neck Surg. 2013 Sep; 149(3):500–5005. https://doi.org/10.1177/0194599813491223. Epub 2013 May 31. PMID: 23728068.
5. Di MY, Jiang Z, Gao ZQ, Li Z, An YR, Lv W. Numerical simulation of airflow fields in two typical nasal structures of *empty nose syndrome*: a computational fluid dynamics study. PLoS One. 2013 Dec 18; 8(12):e84243. https://doi.org/10.1371/journal.pone.0084243. PMID: 24367645; PMCID: PMC3867489.

2012

1. Coste A, Dessi P, Serrano E. *Empty nose syndrome*. Eur Ann Otorhinolaryngol Head Neck Dis. 2012 Apr; 129(2):93–97. https://doi.org/10.1016/j.anorl.2012.02.001. Epub 2012 Apr 16. PMID: 22513047.
2. Di MY, Gao ZQ, Lü W. [Research progress in *empty nose syndrome*]. Zhonghua Er Bi Yan Hou Tou Jing Wai Ke Za Zhi. 2012 Oct; 47(10):873–876. Chinese. PMID: 23302177.

Continued

Table 1.1 PubMed database references: ***Empty nose syndrome*** (ENS) in the title from 2001−November 1, 2022.—*cont'd*

2011

1. Hildenbrand T, Weber RK, Brehmer D. Rhinitis sicca, dry nose and atrophic rhinitis: a review of the literature. Eur Arch Otorhinolaryngol. 2011 Jan; 268(1):17−26. doi: 10.1007/s00405-010-1391-z. Epub 2010 Sep 29. PMID: 20878413. Note: This is the 2nd of 3 exceptions but since in this abstract it is stated as follows: "Since the uncritical resection of the nasal turbinates is a significant and frequent factor in the genesis of dry nose, secondary RA and **ENS (empty nose syndrome)** (definition of abbreviation of ENS added), the inferior and middle turbinate should not be resected without adequate justification, and the simultaneous removal of both should not be done other than for a malignant condition."

2. Modrzyński M. Hyaluronic acid gel in the treatment of ***empty nose syndrome***. Am J Rhinol Allergy. 2011 Mar−Apr; 25(2):103−106. https://doi.org/10.2500/ajra.2011.25.3577. PMID: 21679513.

3. Jang YJ, Kim JH, Song HY. ***Empty nose syndrome***: radiologic findings and treatment outcomes of endonasal microplasty using cartilage implants. Laryngoscope. 2011 Jun; 121(6):1308−1312. https://doi.org/10.1002/lary.21734. Epub 2011 May 6. PMID: 21557228.

4. Freund W, Wunderlich AP, Stöcker T, Schmitz BL, Scheithauer MO. ***Empty nose syndrome***: limbic system activation observed by functional magnetic resonance imaging. Laryngoscope. 2011 Sep; 121(9):2019−2025. https://doi.org/10.1002/lary.21903. Epub 2011 Aug 16. PMID: 22024858.

2010

1. Scheithauer MO. Nasenmuschelchirurgie and "Empty Nose" Syndrome [Surgery of the turbinates and "empty nose" syndrome]. Laryngorhinootologie. 2010 May; 89 Suppl 1: S79−S102. German. https://doi.org/10.1055/s-0029-1246126. Epub 2010 Mar 29. PMID: 20352572.

2. Scheithauer MO. Surgery of the turbinates and "empty nose" syndrome. GMS Curr Top Otorhinolaryngol Head Neck Surg. 2010; 9:Doc03. https://doi.org/10.3205/cto000067. Epub 2011 Apr 27. PMID: 22073107; PMCID: PMC3199827.

2009

1. Chhabra N, Houser SM. The diagnosis and management of ***empty nose syndrome***. Otolaryngol Clin North Am. 2009 Apr; 42(2):311−330, ix. https://doi.org/10.1016/j.otc.2009.02.001. PMID: 19328895.

2. Payne SC. ***Empty nose syndrome***: What are we really talking about? Otolaryngol Clin North Am. 2009 Apr; 42(2):331−337, ix-x. https://doi.org/10.1016/j.otc.2009.02.002. PMID: 19328896

2008 No papers

2007

1. Houser SM. Surgical treatment for ***empty nose syndrome***. Arch Otolaryngol Head Neck Surg. 2007 Sep; 133(9):858−863. https://doi.org/10.1001/archotol.133.9.858. PMID: 17875850.

Table 1.1 PubMed database references: *Empty nose syndrome* (ENS) in the title from 2001—November 1, 2022.—*cont'd*

2006

1. Houser SM. ***Empty nose syndrome*** associated with middle turbinate resection. Otolaryngol Head Neck Surg. 2006 Dec; 135(6):972—973. https://doi.org/10.1016/j.otohns.2005.04.017. PMID: 17141099.

2002—05 No papers

2001

1. Wang Y, Liu T, Qu Y, Dong Z, Yang Z. [***Empty nose syndrome***]. Zhonghua Er Bi Yan Hou KeZa Zhi. 2001 Jun; 36(3):203—205. Chinese. PMID: 12761925.
2. Moore EJ, Kern EB. Atrophic rhinitis: a review of 242 cases. Am J Rhinol. 2001 Nov—Dec; 15(6):355—361. PMID: 11777241 Note: this paper is the 3rd of 3 exceptions but is included because, to our knowledge, this is the first presentation of the term ***"empty nose syndrome"*** in the written medical literature.

Abstracted from the story: "Turbinate reductions are routinely performed around the world, and usually with great success. But some patients say this surgical procedure ruined their lives". In ***Michael Jackson's wrongful death suit***, one of his doctors ***testified*** that Jackson's insomnia could have been a result of ***empty nose syndrome***. Online ENS forums and Facebook support groups are filled with people who say they've been discarded by doctors who told them nothing is wrong—that it's psychogenic, all in their heads. In ***China***, one man who said he had ***empty nose syndrome*** became so enraged that he ***stabbed an otolaryngologist to death.*** Others direct violence toward themselves. When regular ENS commenters go silent online, the community wonders if they're gone for good.

Harmon T. Medical Mystery: ***Empty Nose Syndrome***: (Bold italics added)

CBS News. Aug 30, 2016

https://youtu.be/8Ue4SZihtM4.

(4062 views as of August 2022)

The Medical Science Behind ***Empty Nose Syndrome***. (Bold italics added) December 16, 2018. https://youtu.be/C50JWQkXr3s (9035 views as of August 2022).

ENS Victim Scott Gaffer's Story-a ***Suicide***. (Bold italics added) January 30, 2019.

https://youtu.be/U5h9URck708 (17,249 views as of August 2022)

ENS Victim Dory's Story-a ***Suicide***. (Bold italics added) March 14, 2020.

https://youtu.be/073TilZvc40 (10,325 views as of August 2022)

Empty Nose Treatment at Stanford University. October 24, 2020.

https://youtu.be/pK361MrCYUwdo897.

(3100 views as of March 2023)

The horrifying report of the murder of an ENT surgeon by a patient: Newsday, BBC News. April 6, 2014.

China sees a wave of violence against staff—***Empty Nose Syndrome case—ENT doctor murdered***.

https://youtu.be/ikFlH4CallHerTheOhqbo7o.

(1921 views as of March 2021) (Blue type from original citation and bold italics added)

Note: as of August 2022, when attempting to access this site and the message delivered was: ***"this video isn't available anymore."***

Moreover, the Internet is flooded with numerous patient posts regarding their ENS symptoms along with information and support websites for the "postnasal surgery dysfunction community" including:

https//www.change.org/emptynose

https://www.usasinus.org/empty-nose-syndrome

https://www.nasalcripple.com.

Some other terms and sites acquired from https://www.nasalcripple.com are:

- → Wide nasal cavity syndrome¶
- → Sindrome del naso vuoto [Italian]¶
- → Syndrome du nez vide (SNV) [French]¶
- → Síndrome de la nariz vacía [Spanish]¶
- → sindrome do nariz vacio [Portuguese]¶
- → синдром пустой нос [Russian]¶
- → Boş Burun Sendromu [Turkish]¶
- → lege neus syndroom [Dutch]¶
- → Leer nase syndrom [German]¶
- → متلازمة الأنف فارغة [Arabic]¶
- → תסמונת האף הריק [Hebrew]¶
- → 空鼻症候群 [Chinese]¶
- → 빈코증후군 [Korean]¶

The ENS is an existent authentic reality; it is no longer debatable and it may be more common than the obscure rarity some authors claim.

In 2020, on the **American Rhinologic Society** website, the following quotation appeared:

> *"The exact incidence of ENS is currently unknown. There are still thousands of patients experiencing ENS."*

Yes, ENS patients exist. They are enormously exasperated and often feel betrayed by their surgeon since, by definition, ENS is an iatrogenic syndrome, a secondary atrophic rhinitis, consequent to "aggressive" surgical trauma to their turbinates although denied, refuted, and rejected by some surgeons. The turbinate trauma is generally focused and targeted to the inferior turbinate(s), but not excluding the middle turbinate(s). ENS is meaningful because patients are so miserable physically and so distraught emotionally that tangible acknowledgment by the profession is both consequential and pressing.

Pressing because even today, in the current "enlightened" medical era, patients with ENS are still encountered worldwide, supported by the web sites above, because some surgeons deny the contributing, causative relationship between turbinate trauma and the symptom complex known as ENS. Although exact numbers are unobtainable, nasal operative procedures are carried out today, in the first quarter of the 21st century, in vast numbers,* annually, in the United States of America, as there are over a half a million (500,000) nasal operations, some of which may still result in ENS; therefore, there needs to be a moratorium on the "aggressive" attacks against the nasal turbinates mandating replacement by more conservative turbinate procedures for physiologic reasons and ultimately for the welfare of the patients in our trust.

*Between Plastic Surgery.org and the National Library of Medicine website combined, there are approximately 500,000 to 600,000 nasal septal and cosmetic nasal surgical operations performed annually in the United States of America.

---

3. Nasal physiology: olfaction, breathing ("perfect nasal resistance"), internal nasal valve area, defensive immunoglobulins, cytokines plus T and B lymphocytes

While nasal physiology broadly includes olfaction, it is the primary nasal functions of breathing (respiration) and defense that are wholly wounded leading to the symptoms of ENS. Regarding the major nasal function of breathing, it is important to recognize that the nose is the first portion of the entire respiratory system, which affords an essential and critical upper airway resistance, provided by the ***internal nasal valve area***, which contains the head of the inferior turbinate. Figs. 1.5, 1.6, 1.7 and 1.8.

The internal nasal valve is a three-dimensional structure that includes the head of the inferior turbinate. The other structures composing the internal nasal valve area in addition to the head of the inferior turbinate include the caudal end of the upper lateral cartilage, the nasal septum, and the floor of the pyriform aperture with its mucocutaneous coverings.

This anatomic fact and physiologic conception, of the internal nasal valve as a three-dimensional structure, was announced by the exceptional research of Haight and Cole from the University of Toronto, Canada, over 35 years ago in 1983.[5] This contribution was sustained and verified by the application of this anatomic and functional certainty through the clinical work of surgeons from the Mayo Clinic in 1987,[6] although the awareness of a nasal valve as an anatomic reality was first

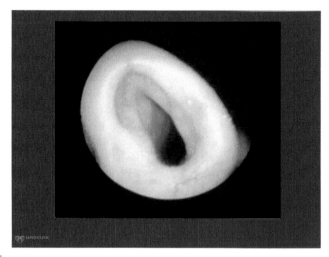

FIGURE 1.5

Uninstrumented base view of the left nostril of a female with a normal nose and a normal "internal nasal valve angle" is easily seen.

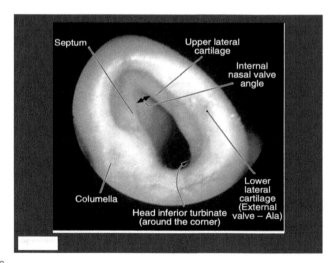

FIGURE 1.6

Photograph is an uninstrumented clinical view of the left side of a female with a normal nose. Many structures of the internal and external nasal valve (lower lateral cartilage and ala) are seen and labeled; the head of the inferior turbinate is part of the internal nasal valve *area*.

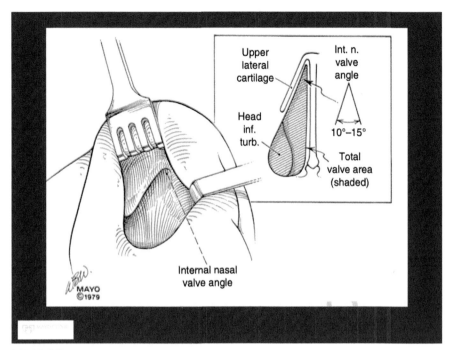

FIGURE 1.7

The *lower left* illustration reveals the clinical internal nasal valve *angle*. In the *upper right* corner of the illustration is the representative conception of the total internal nasal valve *area (shaded area)*. The concept of the entire internal nasal valve area was presented to the profession and verified by Haight and Cole in 1983.[5] The total internal nasal valve *area* includes the upper lateral cartilage (ULC), the septal cartilage (the septal turbinate "swell body" not shown), the floor of the nose, the piriform aperture, the frontal (ascending) process of the maxilla, and the head of the inferior turbinate. The internal nasal valve *angle* is represented as ranging from 10 to 15 degrees, although some other authors have different findings.

Structures of the internal nasal valve area include:

1. Nasal septum (including the premaxillary wings)
2. Upper lateral cartilage (ULC)
3. Piriform aperture
4. Fibroareolar lateral soft tissues
5. Frontal (ascending) process of the maxilla
6. Head of the inferior turbinate
7. Mucosal and cutaneous (skin) "mucocutaneous" coverings of these structures

(Kern and Friedman. By permission of Mayo Foundation for Medical Education and Research. All Rights Reserved).

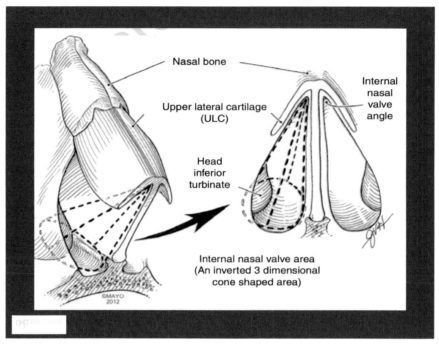

FIGURE 1.8

This illustration depicts the ***internal nasal valve area*** (visualized) as an inverted three-dimensional cone-shaped area. The triangular portion (apex of the cone) fits into the apex of the nasal valve angle, between the nasal septum in the upper lateral cartilage (ULC). The base of the cone fits into a broader area including the floor of the nose (floor of the piriform aperture) and is bounded by the head of the inferior turbinate posteriorly, the premaxillary wing region of the nasal septum medially, and the frontal (ascending) process of the maxilla laterally.

(Kern and Friedman. By permission of Mayo Foundation for Medical Education and Research. All Rights Reserved).

introduced to the literature more than 100 years ago by the anatomist PJ Mink from Utrecht in the Netherlands.[7,8]

We ask you, the reader, the following question, in your personal experience, what is more satisfying, mouth breathing or breathing through your nose (nasal breathing)?

Nasal breathing accounts for approximately 60%–70% of the total respiratory tract resistance and is a higher resistance system than mouth breathing; yet, from our personal experience and according to most patients, nasal breathing is much more satisfying than mouth (lower resistance) breathing.[22]

A specific "perfect nasal resistance" is required for producing the ideal intrathoracic negative pressure gradient, which in turn creates the optimal opening of the peripheral bronchioles enhancing alveolar ventilation, facilitating oxygen and carbon dioxide exchange. Respiration is, after all, the exchange of oxygen and carbon dioxide at the alveolar level. This situation of ideal intrathoracic negative pressure which expedites pulmonary and cardiac venous blood flow return is seriously altered if the head of the inferior turbinate is resected nosediving nasal airway resistance.

Normal nasal airway resistance is essential not only for normal nasal function but also additionally is requisite for optimal and peak pulmonary physiology during both inspiration and during expiration. This fact has been realized by some Italian nasal surgeons for more than a quarter of a century.[9] As has been recently pointed out by Balakin et al.[10] in 2017, understanding nasal airway resistance is crucial as they stated that, "The reduction of aerodynamic resistance observed in the postoperative case may result in disruption of pulmonary functions", as it follows from both Ramadan et al. 1984[11]; and Flanagan and Eccles 1997.[12] Lung hyperventilation may occur in the event breathing depth remains constant, an observation confirmed in literature by Mangin et al.in 2014.[13] Studying nasal aerodynamics by means of computational fluid dynamics (CFD) to understand the ENS symptom of 'paradoxical nasal obstruction', Balakin et al.[10] proposed that a reduction in nasal airflow resistance can modify nasal aerodynamics affecting lung function. "The potential outcome could be changes in the microclimate and sensation and thereby alter the pulmonary function."[10] In a study of lung volumes and arterial oxygenation published in the journal *The Lancet* by Swift and colleagues, using nasal pack occlusion, found that total lung capacity, functional residual capacity, and residual volume *decreased* significantly, which is the equivalent of mouth breathing. All three volumes *increased* back to normal when *nasal* breathing resumed.[14] Therefore, lung volumes are increased back to normal when there is a total *increase* in airway resistance back to normal. In addition, lung volumes are reduced or decreased when there is a total decrease in nasal airway resistance, as in ENS or mouth breathing.

> *"These findings imply that the resistance to expiration provided by the nose helps maintain lung volumes and so may indirectly determine arterial oxygenation."[14]*

After passing through the internal nasal valve, the inspired air exhibits the designed *turbulent* air flow, which heightens intimate contact between the air stream and the nasal mucosa maximizing both heating and moisturizing of the inspired air providing proper warmth and humidity for the flawless exchange of oxygen and carbon dioxide at the alveolar level.

The nasal mucosa is also responsible for significant protective *defensive* functions, which are mechanical, humoral, cellular plus nasal reflexes. The three primary functions of the nose are summarized in Table 1.2. For example, first the vibrissae at

Table 1.2 Three primary functions of the nose.

---

1. Olfaction—Is one of the oldest senses and a component of the defensive system as it provides the organism with odorant identification receptors able to recognize food, prospective mating partners, and possible enemies and other dangers. [34,35]

2. Breathing (respiration)—Regarding the major nasal function of breathing, it is important to recognize that the nose is the first portion of the entire respiratory system, which affords an essential and critical upper airway resistance, provided by the **internal nasal valve area** which contains the head of the inferior turbinate. The nose creates the proper resistance (**'resistor function'—the internal nasal valve area**) for breathing; lung expansion, enhancing venous return, charging the inspired air (**'diffusor function'—turbulent air flow**) with warmth (temperature) and moisture (humidity), enabling idea CO_2 and O_2 exchange to occur optimally at the alveolar level, which is, after all, respiration. [26] The trigeminal nerve mediates the perception of normal nasal airflow by action potentials from the transient receptor potentials melastatin 8 (TRPM8) receptors which are located in the mucosa, goblet cells and vessels, not in the connective tissues. These TRPM8 receptors, the trigeminal "cool" thermoreceptors, are triggered by the wall shearing effects of the inspired air currents cooling the nasal mucosa providing the sense of normal breathing. [33,74,358–360]

3. Defense—The nasal mucosa and submucosa (lamina propria, stroma) have four separate defensive systems including: *mechanical, humoral, cellular,* and various *nasal reflex* defenses. [4]

A. The *mechanical defenses* include vibrissae, the mucus blanket, and the epithelial lining itself.

Nasal cleansing occurs by filtering particles from the inspiratory air by capturing and clearing those particulate particles that precipitate onto the mucosa and removed by ciliary activity. The mucus itself it is composed of a superficial gel layer for trapping foreign particles and a deeper liquid layer that facilitates ciliary motility. Mucociliary transport (MCT) occurs at a rate of 1–2 cm/minute and can be measured using the saccharine test. [4]

B. The *humoral defense system* centers around the immunoglobulins IgA and IgG. IgM also appears in the nasal secretions but at very low levels. All these immunoglobulins are produced in the nasal mucosa by plasma cells and B lymphocytes. Other cells involved in the *humoral defense system* include *histamine, leukotrienes, and prostaglandins*. The *interleukins (IIs)* (a group of cytokines produced in the nasal mucosa) are released during inflammatory events such as rhinitis and rhinosinusitis. These cytokines are released by numerous cells including leukocytes, neutrophils, eosinophils, and fibroblasts. The most important *IIs* include Il-4, Il-5, Il-8, and Il-13. Also included are the antimicrobial secretory proteins lactoferrin (Lf), lysozyme (Ly), and human beta-defensin 1 (hBD-1). [4,15–17]

C. The *cellular defensive system* is a vibrant system living and breathing in the neurovascular bundles located in nasal submucosa (lamina propria, stroma) including the dendritic cells that present foreign proteins to T and B lymphocytes to initiate immune responses. Supplementing the T and B lymphocytes other specific defensive cells include eosinophils, mast cells, basophils, and plasma cells. [4]

Table 1.2 Three primary functions of the nose.—*cont'd*

D. The *nasal reflex system* of defense includes the sneeze and the nasal pulmonary reflex which may induce apnea with laryngeal and bronchial construction as a means of protecting the lower airway. Other lesser-known reflexes that may be protective and defensive include: the diving reflex (apnea and bradycardia), nasocardiac reflex (bradycardia and hypotension), nasovascular reflex (peripheral vasoconstriction) all of which may occur secondary to robust nasal mucosal stimulation secondary nasal tracheal intubation. Lastly there appears to be a genitonasal reflex (obstructive swelling of the nasal mucosa during sexual arousal producing a type of "honeymoon rhinitis").[4]

In summary: Regarding the major nasal function of breathing, the nose is the first portion of the entire respiratory system, which affords an essential and critical upper airway resistance, provided by the **internal nasal valve area** which contains the head of the inferior turbinate. The nasal mucosa and submucosa (lamina propria, stroma) have both humoral and cellular defensive capabilities, and some of defensive functions include olfaction, nasal reflexes including the sneeze, nasopulmonary, nasocardiac and diving reflexes, the vibrissae, mucociliary transport, nitrous oxide, secretory proteins including the antimicrobial proteins lactoferrin (Lf), lysozyme (Ly), and human beta-defensin 1 (hBD-1). Other defensive components include secretory IgA, IgG, leukotrienes, histamine, and prostaglandins along with Ils which are a group of cytokines including Il-4, Il-5, Il-8, and Il-13. The trigeminal nerve mediates the perception of normal nasal airflow by action potentials from the transient receptor potentials melastatin 8 (TRPM8) receptors which are located in the mucosa. These TRPM8 receptors, the trigeminal "cool" thermoreceptors, are triggered by the inspired air currents cooling the nasal mucosa providing the sense of normal breathing.[33,74,358–360] Obviously, there is a vibrant cellular defensive system living and breathing in the neurovascular bundles located in nasal submucosa (lamina propria, stroma) including the dendritic cells that present foreign proteins to T and B lymphocytes to initiate immune responses. Supplementing the T and B lymphocytes, other specific defensive cells include eosinophils, mast cells, basophils, and plasma cells.[4,15–17]

the nostril, then the mucous blanket can mechanically trap foreign elements such as helminths, bacteria, viruses, fungi, pollens, and other particulate matter and with the energetic mucociliary transport system deliver these substances to the posterior pharynx to be swallowed demolished and destroyed. There is, moreover, the physical protection of the nasal pseudostratified ciliated columnar epithelial lining itself, which functions as an effective barrier to external noxious elements. In addition, the nasal mucosa and submucosa (lamina propria, the stroma) have both humoral and cellular defensive capabilities including the antimicrobial proteins lactoferrin (Lf), lysozyme (Ly), and human beta-defensin 1 (hBD-1).[15–17] Added to these three major nasal antimicrobial proteins, there are several other known antimicrobial proteins and peptides, including statherin and secretory phospholipase A2, all have been identified and likely contribute to the total antimicrobial properties of human nasal secretions.[15] Recently, it was suggested that hBD-1 is an important component of the innate immune response, particularly at mucosal surfaces, which are vulnerable to colonization by potential pathogens. Defensins with their antimicrobial and immune properties can both induce inflammation and suppress the inflammatory response through discrete and specific mechanisms. Since these antimicrobial proteins Lf, Ly, and hBD-1 are consistently contained in nasal secretions, the clinician must realize that washing (lavage) these proteins away may interfere with the body's homeostatic mechanism and its ability to protect the nasal mucosa from dangerous bacteria including *Klebsiella ozenae*.

Nasal mucosal cells produce immunoglobulins IgA and IgG, leukotrienes, histamine, prostaglandins along with interleukins (Ils), which are a group of cytokines; some of the important ones include Il-4, Il-5, Il-8, and Il-13. Obviously, there is a vibrant cellular defensive system living and breathing in the nasal submucosa including the dendritic cells which present foreign proteins to T and B lymphocytes to initiate immune responses. Supplementing the T and B lymphocytes, other specific defensive cells include eosinophils, mast cells, basophils, and plasma cells. Remember, the nasal mucosa correspondingly contains abundant seromucinous and goblet cells; furthermore, this submucosa (lamina propria, stroma) features an important network of sensory and autonomic neurovascular bundles with an extraordinarily rich functioning vascular system with an existing dynamic *nasal cycle*.

The autonomic nervous system-controlled nasal cycle allows for the spontaneous congestion and decongestion of the nasal venous sinusoids, so the congested side is the "resting" side of the nose while the decongested side is the "functioning" side. Because of the nasal septum, the total nasal airway resistance remains relatively constant and is calculated at a lower resistance level than either one of the individual right- or left-sided nasal resistance values. How is it possible that the total nasal airway resistance is lower than either one of the individual sides you ask? This is because the calculation of total nasal airway resistance is based on the concept of a parallel circuit and not a series circuit. Consider that nasal airway resistance is not measured, you *calculate* nasal airway resistance by measuring transnasal pressure and nasal air flow during the inspiratory and expiratory respiratory cycle. To calculate nasal airway resistance, nasal airway pressure is divided by nasal air flow. The parallel circuit formula for calculating total nasal airway resistance is the product of the resistance of each right and left side divided by the sum of the right and left side resistance, so the resultant total nasal airway resistance is *less* than either one of the individual sides.

What happens to the patient when the pseudostratified ciliated columnar respiratory epithelium of the nasal mucosa is wounded or the seromucinous and goblet cells are resected? What happens to a patient when the submucosa is impaired, diminished, and damaged by the deft debrider tearing though those delicate neurovascular bundles compressing the precious submucosal spaces with postsurgical choking scar strewn with remnants of frayed and tattered autonomic and sensory neural tissue filaments?

What happens to the patient when the respiratory and the defensive nasal physiologic functions are partially, or in the extreme case totally destroyed; torn asunder as it were, detached by disconnection from the corpus? Is this ablation passed off as a *minor misdemeanor* or is it truly, as demanded by Huizing and de Groot, *a capital nasal crime?*[3,4]

Who is damaged by this mucosal and submucosal punishment? Some surgeons discount the consequences of harming normal nasal physiologic mechanisms or are both unaware of ENS or rebuff the validity of the patient's ENS symptoms and are therefore reluctant to offer understanding and comfort to their patients by acknowledging the existence of ENS or validating their patient's complaints and their plaintive plea for help.[2,18] In medicine, we cure rarely, we aid healing often, and we must be compassionate, always.

With a varied and protean symptomatology, the clinical presentation of ENS may challenge the most astute and experienced clinician, thereby defying diagnosis. Consequently, a principal purpose of this text includes establishing the diagnostic criteria for ENS, examining theories regarding etiology, evaluating effectiveness of current consensus strategies for the management of inferior turbinate enlargement, while stressing prevention of ENS, thereby evading its devastating toll.

Ultimately, this contribution is worthwhile if awareness regarding ENS is raised and scholarship is stimulated among all nasal and rhinoplasty surgeons regarding fundamental nasal airway physiology and the recognition of the debilitating physical and psychological suffering that ENS patients endure. The topics covered in this book are outlined in Table 1.3.

Table 1.3 The *empty nose syndrome* (ENS) chapter outline.

CHAPTER 1 Introduction and overview

A. Introduction and overview

B. *Empty nose syndrome* (ENS) in print media, TV; with ubiquity on the World Wide Web

C. Nasal physiology: Olfaction, breathing ("perfect nasal resistance"), internal nasal valve area, defensive immunoglobulins, cytokines plus T and B lymphocytes

CHAPTER 2 The scope of the *empty nose syndrome* (ENS)

A. Definition: What is the *empty nose syndrome* (ENS)?

B. Symptoms of ENS

C. ENS or atrophic rhinitis? A definition of terms

   1. Primary atrophic rhinitis

   2. Secondary atrophic rhinitis

   3. Differential diagnosis of atrophic rhinitis

Continued

Table 1.3 The *empty nose syndrome* (ENS) chapter outline.—*cont'd*

D. Diagnosis of ENS
E. Iatrogenic wonderland-etiology

CHAPTER 3 Pathophysiology of the *empty nose syndrome* (ENS)

CHAPTER 4 Treatment options for the *empty nose syndrome* (ENS)

A. Medical
B. Surgical
C. Preventing ENS

CHAPTER 5 The turbinates—an overview

A. Historical perspective
B. Turbinate anatomy
    1. Anatomy of the *middle turbinate*
    2. Anatomy of the *inferior turbinate*
C. Physical examination
D. Rhinologic evaluation with assessment tests and biopsy

CHAPTER 6 Brief history of evidence-based medicine (EBM)-David Sackett, MD

CHAPTER 7 The turbinates—management

A. Middle turbinate management
B. Inferior turbinate management
    1. Classification: Inferior turbinate enlargement ("hypertrophy")
    2. Turbinate reduction: Surgical and nonsurgical procedures
        a. Epithelial mucosal *destruction:* Trans mucosal approach (including—partial and complete—total turbinectomy)
            1. Surgical resection-turbinectomy (partial or complete—total)
            2. Electrocautery
            3. Laser therapy
            4. Cryotherapy
        b. Epithelial mucosal *preservation:* Sub mucosal approach
            1. Submucosal soft tissue surgical reduction (conventional "cold knife")
                a. Submucosal soft tissue reduction only
                b. Conchal bone reduction only
                c. Combined: soft tissue and conchal bone reduction
            2. Microdebrider
            3. Radiofrequency
            4. Coblation
            5. Ultrasound
            6. Electrocautery
        c. Complimentary out-fracture (lateralization) techniques
            1. Solitary-isolated and sole intervention
            2. Combined with other procedures
        d. Histopathology

CHAPTER 8 How to find the "best reduction method" for inferior turbinate enlargement ("hypertrophy")?

A. Context with discussion of some specific critical confounding questions
    1. Randomized controlled trials (RCTs) searching for the "best reduction method" from the literature
    2. Future studies—designing the "best study" for finding the "best reduction method"
    3. Thoughts for designing a "best study" for finding the "best reduction method" for treating patients with inferior turbinate enlargement ("hypertrophy")
    4. When are randomized controlled trials (RCTs) NOT needed?
    5. Asking answerable questions and empiricism versus rationalism

Table 1.3 The ***empty nose syndrome*** (ENS) chapter outline.—*cont'd*

   6. Are controlled trials (RCTs) really needed? Can they actually be accomplished in surgery?
      a. Absolute criteria for a valid RCT
      b. Relative criteria for a valid RCT
   7. Evidence first, but what to do when RCT data are limited, incomplete, inconclusive, conflicting, or starkly nonexistent?
   8. What are the influences of "placebo effects" in research and practice outcomes?
   9. What are the ethics of using placebos in *medicine*?
   10. What are the ethics of using placebos in *surgery*?
   11. "*Sham*" surgery, is there an ethical place for research surgical trials or is it forbidden?
   12. What are the limitations, if any, to the doctrine of randomized controlled trials (RCTs)?
   13. Is there an ethical approach to surgical and invasive procedures within randomized controlled trials (RCTs)?
   14. What are the obligations and accountability to our patients regarding surgical *innovations*?
   15. What are the CONSORT requirements and what's their importance for researchers and journals?
   16. What is propensity score matching (PSM) all about?
   17. What about using clinical practice guidelines (CPGs) and associated conflicts of interest (COI)?
   18. What about practice replacement, reversal, and the nature of medical progress?

CHAPTER 9 Children and inferior turbinate reduction

CHAPTER 10 Medical journals: judging the quality of the editors, the peer reviewers, plus the issue of plagiarism

CHAPTER 11 Review, finishing touches, and closure

A. Managing ***empty nose syndrome*** (ENS) Patients
   1. ***Empty nose syndrome*** (ENS) exists
   2. Pertinent nasal physiology
   3. Symptoms of ENS
   4. Etiology of ENS
   5. Pathophysiology of ENS
   6. Preventing ENS
   7. Medical treatment of ENS
   8. Surgical treatment of ENS
B. Evidence-based medicine (EBM)-David Sackett, MD
C. Consolidated standards of reporting trials (CONSORT)
D. Replacement or reversal of a medical practice
E. Managing middle turbinate enlargement
F. Managing inferior turbinate enlargement ("hypertrophy") *Evidence-based proposals*
G. Regarding children
H. Summary, future directions, and closing thoughts
 I. Appendix

This appendix contains seven items: (1) a brief history of Maurice H. Cottle, MD, (2) the ***empty nose syndrome*** 6 questionnaire (ENS6Q), (3) the sino-nasal outcome test 20–25 (SNOT20-25) for ENS, (4) Nasal obstruction symptom evaluation (nose) instrument, (5) the cotton test, and how to perform it, (6) the questionnaire generalized anxiety disorder (GAD-7), (7) the patient health questionnaire-9 (PHQ-9) for depression.

The scope of the empty nose syndrome (ENS)

2

1. Definition: what is empty nose syndrome (ENS)?

The term "empty nose syndrome" (ENS) was coined by the Mayo Clinic team (Stenkvist and Kern) in 1994 when Dr. Monika Stenkvist, visiting surgeon and scientist, observed the noticeably and conspicuously empty nasal cavities on computerized tomography (CT) scans of patients missing almost all identifiable inferior and middle turbinate mucosal structures secondary to surgical resection of the turbinates followed by a multiple *symptom complex arising months to years after their initial surgery* (performed at sites other than Mayo Clinic). Some examples of coronal CT scans found in our practice exhibiting the common findings observed, *not* operated at Mayo Clinic, and diagnosed with the *ENS* are located in Figs. 2.1–2.18.

By definition, ENS is primarily an iatrogenic condition, secondary to turbinate trauma, in which a surgical resection removes various amounts of functioning nasal turbinate mucosal and submucosal (lamina propria, stroma) tissue. ENS may occur secondary to a **n**on-surgical **T**urbinate **R**eduction **A**djunctive **P**rocedure (n-s TRAP), which may also inflict significant turbinate trauma profoundly compromising nasal function. In either case, the patient experiences the distinctive hallmark symptoms of nasal obstruction "congestion," (difficulty breathing, often a "paradoxical obstruction," meaning obstructed breathing usually with "breathlessness" despite a widely patent nasal airway, with a sense of suffocation) and nasal crusting along with various protean symptoms arising months to years following the iatrogenic turbinate trauma.

Specifically and by definition, the term surgery is the medical practice of managing diseases, deformities, and injuries by actually "cutting" into a part of the body while, on the other hand, the procedures of electrocautery, chemocautery, lasers, radiofrequency, coblation, or ultrasound are not surgery in the traditional "strict sense" of "cold knife" cutting, but nonetheless they are currently covered beneath the umbrella of "surgery," although we prefer to label them n-s TRAPs.

Empty Nose Syndrome. https://doi.org/10.1016/B978-0-443-10715-3.00002-0

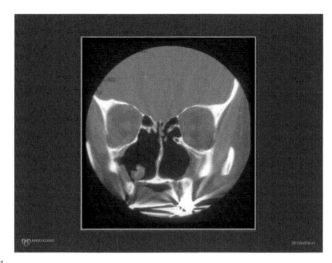

FIGURE 2.1

Coronal CT scan of a patient exhibiting the common findings seen in patients with the *"empty nose syndrome."* There is a cavernous expansion of the intranasal airway with the absence of both middle and inferior turbinates that have been previously surgically resected (removed-not by a Mayo Clinic surgeon) after bilateral total middle and inferior turbinectomies. Note: We do not advocate total or subtotal turbinectomies for benign turbinate enlargement ("hyperplastic").

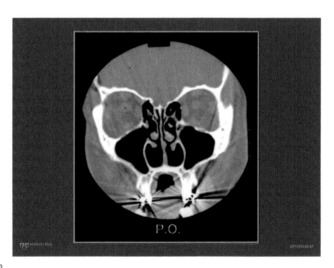

FIGURE 2.2

Coronal CT scan of a patient exhibiting the common findings seen in patients with the *"empty nose syndrome."* There is an absence of almost all of both inferior turbinates that have been previously surgically resected (removed-not by a Mayo Clinic surgeon) after a bilateral subtotal inferior turbinectomies. Note: We do not advocate total or subtotal turbinectomies for benign turbinate enlargement ("hyperplastic").

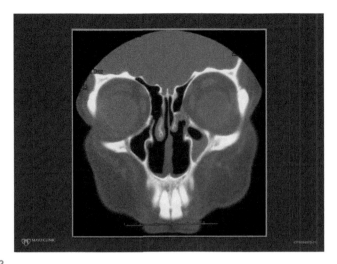

FIGURE 2.3

Coronal CT scan of a patient exhibiting the common findings seen in patients with the *"empty nose syndrome."* There is an absence of both inferior turbinates that have been previously surgically resected (removed-not by a Mayo Clinic surgeon) after a bilateral total inferior turbinectomies. Note: We do not advocate total or subtotal turbinectomies for benign turbinate enlargement ("hyperplastic").

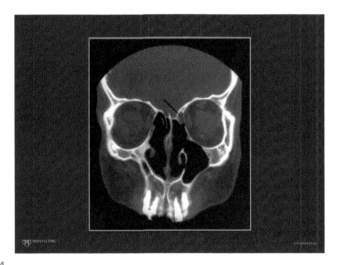

FIGURE 2.4

Coronal CT scan of a patient exhibiting the common findings seen in patients with the *"empty nose syndrome."* There is an absence of almost all of both middle and inferior turbinates that have been previously surgically resected (removed-not by a Mayo Clinic surgeon) after a bilateral middle and subtotal inferior turbinectomies. Note: We do not advocate total or subtotal turbinectomies for benign turbinate enlargement ("hyperplastic").

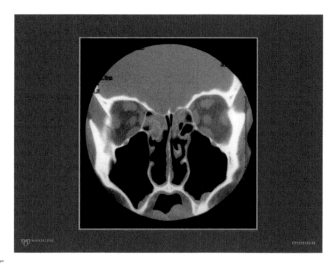

FIGURE 2.5

Coronal CT scan of a patient exhibiting the common findings seen in patients with the *"empty nose syndrome."* There is an absence of the right middle turbinate and almost all of both inferior turbinates that have been previously surgically resected 3(removed-not by a Mayo Clinic surgeon) after a right middle turbinectomy and bilateral total inferior turbinectomies. Note: We do not advocate total or subtotal turbinectomies for benign turbinate enlargement ("hyperplastic").

(Kern and Friedman. By permission of Mayo Foundation for Medical Education and Research. All Rights Reserved).

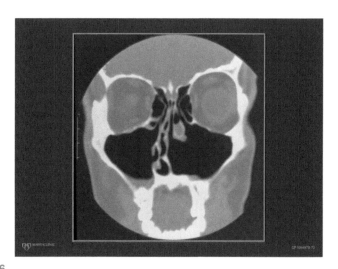

FIGURE 2.6

Coronal CT scan of a patient exhibiting the common findings seen in patients with the *"empty nose syndrome."* There is an absence of the right middle turbinate, an apparent nasal septal deformity, and an absence of both inferior turbinates that have been previously surgically resected (removed-not by a Mayo Clinic surgeon) after a bilateral total inferior turbinectomies. Note: We do not advocate total or subtotal turbinectomies for benign turbinate enlargement ("hyperplastic").

(Kern and Friedman. By permission of Mayo Foundation for Medical Education and Research. All Rights Reserved).

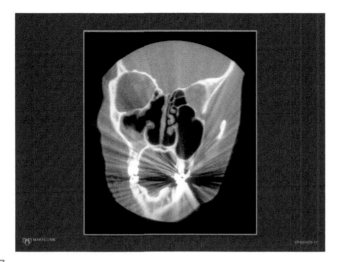

FIGURE 2.7

Coronal CT scan of a patient exhibiting the common findings seen in patients with the *"empty nose syndrome."* There is an absence of the right middle turbinate and almost all of both inferior turbinates, more on the right than the left, that have been previously surgically resected (removed-not by a Mayo Clinic surgeon) after bilateral subtotal inferior turbinectomies. Note: We do not advocate total or subtotal turbinectomies for benign turbinate enlargement ("hyperplastic").

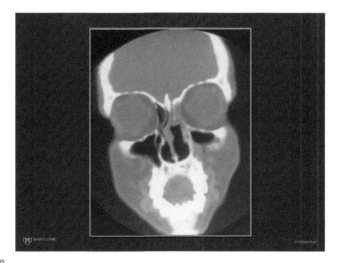

FIGURE 2.8

Coronal CT scan of a patient exhibiting the common findings seen in patients with the *"empty nose syndrome."* There is a nasal septal deformity and what appears to be chronic mucosal changes in the left ethmoid sinus and left maxillary sinus. There is an absence of both middle and inferior turbinates that have been previously surgically resected (removed-not by a Mayo Clinic surgeon) after bilateral total middle and inferior turbinectomies. Note: We do not advocate total or subtotal turbinectomies for benign turbinate enlargement ("hyperplastic").

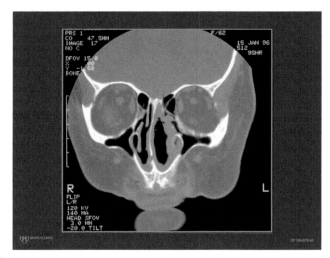

FIGURE 2.9

Coronal CT scan of a patient exhibiting the common findings seen in patients with the *"empty nose syndrome."* There appears to an atrophic change of the right middle turbinate and a reduction (subtotal resection) of the right inferior turbinate. There is an absence of the left middle turbinate and a subtotal reduction left inferior turbinate; they have been previously surgically resected (removed-not by a Mayo Clinic surgeon) after a left middle turbinectomy and bilateral subtotal inferior turbinectomies. Note: We do not advocate total or subtotal turbinectomies for benign turbinate enlargement ("hyperplastic").

(Kern and Friedman. By permission of Mayo Foundation for Medical Education and Research. All Rights Reserved).

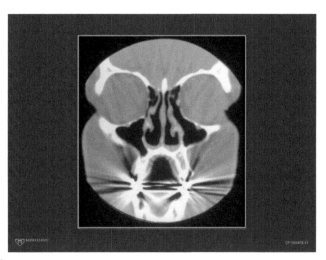

FIGURE 2.10

Coronal CT scan of a patient exhibiting the common findings seen in patients with the *"empty nose syndrome."* Both middle turbinates are absent and a near total reduction (subtotal resection) of both inferior turbinates. They have been previously surgically resected (removed-not by a Mayo Clinic surgeon) after bilateral middle turbinectomies and bilateral subtotal inferior turbinectomies. Note: We do not advocate total or subtotal turbinectomies for benign turbinate enlargement ("hyperplastic").

(Kern and Friedman. By permission of Mayo Foundation for Medical Education and Research. All Rights Reserved).

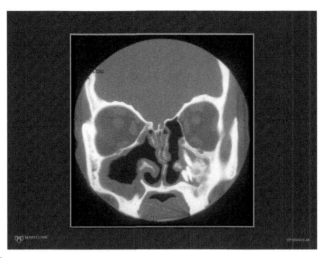

FIGURE 2.11

Coronal CT scan of a patient exhibiting the common findings seen in patients with the *"empty nose syndrome."* The left maxillary sinus "appears" to be filled with bone or another dense material. There is an absence of the left middle and inferior turbinate along with a reduction of the right middle and inferior turbinates. They have been previously surgically resected (removed-not by a Mayo Clinic surgeon) after left middle and inferior turbinectomies and right subtotal middle and inferior turbinectomies. Note: We do not advocate total or subtotal turbinectomies for benign turbinate enlargement ("hyperplastic").

(Kern and Friedman. By permission of Mayo Foundation for Medical Education and Research. All Rights Reserved).

2. Symptoms of the empty nose syndrome (ENS)

One of the characteristic symptoms of ENS includes a "paradoxical sense of nasal airway obstruction."[18–20] The paradox lies in the patient's perceived sense of problematic nasal breathing despite a widely patent nasal cavity following varying amounts of mucosal and submucosal turbinate tissue resection or submucosal injury subsequent to an n-s TRAP. The diagnosis of ENS is challenging because the patient may experience a long lag time (unpredictably varying from months to years) before symptoms appear, which are almost always nasal airway obstruction ("congestion") and associated nasal crusting and postnasal discharge, while many symptoms are assorted, protean, and inconsistent, but what is consistent and unifying is the fact, by definition, that almost every patient with ENS has had a previous documented nasal turbinate operative resection or n-s TRAP. These ENS patients experience many specific symptoms listed in Table 2.1. Some findings seen in ENS patients

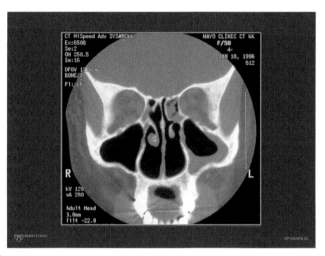

FIGURE 2.12

Coronal CT scan of a patient exhibiting the common findings seen in patients with the *"empty nose syndrome."* There is a reduced left middle turbinate and an absence of the left inferior turbinate along with an absence of the right inferior turbinate. They have been previously surgically resected (removed-not by a Mayo Clinic surgeon) after bilateral inferior turbinectomies and a left subtotal middle turbinectomy. There are inflammatory changes in the ethmoid sinuses, greater on the left than the right with inflammatory changes in the left maxillary sinus. There appears that the "bilateral antrostomies" have closed with soft tissue, scar. Note: We do not advocate total or subtotal turbinectomies for benign turbinate enlargement ("hyperplastic").

(Kern and Friedman. By permission of Mayo Foundation for Medical Education and Research. All Rights Reserved).

on intranasal exam range from atrophy, crusting, to absent turbinate tissue as viewed in Figs. 2.19–2.24.

3. Empty nose syndrome or atrophic rhinitis? A definition of terms

1. Primary atrophic rhinitis
2. Secondary atrophic rhinitis
3. Differential diagnosis of nasal atrophy

Conceptually, there is some controversy as to whether ENS should be considered an iatrogenic entity with a *secondary atrophic rhinitis* or whether *atrophic rhinitis* should be considered its own distinct clinical entity unrelated to surgical intervention. Chhabra and Houser contend that ENS must be viewed separately from

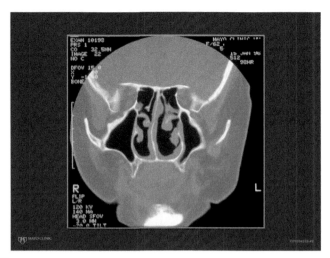

FIGURE 2.13

Coronal CT scan of a patient exhibiting the common findings seen in patients with the *"empty nose syndrome."* The middle turbinates are smaller on the right than the left, and both inferior turbinates have been subtotally reduced. They have been previously surgically resected (removed-not by a Mayo Clinic surgeon) after bilateral subtotal middle turbinectomies and bilateral subtotal inferior turbinectomies. Note: We do not advocate total or subtotal turbinectomies for benign turbinate enlargement ("hyperplastic").

(Kern and Friedman. By permission of Mayo Foundation for Medical Education and Research. All Rights Reserved).

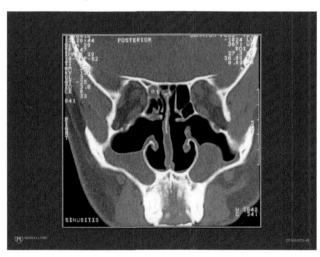

FIGURE 2.14

Coronal CT scan of a patient exhibiting the common findings seen in patients with the *"empty nose syndrome."* Both middle turbinates are absent, and both inferior turbinates are almost totally nonexistent. They have been previously surgically resected (removed-not by a Mayo Clinic surgeon) after bilateral total middle turbinectomies and bilateral subtotal inferior turbinectomies. Note: We do not advocate total or subtotal turbinectomies for benign turbinate enlargement ("hyperplastic").

(Kern and Friedman. By permission of Mayo Foundation for Medical Education and Research. All Rights Reserved).

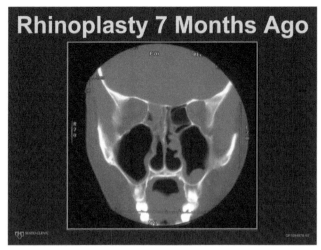

FIGURE 2.15

Coronal CT scan of a patient exhibiting the common findings seen in patients with the *"empty nose syndrome" after a previous rhinoplasty* with the absence of both inferior turbinates and the right middle turbinate and a possible subtotal reduction of the left middle turbinate. This rhinoplasty operation was performed at another institution and not at Mayo Clinic. For the record, we adamantly and categorically denounce inferior turbinectomy as part of a routine rhinoplasty operation.

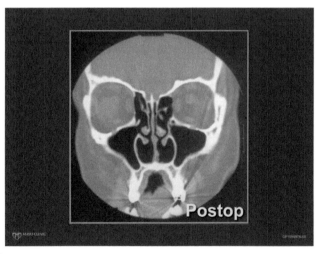

FIGURE 2.16

Coronal CT scan of a patient exhibiting the common findings seen in patients with the *"empty nose syndrome" after a previous rhinoplasty* with almost a total absence of both inferior turbinates. This rhinoplasty operation was performed at another institution and not at Mayo Clinic. These inferior turbinates have been surgically resected (removed-not by a Mayo Clinic surgeon) after bilateral subtotal inferior turbinectomies. For the record, we adamantly and categorically denounce inferior turbinectomy as part of a routine rhinoplasty operation.

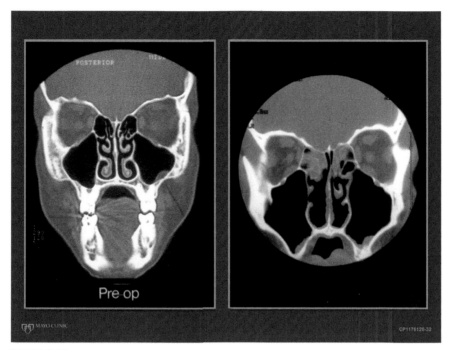

FIGURE 2.17

Coronal CT scan of a patient exhibiting the common findings seen in patients with the *"empty nose syndrome" after a previous rhinoplasty performed elsewhere.* The CT scan on the left is preoperative. The CT scan on the right is after a rhinoplasty operation performed at another institution and not at Mayo Clinic. There is an absence of the right middle turbinate and almost total absence of both inferior turbinates. The right middle turbinate and both inferior turbinates have been surgically resected (removed-not by a Mayo Clinic surgeon) after right middle turbinectomy and bilateral total inferior turbinectomies. For the record, we adamantly and categorically denounce inferior turbinectomy as part of a routine rhinoplasty operation.

(Kern and Friedman. By permission of Mayo Foundation for Medical Education and Research. All Rights Reserved).

atrophic rhinitis despite "similarities in the symptoms," especially the symptoms of "paradoxical nasal airway obstruction, congestion, dryness, and crusting."[21] They argue that ENS, unlike atrophic rhinitis, is not always associated with obvious visible nasal mucosal atrophy, and that ENS is exclusively iatrogenic in origin and does not have a clear link to pathologic organisms.[18,20] Other authors agree that the atrophy and dryness of the nasal mucosa seen in ENS can occur either subsequent to a surgical turbinate reduction or following a n-s TRAP.[18,21,22]

We agree, in part, with Chhabra and Houser[21] that ENS is almost always and exclusively iatrogenic in origin and that ENS is not always associated with obvious nasal atrophy. We consider ENS as a subcategory of atrophic rhinitis, a *secondary atrophic rhinitis.* Primary atrophic rhinitis is almost exclusively associated with the bacterial infections of *Klebsiella pneumoniae ozaenae.* For clarity, recognize

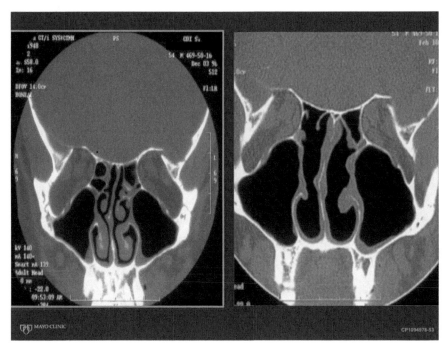

FIGURE 2.18

Coronal CT scan of a patient exhibiting the common findings seen in patients with the
"empty nose syndrome" after a previous rhinoplasty performed elsewhere. The CT scan
on the left is preoperative. The CT scan on the right is after a rhinoplasty operation
performed at another institution and not at Mayo Clinic. Both middle turbinates are
absent. The right inferior turbinate is absent, and the left inferior turbinate is almost totally
absent. These turbinates have been surgically resected (removed-not by a Mayo Clinic
surgeon) after bilateral middle and inferior total turbinectomies. For the record, we
adamantly and categorically denounce inferior turbinectomy as part of a routine
rhinoplasty operation.

*(Kern and Friedman. By permission of Mayo Foundation for Medical Education and Research. All Rights
Reserved).*

that ozena is a type of primary atrophic rhinitis caused by the bacterial infection of
Klebsiella pneumoniae ozaenae.

Another Klebsiella infection is called rhinoscleroma, which can present similarly to ozena in its earliest stage. Rhinoscleroma is caused by *Klebsiella pneumoniae rhinoscleromatis*, and it is important to realize that this infection is chronic
and the gram-negative rods, particularly Klebsiella, are increasingly resistant to
antibiotics.[23]

For comprehensive clarity, we classify ENS as a *secondary atrophic rhinitis.* Previous terminologies found in the literature for atrophic rhinitis unfortunately added

Table 2.1 The various and fluctuating symptoms seen in the empty nose syndrome (ENS).

1. Paradoxical nasal airway obstruction (nasal "congestion," difficult nasal breathing usually with "breathlessness," often with a sense of suffocation)
2. Nasal crusting, nasal dryness ("rhinitis sicca"), bleeding (varying degrees of epistaxis)
3. Inability to feel nasal airflow
4. Foul (fetid) odor (often noted by others) with thick nasal discharge and postnasal "drip"
5. Anosmia or hyposmia
6. Headache
7. Localized nasal facial pain (posttraumatic neuropathic pain)
8. Disturbed sleep (with secondary symptoms of fatigue and lethargy)
9. Aprosexia nasalis (inability to concentrate)
10. Psychological alterations (anxiety, clinical depression, suicidal ideation)
11. Disturbance in the sense of "well-being"
12. Impaired quality-of-life

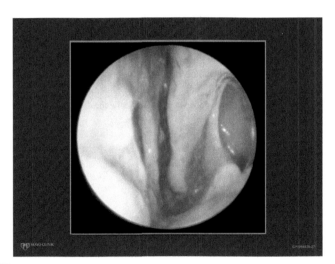

FIGURE 2.19

Endoscopic intranasal view of a patient exhibiting the common finding of extensive intranasal atrophy (*secondary atrophic rhinitis*) often seen in patients with the *"empty nose syndrome."* Note the previously performed subtotal resection of the left inferior turbinate as well as the left inferior meatal antrostomy with mucopurulent material exuding from the maxillary sinus onto the nasal floor. The perforation of the nasal septum is also visible. The previous surgical operation was performed at another institution and not at Mayo Clinic.

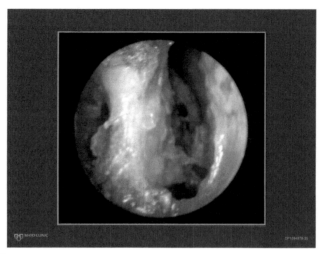

FIGURE 2.20

Endoscopic intranasal view of a patient exhibiting the common finding of extensive intranasal crusting and atrophy (*secondary atrophic rhinitis*) often seen in patients with the *"empty nose syndrome."* Note the absence of the inferior turbinate on the left and the large perforation of the nasal septum. The previous surgical operation was performed at another institution and not at Mayo Clinic.

(Kern and Friedman. By permission of Mayo Foundation for Medical Education and Research. All Rights Reserved).

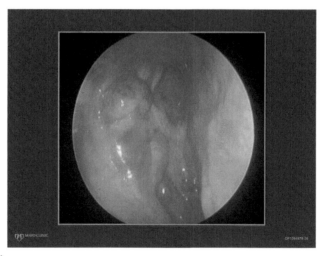

FIGURE 2.21

Endoscopic intranasal view ("empty" right nasal chamber) in a patient exhibiting the common gross findings resulting from a previous *total inferior turbinectomy* and commonly seen in patients with the *"empty nose syndrome."* The previous *total inferior turbinectomy* was performed at another institution and not at Mayo Clinic.

(Kern and Friedman. By permission of Mayo Foundation for Medical Education and Research. All Rights Reserved).

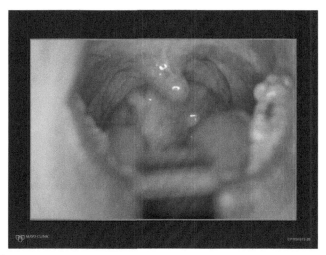

FIGURE 2.22

Intraoral view of a patient exhibiting the common finding of mucopurulent postnasal discharge commonly seen in patients with the *"empty nose syndrome."*

(Kern and Friedman. By permission of Mayo Foundation for Medical Education and Research. All Rights Reserved).

to the perplexing puzzle by using the terms atrophic rhinitis, rhinitis sicca, ozaena, ozena, nasal atrophy, primary and secondary rhinitis atrophicans, rhinitis atrophicans, and dry nose among others, interchangeably at times, utterly without precise definition, differentiation or distinction among the various subclassifications of atrophic rhinitis. The principal purpose of discussing atrophic rhinitis, at this juncture, is to clearly eliminate any misunderstandings by offering a precise terminology. With this definition of terms, atrophic rhinitis is specifically classified into (1). *primary atrophic rhinitis* and (2). *secondary atrophic rhinitis*.

3.1 Primary atrophic rhinitis

Primary atrophic rhinitis is often called ozena, which is merely the descriptive Greek term meaning "stench" (strong unpleasant odor). *Primary atrophic rhinitis* has decreased in incidence in the Western world during the past 100 years, which is likely due to advanced hygiene and the liberal use of antimicrobials for chronic nasal infections. While the exact etiology of *primary atrophic rhinitis* is still unknown, what is known is that almost all of these *primary atrophic rhinitis* patients have culture-positive bacterial infections with *Klebsiella pneumoniae ozaenae*.[18,23] There is progressive atrophy of the nasal mucosal elements including the epithelium, the submucosal glandular and vascular structures along with osteoclast infiltration of the bony concha of the turbinates. The pseudostratified ciliated respiratory epithelium of the nasal mucosa is replaced by squamous metaplasia along with atrophy of the seromucinous and goblet cells along with scarring of the submucosal (lamina propria, stroma). The submucosal vasculature is not only diminished in quantity but also there is definitive evidence of endarteritis.[18] The fact that mucociliary transport has been compromised, along with a reduced number of glandular elements, the

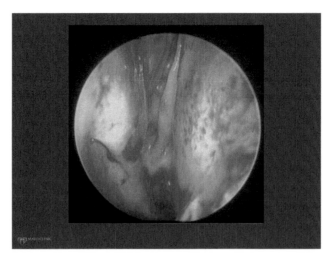

FIGURE 2.23

Endoscopic intranasal view of a patient exhibiting the common finding of intranasal atrophy, with some suggested evidence of mucopurulent material posteriorly after a previously performed *right partial (subtotal) inferior turbinectomy* often seen in patients with the *"empty nose syndrome."* The previous *right partial (subtotal) inferior turbinectomy* was performed at another institution and not at Mayo Clinic. If a biopsy was performed at the head of the right inferior turbinate remnant, then squamous metaplasia would be found replacing the normal pseudostratified ciliated columnar respiratory epithelium.

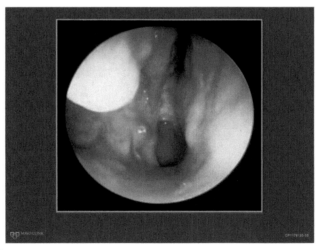

FIGURE 2.24

Endoscopic intranasal view of a patient exhibiting the common finding of intranasal atrophy after a previously performed *right total inferior turbinectomy* often seen in patients with the *"empty nose syndrome."* The previous *right total inferior turbinectomy* was performed at another institution and not at Mayo Clinic.

secretions are thickened, forming crusts, encouraging bacterial multiplication, while the products of bacterial metabolism release a noxious gas perceived as a vile fetid odor. On the other hand, patients with a *secondary atrophic rhinitis* **rarely** demonstrate positive cultures for *Klebsiella pneumoniae ozaenae*. Most assuredly, *primary atrophic rhinitis* is a debilitating nasal mucosal and submucosal progressive disorder with a constellation of conspicuously prominent "hallmark" symptoms, which are especially and particularly analogous to ENS including:

a. Nasal airway obstruction
b. Nasal dryness, nasal crusting, and bleeding (varying degrees of epistaxis)
c. Foul (fetid) odor (often noted by others) with thick nasal discharge
d. Anosmia
e. Headache
f. Localized facial pain
g. Psychological alterations including depression

What is almost universal and remarkable in patients with *primary atrophic rhinitis* is the wide-open intranasal airway; yet, the patient often paradoxically complains of nasal airway obstruction (difficulty breathing despite the broadly patent nasal airway). In essence, *primary atrophic rhinitis* is of unspecified etiology, with a spontaneous onset, and a slowly progressive relentless course consistently associated with the bacteria *Klebsiella pneumoniae ozaenae*.

3.2 Secondary atrophic rhinitis

Secondary atrophic rhinitis, as the term implies and by definition, develops subsequent to either a *surgical* or *nonsurgical* nasal trauma or may occur as a nasal manifestation of a systemic illness or rationally subsequent, secondary, to the inexorable aging process. *Secondary atrophic rhinitis* patients consistently have predisposing factors for developing their symptom complex including surgery for turbinate volume reduction to alleviate nasal breathing obstruction, which may induce the ENS producing a *secondary atrophic rhinitis*. This *secondary atrophic rhinitis* does not occur instantaneously but only materializes months to years following the initial surgical intrusion and trauma. There is a vast list of both surgical and nonsurgical adjunctive procedures designed to improve nasal breathing by treating enlargement ("hypertrophy") of the inferior turbinate, which may in turn spawn a *secondary atrophic rhinitis*. Based on our observations and experience with hundreds of ENS patients, any of the surgical procedures listed in Table 2.2 can produce ENS.[18] Principally, the surgical turbinate reduction procedures of the turbinates have regularly been undertaken *without* any preoperative functional physiological testing.

The adjunctive procedures which we term: n-s TRAPs are listed in Table 2.3.[25,26]

Table 2.4 Summarizes various treatment modalities created and crafted for inferior turbinate enlargement ("hypertrophy") collected and presented by Hol and Huizing in 2000 dating back to the middle of the 19th century.[25] With the passage of

Table 2.2 Surgical turbinate reduction procedures (inferior and or middle) able to produce the empty nose syndrome (ENS).

1. Total turbinectomy
2. Partial turbinectomy (inferior and or middle)
3. Crushing and mucosal trimming procedures
4. Posterior inferior turbinate tip resection
5. Submucosal tissue resection-inferior turbinate (broadly called turbinoplasty)
6. Submucosal resection of the conchal bone (broadly called turbinoplasty)
7. Combined resection of submucosal tissue and conchal bone (broadly called turbinoplasty)

Table 2.3 Non-surgical Turbinate Reduction Adjunctive Procedures (n-s TRAPs).[a]

1. Thermal coagulation (electrocautery)
2. Chemocoagulation
3. Injection of corticosteroids, sclerosing agents
4. Cryosurgery
5. Laser surgery
6. Radiofrequency ablation
7. Coblation (derived from "controlled ablation" meaning tissue removal in a controlled manner or "cold ablation" meaning tissue removal by a reduced or "colder" temperature)
8. Ultrasound

[a] Specifically, and by definition, the term surgery is the medical practice of managing diseases, deformities, and injuries by actually "cutting" into a part of the body, while, on the other hand, the procedures of electrocautery, chemocautery, lasers, radiofrequency, coblation, or ultrasound are not surgery in the traditional "strict sense" of "cold knife" cutting, but nonetheless they are currently covered beneath the umbrella of "surgery," although we prefer to label them: "**n**on-**s**urgical" **T**urbinate **R**eduction **A**djunctive **P**rocedure (n-s TRAP).

time, we added radiofrequency (2004) and ultrasound (2010) to the list of treatment options for inferior turbinate enlargement ("hypertrophy").

3.3 Differential diagnosis of nasal atrophy

There are a number of systemic illnesses that the physician needs to be interested in, such as lymphoma, with epistaxis, also termed midline destructive lesions with various additional names such as idiopathic midline granuloma or lethal midline granuloma or polymorphic reticulosis because these systemic diseases may have an initial rhinologic presentation, which is designated a nasal manifestation of a systemic disease. For example, a granulomatous disorder such as sarcoidosis, or

Table 2.4 History of treatments for Inferior Turbinate Enlargement (hypertrophy).[4,25]

---

1. Thermal coagulation, electrocautery 1845–1880
2. Chemocoagulation, chemotherapy 1869–1890
3. Turbinectomy 1882
4. Lateralization, lateropexia (out-fracture) 1904
5. Submucous resection of the turbinate bone 1906–1911
6. Crushing + trimming, partial resection 1930–1953
7. Injection of corticosteroids 1952
8. Injection of sclerosing agents 1953
9. Vidian neurectomy 1961
10. Cryosurgery 1970
11. Laser surgery 1977
12. Turbinoplasty 1982
13. Powered instruments (shaver, microdebrider) 1994
14. High radiofrequency radiation 1998
    With the passage of time, we added to their list:
15. Radiofrequency 2004 (Nease and Krempl)[26]
16. Ultrasound 2010 (Gindros et al.)[27]

---

mycobacterial tuberculosis, leprosy or syphilis*, or other rarer infectious diseases may present with nasal obstruction, crusting, epistaxis, anosmia, and face pain.

Syphilis is the well-known infectious disease produced by the spirochete Treponema pallidum. *Because of its diverse, and at times confusing, clinical and histopathologic portrait, syphilis may appear in any of three specific phases: primary syphilis presents as an ulceration (chancre), secondary syphilis has a variable histology and may be easily misinterpreted, while tertiary syphilis presents as a necrotizing granulomatous inflammation.*

Autoimmune diseases such as granulomatosis with polyangiitis (formerly known as Wegener's granulomatosis) may present with nasal obstruction, nasal crusting, foul (fetid) odor, and epistaxis. Other autoimmune diseases including relapsing polychondritis have the nasal manifestations of nasal atrophy with crusting and epistaxis and may coexist with an underlying malignant disease. Another autoimmune disease, eosinophilic granulomatosis with polyangiitis (necrotizing vasculitis) formerly Churg-Strauss syndrome can present with nasal obstruction (difficulty breathing), nasal crusting, and epistaxis. Sjogren's syndrome is a progressive autoimmune inflammation with nasal manifestations of nasal airway obstruction, dryness, crusting, epistaxis, and hyposmia. In considering the differential diagnosis of ENS, physicians and surgeons must also consider the possibility of an underling systemic disorder or medication-induced nasal dryness and associated difficulty

Table 2.5 Differential diagnosis of nasal atrophy.

A. *Primary atrophic rhinitis*
B. Secondary atrophic rhinitis
    1. Empty nose syndrome (ENS)
    2. Lymphoma also called:
       a. Idiopathic midline granuloma
       b. Lethal midline granuloma
       c. Polymorphic reticulosis
    3. Granulomatous
       a. Leprosy
       b. Rhinoscleroma, gram-negative bacilli, *Klebsiella pneumoniae rhinoscleromatis*
       c. Sarcoidosis
       d. Tertiary syphilis (necrotizing granulomatous inflammation) [a]
       e. Tuberculosis
    4. Autoimmune
       a. Granulomatosis with polyangiitis (formerly Wegener's granulomatosis)
       b. Eosinophilic granulomatosis with polyangiitis (formerly Churg-Strauss syndrome)
       c. Relapsing polychondritis
       d. Sjogren's syndrome
    5. Rhinitis of "aging" (also known as "geriatric" rhinitis, "senile" rhinitis)
    6. Surgical and nonsurgical turbinate trauma
    7. Other

[a] *Syphilis is the well-known infectious disease produced by the spirochete Treponema pallidum. Because of its diverse, and at times confusing, clinical and histopathologic portrait, syphilis may appear in any of three specific phases: primary syphilis presents as an ulceration (chancre), secondary syphilis has a variable histology and may be easily misinterpreted, while tertiary syphilis presents as anecrotizing granulomatous inflation.*

Table 2.6 Diagnostic workup for intranasal atrophic changes.

1. "Routine" blood studies
2. Sedimentation rate
3. C-reactive protein
4. Antineutrophil cytoplasm antibodies (c-ANCA)
5. Additional serologic assays as indicated
6. General bacterial culture and sensitivity
7. Analysis for acid-fast bacillus
8. Culture for fungi and anaerobes
9. Intranasal tissue biopsy

with nasal breathing. Table 2.5 is a list of the probable (most likely) differential diagnosis of a patient with nasal atrophy.

All of these disorders must be considered in the differential diagnosis of nasal atrophic changes (nasal atrophy) observed on the physical examination and correlated with the patient's symptomatology, which may require some of the following studies depending on your clinical suspicion, remembering that intranasal tissue biopsy is usually, but not always, diagnostically decisive.

A summary of the diagnostic workup for intranasal atrophy is seen in Table 2.6.

Consultation with colleagues in internal medicine, infectious disease, and rheumatology may be helpful. While *secondary atrophic rhinitis*, in this classification, is more commonly encountered in the Western world than *primary atrophic rhinitis*, both disorders share overlapping symptoms with entirely different etiologies.

In summary, the physician and surgeon can distinguish between *primary and secondary atrophic rhinitis* as follows: *primary atrophic rhinitis* is defined when the "hallmark" symptoms occur *without* a definite antecedent cause or trigger in the *absence* of surgical or nonsurgical nasal trauma, (n-s TRAPs) without any evidence of granulomatous or inflammatory autoimmune diseases, with a *positive culture* for *Klebsiella pneumoniae ozaenae.*

Secondary atrophic rhinitis frequently has a definitive and indisputable antecedent cause such as surgery, systemic illness, or the aging process together with bacterial culture findings almost always *negative* for *Klebsiella pneumoniae ozaenae.* Overall, *primary atrophic rhinitis* is a debilitating chronic disorder heralded by a constellation of symptoms with an abnormally patent nasal airway with the patient complaining of nasal airway obstruction. Diagnosis is aided by history, physical examination, classic symptomatology confirmed with imaging studies, tissue biopsy with histology, and culture positive for *Klebsiella pneumoniae ozaenae*, while considering an extensive differential diagnosis and ruling out systemic illness. It must also be acknowledged that changes in the nasal mucosa may be part of the inexorable aging process.

With an ever-increasing elderly population, newly descriptive terms have been introduced into the literature such as "geriatric" rhinitis, "senile" rhinitis, or the rhinitis of "aging," all of which are describing the atrophic nasal mucosal changes secondary to a loss of submucosal seromucinous and goblet cells, decrease of collagen, and an alteration in mucosal microvascular blood flow. Certainly, the rhinitis of "aging" is an example of *secondary atrophic rhinitis.* Senior citizens often have thin atrophic nasal mucosa and symptoms of nasal crusting, thickened nasal secretions, nasal obstruction, and a decreased olfactory acuity. Complicating issues include the fact that many older patients are medicated with diuretics, beta blockers, and psychological medications that have known side effects including nasal dryness and difficulty breathing secondary to nasal airway obstruction. A list of various medications with the side effect of dry nose is seen in Table 2.7.

Based on a literature review, and our own combined clinical experience, the evidence is undeniable that ENS is an iatrogenic disorder with *secondary atrophic*

Table 2.7 Various medications with the side effect of dry nose.

1. Doxepin (tricyclic antidepressants)
2. Methyldopa (antiadrenergic) for hypertension
3. Sympathomimetics (local-topical)
4. Antihistamines (first generation)
5. Retinoids (1%–10%)

rhinitis. This *secondary atrophic rhinitis* develops subsequent to the *surgical* resection of functioning turbinate tissue or *nonsurgical*-induced mucosal damage resulting from an adjunctive procedure to the turbinates (n-s TRAP) There are many physiological reasons to explain why some patients undergoing a turbinate procedure experience mucosal damage secondary to either an "excessive invasive" surgical resection or a "minimally invasive" n-s TRAP. These patients can subsequently develop symptoms of ENS, as nasal mucosal atrophy ensues into the future and perhaps exacerbating the aging process. Aside from a paradoxical sense of nasal airway obstruction, dryness, and crusting, psychiatric manifestations (clinical depression and or anxiety with suicidal ideation) are found in both the ENS and other patients with a *secondary atrophic rhinitis.* In a Mayo Clinic study, among the 242 atrophic rhinitis patients (*primary atrophic rhinitis n* = 45, without a history of nasal surgery, *secondary atrophic rhinitis*, with a history of nasal turbinate surgery *n* = 197), more than half (52%) experienced an associated reactive depression, evidenced by positive findings of the Minnesota Multiphasic Personality Inventory (MMPI) instrument.[18]

Given the difficulty characterizing ENS, the incidence or probability of developing ENS after a turbinate procedure is unknown, unpredictable, and usually unable to be conveyed to the patient preoperatively. Another drawback to tracking the disease is that ENS manifestations, signs and symptoms, may occur shortly after the turbinate procedure, or may require months or even years to evolve progressing to become symptomatic and consistent with a *secondary atrophic rhinitis* picture.[18,21] In 1985, almost 10 years prior to defining ENS, Moore et al.,[2] from the University of Nebraska, found an overwhelming majority of patients at three to five years subsequent to a bilateral total inferior turbinectomy experiencing symptoms that now would be consistent with ENS. In the same cohort of patients seen at two years following initial surgery, very few patients had any symptoms suggestive of ENS.[2] As previously stated, these findings led their team to denounce total inferior turbinectomy, warning the profession that symptoms may not become obvious pending the passage of years following the initiating surgery. We should recognize and acknowledge patient complaints regarding nasal symptoms even if they occur many years after nasal procedural interventions. It may take an unspecified aggregate of time, for any given individual, at times measured in years, before the breathing and defensive nasal functions devolve into symptomatic blatant ENS. Again, realize that there are numerous medications that may generate a side effect of dry nose are seen in Table 2.7.

4. Diagnosis of ENS

The variety and intensity of symptoms seen in ENS cannot be predicted based upon the gross amount of nasal turbinate tissue surgically resected, removed, or damaged following any one of a number of turbinate reduction procedures. The bedrock of medical diagnosis is the history and physical examination findings, and remains unwavering in our practice, the massive majority of patients with ENS presented with a history and findings of previous trauma (surgical and nonsurgical) to the nasal turbinates. These findings included surgically absent, reduced, or damaged turbinate mucosal tissue which secondarily initiated a disruption of the normal functioning nasal mucosa. When thinking about the nasal mucosa, recall that the nasal mucosa encompasses the entire pseudostratified ciliated respiratory nasal epithelium including the subepithelial submucosa (lamina propria, stroma) neurovascular and active glandular secreting structures. The neurological connections include both a sensory and the autonomic nervous systems. If we consider the nasal mucosa as the "organ of the nose," any operative procedure or disease process that disturbs the functioning nasal mucosa may theoretically provoke and trigger ENS, as an example of *secondary atrophic rhinitis*. This includes surgeries that "significantly" damage the nasal mucosa (including partial or complete turbinate resection), in addition to relatively "minor" procedures producing ENS symptoms, which have been reported following laser turbinate reduction.[18] "Damaged mucosa" does not simply and exclusively include nasal turbinate mucosal resection. We, as well as others,[18-27] have repeatedly observed patients with severe ENS symptoms in the absence of any removal of nasal mucosa but who suffered symptomatic damage from "simple" or "minor" turbinate procedures including the listed n-s TRAPs seen in Table 2.3.[25,26] The sine qua non for diagnosing ENS is evidence of the classic symptoms subsequent to a documented history of a preceding nasal surgical or nonsurgical intervention with removal or traumatic impairment of the nasal turbinates seen in Table 2.1. Complicating the diagnosis of ENS is the fact that these ENS symptoms may not appear until a lengthy number of months or even years ensue after the initial nasal traumatic intervention and these symptoms may be experienced by patients with other disorders.[18,28-30] Accordingly, a differential diagnostic challenge is presented to the clinician attempting to accurately diagnose ENS patients and summarized in Table 2.5.

In the past few years, several validated tests have been introduced to aid in diagnosing ENS. The first is the Empty Nose Syndrome 6 Questionnaire (ENS6Q) questionnaire, which is a validated survey specifically designed to support the diagnosis of ENS.[31] This ENS6Q contains many common, but far from comprehensive, ENS symptoms including:

1. Nasal suffocation
2. Nasal burning
3. Nasal openness
4. Nasal crusting
5. Nasal dryness
6. Impaired air sensation through the nasal cavities

The second validated test is termed the "cotton test." In this test, a piece of dry cotton is introduced into the nose adjacent to the head of the inferior turbinate and remains in place for approximately 30 min. The patient performs the ENS6Q test before, during, and after the "cotton test," and if they experience improvement, evaluated on a 5-item transition score, then a diagnosis of ENS is strengthened and theoretically, at least, a "beneficial" surgical intervention might be considered.[32]

Recently, in 2020, Gill and associates[33] noted an increased interest in ENS as a legitimate "physiologic disease entity" obliging clinicians to become familiar with current diagnostic tools, thereby allowing ENS validation. The reality of being able to diagnose ENS ultimately leads physicians toward intelligent management of distressed ENS patients, many of whom (up to 66%) suffer significant psychological anguish requiring compassionate, time-consuming counsel. Many of the Mayo patients (125/242,52%) were also diagnosed with psychological pain especially depression as evidenced by the MMPI and/or in consultation with a Mayo Clinic psychiatrist.[18]

The ENS6Q may supplement the history coupled with the intranasal examination that supports attaining a reasoned diagnosis of ENS. The in-office "cotton test" may be helpful to identify patients who might conceivably experience symptomatic improvement from a turbinate "replacement" graft or implant. Recognize that the CT scan, computational fluid dynamics, and intranasal trigeminal nerve function testing presently are *insufficient* to corroborate and confirm the diagnosis of ENS.[31]

5. Iatrogenic wonderland-etiology of ENS

For our group,[18] and others[2–4,18–28], the etiology of ENS remains clearly and undoubtedly a *secondary atrophic rhinitis*, that is secondary to a preceding nasal surgical turbinate reduction procedure on the inferior and or the middle turbinate Table 2.2. ENS may also occur with nasal mucosal trauma secondary to one or more n-s TRAPs. Table 2.3. All of the symptoms in patients with the ENS are subsequent to disturbances of one or more of the three primary physiologic nasal functions of olfaction, breathing (respiration), and defense summarize in Table 2.2.

As previously cited, there are a number of systemic illnesses that the physician needs to be cognizant of because the symptomatic complaints of difficulty breathing, crusting, epistaxis with the findings of atrophic mucosal changes may appear as a *secondary atrophic rhinitis* which necessitates thinking of the differential diagnosis of nasal atrophy as outlined and summarized in Table 2.5. Several of these systemic illnesses presenting with nasal manifestations are critical to accurately diagnose since some of these disorders may be deadly.

Pathophysiology of the empty nose syndrome (ENS)

3

Although scientific research regarding nasal physiology, the essence of nasal function, has increased considerably, there are, according to the literature, *still insufficient preoperative objective studies to guide surgical practice.* Germane to the state of development of scientific advancement in measuring nasal physiological function, it is noted that the eminent scientist Lord Kelvin (Sir William Thompson 1824−1907) remarked:

> *"I often say that when you can measure what you are speaking about, and express it in numbers, you know something about it; but when you cannot measure it, when you cannot express it in numbers, your knowledge is a meagre and unsatisfactory kind; it may be the beginning of knowledge, but you have scarcely in your thoughts advanced to the state of Science, whatever the matter may be."* *

*Popular Lectures and Addresses (PLA), 1891−1894, Volume 1 of three volumes, "Electrical Units of Measurement," 1883-05-03 by Lord Kelvin.

Often the nasal surgeon determines the functional capacity of the nasal "organ" by observation and subjective patient reporting alone, as evidenced by the *abundant absence* of objective testing data in the majority of papers in the literature dealing with almost any aspect of nasal surgery. The justification of this "observational" practice stems from a number of factors. Although some objective nasal functional tests are available, few are *routinely* used by practicing surgeons. In addition, there is an associated absence of medical or patient community pressure demanding functional testing prior to any nasal surgery including rhinoplasty. Who among us, but the most imprudent and cavalier would perform otologic surgery without a preoperative audiogram? In reality, patients present for rhinoplasty or for complaints of nasal airway subjective obstructive symptoms (difficulty breathing) and surgeons willingly operate based on the patient's subjective symptoms coupled with their "observational" assessment alone. The "success" of the surgery simply relies upon the patient's subjective sense of change in their nasal airway function, and the surgeon's physical examination or photographic comparison. There has been objective, evidence-based data to support a correlation between the patient's subjective sense of nasal breathing improvements following internal nasal valve surgery and the surgeon's observational findings on clinical examination.[36,37] Surgeons cite these papers as credible scientific evidence supporting a long-held belief that the combination of the patient's *subjective* sense of nasal breathing and the surgeon's findings on careful history and physical examination is sufficient to achieve high-quality outcomes from functional nasal breathing surgery.

When it comes to turbinate surgery, however, there is presently no agreed upon "right amount" of functional tissue to be removed or preserved. Patients may develop symptoms of empty nose syndrome (ENS) following *qualitative functional changes* to the turbinate mucosa consequent to chemocautery, laser therapy, cryosurgery, radiofrequency, coblation, and submucosal cauterization, even when the "observed" amount of turbinate tissue remains fundamentally unchanged.

Does this situation shout for some functional testing of nasal physiologic mechanisms as part of routine "preoperative" patient evaluation?

Recall Lord Kelvin, "… but when you cannot measure it, when you cannot express it in numbers, your knowledge is a meagre and unsatisfactory kind; it may be the beginning of knowledge, but you have scarcely in your thoughts advanced to the state of Science, whatever the matter may be."

The question arises, how does damage to the nasal mucosa generate each and every one of the various protean symptoms seen in ENS?

A recent computerized tomography (CT) study examining the volume of turbinate tissue remaining in ENS patients versus a control group demonstrated a significant correlation between symptoms of nasal dryness, facial pain, posterior nasal "drip," and nasal discharge with small inferior turbinate volume (size) compared with normal sized (volume) turbinates in the control group. The study also identified an impaired quality-of-life for these ENS patients and discovered that the mean time to diagnosis of ENS from the time of initial surgical turbinate reduction was *over 6.5 years*.[28] That delay or latency time can be measured in years, which is similar to the findings of others.[2,18] Despite these valued findings, currently there are no objective criteria indicating the amount or volume of turbinate tissue removal or residual mucosal remnants that specifically induces ENS.

Regarding the symptom of pain, some researchers have hypothesized that a large contributor of pain seen in ENS is neural damage, akin to "phantom limb" pain, in the turbinate tissue (parenchyma) with abnormal neural regrowth.[31] The support for this reasoning comes from studies demonstrating the absence of trigeminal responses in ENS patients, localization of nerve growth factor to the turbinates, and the abundance of mechanoreceptors, thermoreceptors, and nerve endings in the nasal cavity.[38–40] Nerve injury, secondary to resection trauma, may result in a neurogenic pain syndrome, "Phantom Turbinate", likely due to sprouting of pain (A) fibers after a traumatic injury.[41] The simple alteration in degree and type of sensation may be enough to create a "different" and "bothersome" sensation for the patient that continues as a constant and persistent irritant.

A substantial decrease in nerve growth factor or paucity of sensory receptors could result in the diminished sensation of airflow.[39] Studies have shown that the lining of the nasal vestibule is more sensitive to airflow than any other region of the nasal cavity.[40] Since a turbinate procedure reduces the amount of viable and functioning tissue, the sense of stuffiness or difficulty breathing experienced by most ENS patients may be in part explained by the damage to trigeminal nerve endings and the decrease of growth mediators.[19] In ENS, there is disruption of the normal nasal aerodynamics. Physiological studies have shown that lung volumes are expanded with increased nasal resistance, but with reduced nasal resistance, as in ENS or with mouth breathing, lung volumes are decreased.[40]

Computational models have demonstrated that surgery disrupting turbinate tissue clearly causes changes to nasal airflow from an evenly distributed normal airflow over the entire nasal cavity to an abnormal uneven airflow distribution with minimal mucosal contact.[41−43] Given the fact that patients experiencing ENS have wider nasal passages with decreased oronasal resistance, as their lung volumes and, indirectly, arterial oxygenation is decreased, after turbinate reduction, results in disordered breathing and a sense of suffocation.

Why would this sense of suffocation occur? Because the nose normally creates optimal resistance and efficient air-conditioning, adjusting inspired air to allow for optimal warmth (temperature) and moisture (humidity) permitting optimal exchange of carbon dioxide and oxygen at the alveolar level, removal of the middle and inferior turbinates reduces the efficiency of these essential functions.[44−48]

Ten ENS patients studied at the University of Ulm in Germany demonstrated lower air temperatures at the nostrils, and lower absolute humidity throughout the nasal cavity, compared to controls.[49] The disturbed airflow and the reduced ability to warm and humidify the inspired air could explain the crusting and the sensation of dryness in these patients. Moreover, breathing is adversely affected by the inability to adjust the temperature and humidity of the inspired air due to the *nasopulmonary reflex*, afferent nerve impulses in the trigeminal nerve with efferent nerve impulses in the vagus nerve, which is elicited when temperature-sensitive mucosal nerve endings are activated, producing bronchospasm in response to dry and or cold air.[50,51]

There are known physiologic and pathologic conditions that have a direct or indirect impact on nasal aerodynamics. These factors, combined with the effect of a wider nasal airway on airflow after a turbinate procedure, may allow understanding as to why some patients develop ENS and others do not. The relationship between nasal form and function is one such consideration. Studies have shown that airflow characteristics vary from person to person based on anatomic variables such as nostril orientation (shape), turbinate configuration, overall nasal airway length, and internal nasal valve area dimensions.[52−56] Since individuals with different nasal geometries such as the long, narrow high-arched (leptorrhine) nose compared to the short broad (platyrrhine) nose may have completely different experiences after turbinate reduction resulting from variations in turbulence and airflow rates, which ultimately determine the amount of air−mucosal contact. However, nasal anatomy may only be relevant in certain climates. Payne pointed out that ENS seems to occur in certain geographic regions more frequently than others.[55] Given the important air modifying (adjusting temperature and humidity) function of the nose, patients with certain nasal anatomy undergoing a turbinate reduction procedure would have a different outcome depending on their specific geographic location.

Other important factors related to the development of ENS concern the altered airflow dynamics secondary to portions of functioning turbinate tissue (if any) remaining after surgical resection in addition to the presence of any underlying disease process.[56] For example, an underlying disease process such as allergic rhinitis could mitigate the effects of turbinate loss due to persistent hypertrophy or an increased ability to warm or humidify inhaled air.[56,57] Another contributing factor to the development of ENS is atrophy of the nasal mucosa from chronic inflammation. A recent study presented patients with normal CT scans prior to inferior turbinectomy only to have mucosal thickening with maxillary and ethmoid sinus opacity on CT scans postoperatively.[58] The resultant mucosal thickening was independent of sinusitis. Specifically, patients with unilateral sinusitis showed no difference in mucosal thickening between the affected and unaffected nasal cavities, whereas patients with ENS had increased mucosal thickening ipsilateral to the operated side.[59] The nasal mucosal changes after intervention may be secondary to disruptions in airflow dynamics with or without mucosal inflammation resulting in squamous metaplasia. In terms of airflow dynamics, research has shown that, in rabbits with one nostril surgically closed, increased airflow in the open nostril leads to repeated cycles of ciliary damage and repair.[59] In patients with a "deviated" nasal septum, the nostril with increased airflow often becomes inflamed and shows impaired mucociliary clearance with an associated decrease in glandular acini density.[60] It is well documented that chronic inflammation leads to metaplasia, changing the normal respiratory epithelium to a nonciliated squamous epithelium.[18,60] Intranasal biopsy reveals squamous metaplasia from an ENS patient seen in our practice, Fig. 3.1.

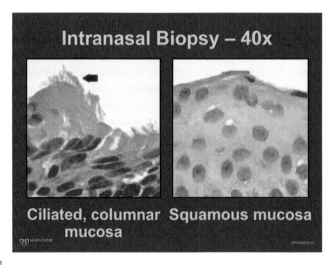

FIGURE 3.1

On the left, normal ciliated (*arrow*) columnar respiratory epithelium of the nasal mucosa. On the right, squamous metaplasia of the intranasal mucosa often seen in patients with the *"empty nose syndrome."*

(Kern and Friedman. By permission of Mayo Foundation for Medical Education and Research. All Rights Reserved).

Damage to normal pseudostratified ciliated respiratory nasal mucosa can lead to squamous metaplasia, which in turn inhibits normal nasal defensive and respiratory function due, in part, to disturbed nerve endings contributing to the diminished airflow sensation frequently reported by ENS patients.[56]

Moreover, since the mucociliary apparatus is destroyed and replaced by squamous metaplasia, bacteria can flourish and multiply, no longer swept away by physiologic ciliary action, thereby accounting for the malodorous (fetid) nasal discharge experienced by many ENS patients. While most of the symptoms of ENS are understood based on disturbed physiology and explained in the existing literature, the profound psychological comorbidities seem less explainable.

Payne speculates that ENS "could be likened to other phenomena where there seems to be a correlation between psychosocial distress and disease tolerance, such as tinnitus" or that it could be the result of a preexisting "nasal neuropathy" that is exacerbated by a turbinate procedure.[55] It may be useful to test some of the proposed ideas, such as giving ENS patients who experience facial pain a trial of gabapentin as Payne advises; however, more data must be gathered on psychological factors. As mentioned previously, the Mayo group found that 52% of their 242 patients experienced depression established on the Minnesota multiphase personality inventory (MMPI) or with psychiatric evaluation.[18] Often these patients feel a loss of control in their lives and psychological depression ensues. The emotional issues need further exploration to better understand how to treat and support these patients.[61,62] To add affront to grievance, patients have regularly informed us that they were callously dismissed by their treating surgeons; frequently told that their physical problems were psychologically based. These denials of a patient's suffering are grim verdicts for our patients to both hear and digest which often exacerbates their psychological distress heightening their determination to find a specific medical or surgical resolution or press for a tangible explanation for their desolation.

Treatment options for ENS

4

1. Introduction

A. Medical
B. Surgical
C. Preventing empty nose syndrome (ENS)

Unfortunately, currently there are no curative or even restorative therapies for ENS.

Realistic management is obliged to provide emotional support by compassionate attentive listening along with controlling and relieving as many of the patient's debilitating symptoms as feasible. Available treatments range from conservative medical measures to surgical interventions, although nothing that we know of today can renew, restore, or recreate the damaged or resected nasal mucosa. Short of stem cell rejuvenation the question remains, how do you create a new and functional nasal turbinate? Hope nonetheless exists that research in the realms of stem cell and tissue engineering will deliver potential future possibilities for our patients. Prevention is always the most prudent choice, of course.

1.1 Medical

Evidence in the literature plus our own experience suggests that certain medical treatments are enormously effective in reducing some of the distressing nasal symptoms, especially the crusting seen in almost all of these patients. Topical moisturizing and malodor control agents, including oil of sesame with rose geranium, which we have used for many years has been useful in helping ease a patient's discomfort.[18] Manuka honey* which we have not used may offer promise based on the recent, 2017, publication from the Department of Otolaryngology-Head and Neck Surgery, University of Washington, Seattle, Washington noted below.

* Lee VS, Humphreys IM, Purcell PL, Davis GE. Manuka honey sinus irrigation for the treatment of chronic rhinosinusitis: a randomized controlled trial. Int Forum Allergy Rhinol. 2017 Apr;7(4):365—372. doi: 10.1002/alr.21898. Epub 2016 Dec 9. PMID: 27935259

"Conclusion: In patients with active chronic rhinosinusitis (CRS) and prior sinus surgery, both Manuka honey (MH) and saline improved outcomes, but there was no statistically significant difference between these groups. However, in the subset that did not receive oral antibiotics/steroids, culture negativity was statistically better on MH, suggesting that MH alone may be effective for acute exacerbations of CRS."

The work of Brown and Graham clearly demonstrated that positive pressure nasal irrigations, although underutilized, can be very effective, especially the finding that *hypertonic* saline irrigations are superior to *isotonic* saline in reducing symptoms. Nasal irrigation (lavage), using a bulb syringe is a pressure method, a "power" wash, that is more effective compared to the nebulizer (spray) method to introduce the irrigation solution especially when mucociliary transport mechanisms are disrupted.[63] Nasal irrigation (lavage is more successful than sprays) is effective by physically removing thickened mucus debris (crusts), bacteria, and the inflammatory mediators, which can interfere with normal mucociliary (ciliary beat frequency) activity.[63]

Table 4.1 summarizes the nasal mucosal moistening agents used in the medical management of patients with ENS and other instances of primary and secondary atrophic rhinitis.

A useful nasal lavage solution (home recipe) as suggested by Brown and Graham from the University of Iowa is presented in Table 4.2.

Saline irrigations with and without antibiotics, most notably Wilson's solution (80 mg of gentamicin a liter of saline), is often helpful. Wilson solution is first utilized as a 30-cc lavage, not nebulized, three times daily and as symptoms improve reduced to twice daily, then once daily, or on alternate days as necessary. The temporary reversible use of cotton obstruction of the nasal cavity has been helpful in moisturizing the nasal mucosal interior while providing some increased resistance to breathing. This strategy has been helpful for some of our patients in the past.

Table 4.1 Nasal mucosal moistening agents.

A. Nasal lavage[a] ("power washing" is superior to nebulization) with saline solution
    1. NaCl **hypertonic** solution (superior to isotonic solution)
B. Nasal sprays
    1. Dexpanthenol 5% for "Rhinitis Sicca"
    2. Liposomal[b] for "Rhinitis Sicca"
    3. Sesame oil with Rose Geranium[c] (lubrication and odor control)
    50 cc Sig. 2 sprays each nostril bid

---

[a] Note: In general, nasal lavage is superior to nasal spray for the **removal** of crusts, debris, bacteria, inflammatory mediators and introducing topical nasal medication(s) in ENS patients.
[b] Note: Based on work of: Hahn C, Böhm M, Allekotte S, Mösges R. Tolerability and effects on quality of life of liposomal nasal spray treatment compared to nasal ointment containing dexpanthenol or isotonic Na Cl spray in patients with rhinitis sicca. Eur Arch Otorhinolaryngol. *September 2013;270(9):2465—72.*
[c] Note: Based on the Mayo Clinic pharmacy proprietary formulation, Rochester, Minnesota.

Table 4.2 Nasal lavage solutions (home recipe) from the University of Iowa.

Liquid	Salt	Baking soda	Final tonicity
Four cups (1 quart) H_2O BOILED 5 Min	1 1/2 tsp.	None.	0.9%

Modified from: Brown CL, Graham SC. Nasal irrigation: good or bad? Curr Opin Otolaryngol Head Neck Surg. 2004;12:9–13.
"Home recipes" versus manufactured powders/solutions
The section on Practical points is quoted directly from Brown and Graham. [63]

"Solutions too cold or too hot are not ideal. The careful use of microwaves can be helpful. Nasal irrigations can be performed over a kitchen sink, over the bathroom basin, or in the shower. The shower provides a ready source of nonsterile water at a chosen temperature. Patients administer the solution with a bulb syringe after instruction by the nursing staff. Demonstrations and handouts are provided." [63]

This "Home recipe" **(Table 4.2)** *generally consist of boiled water, which is cooled before use, mixed with nonionized salt. Table salt is generally* **not** *recommended because it contains additives. Baking soda may be used to buffer the solution but is not essential. Solutions are generally kept in the refrigerator before being discarded after several days. In a recent study, a randomized, controlled trial looking at patients with two episodes of acute sinusitis or one episode of chronic sinusitis per year for 2 consecutive years. Fifty-two patients received hypertonic saline, whereas 24 patients did not receive any irrigations. When using* **hypertonic nasal irrigations,** *improvements in quality-of-life and overall symptom severity scores* **were statistically significant.** *Steroid nasal spray use was also decreased.*

Evaluation at a pain management center with therapeutic use of pain medications administered by those physicians expert in pain control could be considered for patients suffering facial pain and headache.

Psychological support with a compassionate respectful referral to a psychiatrist or other interestedmental health professionals has been valuable inmanaging the anxiety and depression experienced by a sizable share (over 50%) of these patients.[18,62]

Offering a summary of the treatment strategies and diagnostic tools for the *ENS,* Gill and associates observed that, "Nasal humidification, patient education, and treatment of possible concomitant medical conditions (e.g., depression) constitute first lines of treatment."[33]

1.2 Surgical

The goal of surgical procedures has been to reduce ENS airway symptoms by narrowing the nasal cavity in an attempt to reconfigure nasal airway anatomy and reestablish "normal" nasal airway resistance. A diverse assortment of materials has been attempted to reestablish a "normal" nasal airway with varying degrees of success. That's the challenge, how to create a turbinate analog? One of the answers was the use of injectables such as hyaluronic acid (HA) and autologous stromal vascular fraction (SVF). Recently, Modrzyński injected HA submucosally resulting in an increased sensation of nasal airflow and decreased crusting and dryness for less than a year ($n = 3$).[64] Since the effects of HA are temporary, repeat injections are required to sustain relief.

Caution with injections of fillers must be exercised as vascular obstructive incidents and infections are known complications that could be symptomatically and emotionally devastating plus painful to the patient. Others have utilized autologous cartilage grafts from various donor sites including the nasal septum, conchal and rib cartilage. These autologous septal, conchal, and costal cartilage grafts have been found, in ENS, to decrease pain (nasal and facial), reduce the sensation of extreme airflow, lessen nasal crusting, and decrease the feeling of nasal obstruction.[18,65] The cartilage graft donor site comorbidities are a cause for disquiet particularly because as Jang et al. noted there may not be enough conchal or septal cartilage available to produce the required volume to reduce the symptoms.[65]

Recently, a study showed that costal cartilage may be superior to conchal cartilage in the treatment of ENS—statistically significant improved SNOT-25 scores were obtained for both conchal and rib cartilage implants, and suggested reasons for this difference included the increased availability, volume, and strength of rib cartilage as compared with conchal cartilage.[65] Allografts of acellular dermal implants have also been shown to be somewhat effective, with noted improvements in breathing sensation, reduction in nasal crusting, improved sleep, and alleviating some of the psychological stress including depression or anxiety.[19,62,64,65] For patients experiencing pain, Houser noted that dermal implants are not particularly helpful.[20] Alloplastic implant materials are unproven but have been used for ENS including: alloplastic implants of Plastipore, hydroxyapatite, Medpor, and beta-tricalcium phosphate.[66–69]

A new study comparing silastic with alloderm implants found no significant difference between the two materials since patients in both groups showed objective and subjective symptomatic improvement.[70] Unfortunately, most of these studies are limited by small sample size and varied outcome measures. The idea of engaging regenerative treatments using stem cells as a therapeutic management option for ENS patients has been considered with two studies showing mixed results. Kim and colleagues evaluated the effectiveness and safety of the autologous stromal vascular fraction (SVF) in the treatment of nine ENS patients. Although the SVF treatments act to decrease the inflammatory cytokine levels in the nasal mucosa, a single SVF injection was not effective in terms of symptom improvement and patient satisfaction.[71]

New research, in 2015, by Xu et al., using adipocyte-derived stem cells (ADSCs) has provided ENS patients with renewed hope for the future. These ADSCs produce and secrete cytokines that support tissue growth while dampening mucosal injury. The nasal mucociliary activity was significantly improved in the 28 ENS study patients, and there was noted improvement in the symptom of nasal obstruction as tissue inflammation was reduced significantly.[72] Further trials, preferably randomized controlled trials, are clearly compulsory to identify the most practical and useful regenerative treatment modality for patients with ENS.

Leong performed a literature review of various surgical interventions in which implanted materials were applied to the nasal sidewalls of ENS patients. He included eight studies and reported on the aggregate data collected on 128 ENS patients. His analysis, using the reported SNOT-20 and SNOT-25 scores at 3 months and 12 months posttreatment, found that 21% of patients in the various studies reported only marginal subjective improvements.[73]

Since not all surgical interventions resulted in patient benefit, Leong cautioned and advised us to require larger numbers and lengthier follow-up periods with uniform outcome measures before determining the utility of any surgical therapeutic intervention and before deciding which specific surgical intervention is superior and most beneficial for the patient.[73]

Anecdotally, in our practice, we have seen many patients treated surgically with implants, at other institutions, who have returned disappointed complaining of persistent or worsening; escalation of symptoms. Even more unsettling are those patients who after implant surgery experience intensified and increased psychological distress. Aggravated anxiety and "nasal focus" have been typically found among patients whose hopes and expectations are heightened leading into a surgical intervention aimed at reversing or ameliorating the ENS symptoms, only to be disheartened by the discouraging postoperative outcome. Many ENS patients experience emotional suffering with abundant anxiety and discernible depression; it is our responsibility as treating physicians and surgeons to genuinely and sympathetically counsel our patients, as the "guardians of reality"; not discounting our patient's symptoms but listening intently and offering realistic therapeutic options and never the mirage of "cure."[18,62,73-75]

Regarding an update on the treatment strategies for ENS, Gill and colleagues in 2019 stated that, "Although injectable implants to augment turbinate volume show promise as a therapeutic surgical technique, there is ***insufficient data to fully support their use*** at this time."[76] (Bold italics added) Additional procedures hold promise and are described in Chapter 11. A comprehensive list of surgical operations are described in Chapter 11.

1.3 Preventing ENS

In life, as in nasal surgery, especially concerning inferior turbinate surgery, "it's not what you take, it's what you leave behind that matters."

Regardless of turbinate treatment strategies advocated by some surgeons, it is clear that the optimal turbinate management lies in the *prevention* of ENS. It is our experience and that of others, preservation of the nasal mucosa is the authoritative imperative to elude the catastrophic calamity of ENS. Unfortunately, it is unknown, at the present moment, as to the precise amount of nasal mucosa and submucosa that must be preserved during intranasal turbinate procedures to prevent ENS. As a consequence, we should *always minimize* turbinate manipulation with attendant mucosal and submucosal damage, including radical excision of the turbinates only when absolutely obligatory. We all realize that radical turbinectomy is indispensable for inverting papilloma, certain malignant tumors and may be requisite for teenage boys with juvenile angiofibroma.

Our maximum turbinate preservation position has been ferociously argued against by a cavalcade, in our opinion, of *"cavalier"* surgeons two of whom are well-known proponents of total turbinectomy from their writings, Eugene Courtiss, MD and Dov Ophir, MD. One of us (EBK) has had the opportunity to publicly debate, each one on separate occasions, challenging their denial of any explicit or pivotal relationship between total inferior turbinectomy, with its cataclysmic physiological wreckage, and its proficient propensity for precipitating ENS.

How often is the impact of altering nasal breathing mechanics, injuring the nasal defenses, damaging the nasal cycle and a plethora of nasal reflexes, or the likelihood of inducing a posttraumatic amputation pain syndrome considered before nasal surgical intervention? How often are objective nasal functional testing methods available or obtained prior to or following nasal surgical intervention in our "modern 21st century era"? We do not know the answer to these questions; however, if the literature is accurate, we reason that nasal physiologic measurements prior to nasal surgery are quite infrequent in our country. Because of the unique variability of a given individual's response or a person's "host resistance" to nasal mucosal trauma, which is arbitrary, unpredictable, and unmeasurable, surgery on the turbinates, especially the inferior turbinate, to improve nasal airway breathing, must be very "conservative" inflicting the "minimal" trauma and should be directed to the head of the inferior turbinate, which is the posterior portion of the internal nasal valve area, the most critical site for nasal breathing.

Since none of the current ENS treatment options can resolve all of the symptoms of ENS nor can resected or damaged nasal mucosa ("organ of the nose") be replaced, repaired, or restored. Based on our current understanding of the iatrogenic nature and the pathophysiology of ENS, it is clear from the literature, linked with our own involvement with hundreds of ENS cases, for more than a quarter-century, that wide-ranging extensive evidence assuredly exists that total inferior turbinate resection for nonmalignant disease should be *condemned,* in concert with Moore et al.,[2] and that nasal mucosal trauma must be avoided at best or minimized at least.

Because it is unclear the degree of nasal mucosal or submucosal injury in any particular individual that will significantly disturb nasal function(s), especially breathing (respiratory) and defense, which are capable of producing ENS; we exercise remarkable restraint when considering turbinate management and offer some options when managing the turbinates in Chapter 7 The Turbinates-Management.

So, we conclude this section on the prevention of ENS with the repetitive chorus of Prevention, Prevention, and more Prevention of iatrogenic ENS through the avoidance of "excessive" turbinate reduction, which remains an imperative in preventing the plague and torment of ENS. Finally, in a thoughtful 2019 paper by Gill and colleagues discussing the pathophysiology of ENS and reviewing the medical and surgical treatment approaches for ENS patients, they concluded that the ***prevention*** of iatrogenic ENS "… ***is through avoidance of excessive turbinate reduction*** …"[76] (Bold italics added)

The turbinates—an overview

5

1. Historical perspective*

To the best of our knowledge, it was a New Yorker, William M. Jarvis, MD who in 1882 described three cases of utilizing a snare to affect a partial turbinectomy in which he stated: "I have selected two cases of posterior turbinated hypertrophy and one of anterior hypertrophy from a number of the kind, as best illustrating certain points to be fully considered in my conclusions. The Écraseur** used by me to remove these growths was shown to the American Laryngological Association in 1880." In his description, he said that: "I removed the gelatinous polyps from both sides of the nose using the écraseur. I then snared postinferior turbinated hypertrophy occupying the left postnasal opening and drew the wire loop tightly around the growth."[77]

*Authors note: We have chosen to be historically inclusive, perhaps excessively expansive, at the risk of being "overly comprehensive" in presenting the "other side" of the "turbinate debate" in their own words from their own writings, which supports our preference for conservative tissue sparing principles when compared to aggressive tissue resection with seemingly little regard for the functional, physiologic, activities of the nasal respiratory mucosa, including the epithelial layer and the deeper submucosal stromal tissues. To fathom the depth of the acerbic aspects of the "turbinate debate," especially regarding inferior turbinate management, we believe this in-depth historical perspective is required, virtually commanding.

** Note: Écraseur translated from the French language as "crusher."

At the dawn of the 20th century, most surgeons were promoting total inferior turbinectomy not only for nasal airway obstruction but astoundingly also for hearing impairment and tinnitus. T. Carmalt Jones presented at a meeting of the British Medical Association and notes from that meeting were presented in the distinguished and dignified medical journal *The Lancet* in 1895 which cited his presentation as follows:

"Removal of hypertrophied inferior turbinals and moriform growths should be practiced in cases of deafness and tinnitus where the auditory nerve was in a healthy condition." He had operated in upwards of 500 cases. Notes were read of twelve cases of deafness or tinnitus in which turbinotomy had been performed. *"Eleven of these were cases of deafness and tinnitus combined. Relief to both conditions was afforded in eight cases; slight relief to deafness only in one. In two there was no relief at all. A discussion followed."*[78]

Two months later at the Fifth International Congress of Otology, another physician with the identical surname as T. Carmalt, Dr. MacNaughton Jones presented a paper which was also covered in *The Lancet* and titled: *"Turbinale Hypertrophy and its Deafness Relations, especially with regard to Operation Turbinotonrie."* This chronicle was translated from the French and was introduced by Dr. MacNaughton Jones and was respectably described in the journal as follows:

"Dr. MacNaughton Jones gave a masterly review of the subject as dealt with by previous otologists, and summed up by some of his own conclusions: "Turbinal hypertrophy must be regarded as a serious complication of deafness and the cognate aural affections; in those cases, in which it precedes the aural symptoms we may justly regard it as being their principal cause." Dr. Jones resumes:

"In all cases in which this hypertrophic change is discovered active therapeutic measures, of which galvano-cauterisation is the chief, ought to be put in practice to reduce it. Turbinotomy is indicated and ought to be reserved for those cases in which, whether in consequence of the bulk or of the nature of the growth, it is vain to expect improvement from any other treatment."[79]

Of course, turbinate enlargement or "hypertrophy" is neither the cause nor a complication of hearing loss. Fortunately, and for the most part, dazed blunders and egregious errors in thinking by esteemed experts, for the most part, have remedied itself through scientific studies, since the late 19th century.

A mere five years later, in 1900, CR Holmes published an article in *The New York Medical Journal* where he acknowledged the status of the **nose as a significant organ system** and that **minimal resection of the inferior turbinate was superior to** "extensive destruction," **which** "**generally leads to dryness of the pharynx.**" Which we can probably assume that "dryness of the pharynx" is a form of atrophy, a secondary atrophic rhinitis.[80] (Bold italics added)

Dr. Holmes astutely continued:

"The object of every operation is to restore as nearly as possible the parts to a normal condition, and in operating we should not only consider the immediate but also the remote effects. ***In operating upon the nose, we must remember that it is a very important organ,*** *whose function is to partly filter, moisten, and warm the air before it enters the pharynx, larynx, and lungs. Too extensive destruction these bodies generally leads to dryness of the pharynx and inability of the patient to effectually expel the nasal secretion by forcible blowing of the*

*nose, which is another source of annoyance…" "**In all cases, aim to remove as little of the edge of the inferior turbinated** as is consistent with the restoration of sufficient breathing space, and save as much of the anterior end of the bone as possible…"[80]* (Bold italics added)

The renowned rhinologist, Dr. Otto T. Freer of Chicago, in the early part of the 20th century, recognized along with CR Holmes that *radical procedures of the inferior turbinate were both irresponsible and unwise.* In a paper written in 1911, Freer indicated that:

*"In order to avoid the creation of the bad stump embodying the objections mentioned and with the idea of sufficiently **preserving the physiologic function** of moistener of the inspired air, possessed by the turbinated body, I gradually devised the operative method here described and have employed for several years with great satisfaction. It reduces the turbinated body to any size desired and insures covering of the cut surface by a flap."[81]* (Bold italics added)

Dr. Freer observed the introduction of radical turbinate operations replacing the unpredictable results with cauterization, and yet he reports that he has never seen a case of atrophic rhinitis:

*"Rhinologists, therefore, have in a large measure abandoned cauterization for intumescence and have adopted the more radical procedure turbinotomy instead the turbinate being wholly almost cut away with the saw, scissors, or punch. I have not, however, after turbinotomy performed even in this crude manner, found the permanent chronic scabbing described by some authors and have found that in time the stump always heals over smoothly; **nor have I ever seen atrophic rhinitis** as a consequence of even the complete removal of an inferior turbinate, atrophic rhinitis being a distinct pathological process which cannot be surgically created."[81]* (Bold italics added)

Despite the brilliant observational powers of the dazzling Otto T. Freer, his statement that atrophic rhinitis cannot be surgically created likely refers to ozena, as we now know, from hundreds of cases that secondary atrophic rhinitis can be "surgically created" secondary to radical excision that may not appear for some many years after the initial surgery.[2-4,18-28] Freer proceeded to describe his technique for excising the conchal bone while preserving the mucosa with an inferior turbinate mucosal flap. This mucosal flap preservation occurs all the while performing a longitudinal resection of as much of the conchal bone as possible at its root. Sadly, Freer does not offer any patient data and concludes the paper with:

"The longitudinal resection I have described here has been successfully employed by me for a number of years and I recommend it as a tried and completed procedure."[81]

In 1914, just a few years after Dr. Freer's inferior turbinate conchal bone excision with mucosal flap preservation, Dr. Albert Mason of Georgia also recognized along with CR Holmes the requisite prerequisite for ***preserving the physiologic function*** of ***the nose*** as he wrote a plaintive plea for conservation of the inferior turbinate mucosa:

*"In the first place, 'damage to mucous membrane' is certainly much greater in turbinotomy than in submucous resection. In the former, a large area is completely removed, while in the latter, the linear incision heals with practically no destruction of the nasal mucous membrane. Furthermore, the **mucous membrane covering the inferior turbinate is the most important functionating part of the nose, and for this reason should be left alone, when possible."*** (Bold italics added)

Dr. Mason added that:

*"I have also seen a condition resembling **atrophic rhinitis** follow the removal of part of the turbinate. Patients, upon whom turbinotomies had been done some time previously, complain of a dryness of the nose and throat, but have never seen or heard of a case developing a dryness after a submucous resection."* ***"In conclusion, I plead with you, both rhinologist and general practitioner, to respect the function of the inferior turbinate and to save it when possible to do so."***[82] (Bold italics added)

Obviously, Dr. Mason observed the deleterious consequences of injury to the nasal mucous membrane of the inferior turbinate resulting in *secondary atrophic rhinitis*. Realizing and articulating that the nasal mucous membrane is the most important functioning portion of the nose obliging preservation. Evidently, even in the first quarter of the 20th century, enough cases were discussed or reported that warned the profession of adverse sequelae after an aggressive inferior turbinate injury with secondary atrophic rhinitis. In addition to *secondary atrophic rhinitis*, surgeons had to contend with the terrorizing experience of intraoperative and or postoperative hemorrhage after aggressive turbinate resections. Dr. Mason reported that he never detected a case of atrophic rhinitis when only the conchal bone of the inferior turbinate was removed but the nasal mucous membrane was preserved.[82]

Dr. William Spielberg of New York City influenced by Freer and Dr. W. Stuart Low further discussed resection of the conchal bone of the inferior turbinate, with turbinate mucosal preservation. Dr. Spielberg realized that adverse sequelae could occur when excessive mucosal tissue of the inferior turbinate is removed. Quoting directly from his 1924 paper as follows:

*"The chief objection to many of the operations as at present performed on the nasal passages in general and the inferior turbinate in particular for the alleviation of nasal obstruction, **is that frequently to much tissue was removed**. This holds true for such operative procedures as cauterization, partial amputation, or the so-called clipping of the inferior turbinates, the spoke shave operation, Ballenger's swivel knife operation, the flap resection operation of Otto T. Freer. The submucous anterior turbinectomy operation first described by W. Stuart Low*

and apparently later (1911) modified, but not very much improved by Freer,
comes closest in the opinion of the writer, to the ideal manner in dealing surgi-
cally with an hypertrophy of the inferior turbinate." (Bold italics added)

Dr. Spielberg presented details of a limited submucous resection operation of the conchal bone all the while preserving the nasal mucosa. He presented details regarding 20 patients (9 females, 11 males) with follow-up from one month to six months, age range from 16 to 56 years and 19 were pronounced cured while his last patient's result was less than cured but nonetheless graded as "good."[83]

The eminent otologist Howard House of Los Angeles, California, continued the tradition of submucosal resection of the inferior turbinate conchal bone with preservation of the precious functional nasal mucosa and submucosa of that same inferior turbinate.

"The success of this operation depends upon removing the thickened anterior
portion of the inferior terminal bone with a minimum amount of trauma to the sur-
rounding mucosa."[84]

Using a postoperative questionnaire in the entire study population ($n = 102$), House found complete (100%) relief of nasal airway obstruction in 47 patients (46%) and 75% relief in 19 patients (18%). He concluded that the majority of patients ($n = 102$) who underwent submucous resection of the anterior one-third of the inferior turbinate conchal bone had a favorable response with 64% of patients having 75%−100% relief of nasal airway obstruction at 2 years after surgery. Another 14 patients (14%) had 50% relief of nasal airway obstruction, and 5 patients (5%) had 25% relief, no relief in 14 patients (14%) while 3 patients (3%) were made worse. The operation reduced the size of the anterior head of the inferior turbinate with a minimal of interference to nasal physiology.[84]

In 1973, Hunter Fry published in the *Australian and New Zealand Journal of Surgery* an article entitled, "Judicious turbinectomy for nasal obstruction."[85] With that title one would plausibly anticipate that the "conservative" approach advised by Holmes,[80] Freer,[81] Mason,[82] Spielberg,[83] or House[84] would have reached the shores of the island country Australia, even by an extremely dawdling boat; however, Fry plunges precipitously and abruptly into total inferior turbinate resection, turbinate termination by the stealth of steely scissors. The quotation from his work listed under the section titled *Technique* reads quietly and unassumingly:

"The inferior turbinate is reduced with turbinectomy scissors."[85]

Addressing the middle turbinate, he continues:

"The middle turbinate is reduced by Hartman's conchotome, or sometimes by
Luc's forceps when there is no room to spare and a septoplasty has not been car-
ried out (which assists exposure of the middle turbinate)."

Fry, in the *Conclusions* of his paper, writes:

"The operation of surgical reduction of the turbinates has been found to be a most satisfactory and necessary procedure for the relief of nasal obstruction. It can be relied on to relieve nasal obstruction and its complications. In the last year post-operative bleeding has not been a significant problem. The writer has not seen any cases of rhinitis sicca in his own patients."[85]

Of his abbreviated list of 8 references include: 2 "personal communication," 1 "not published" and symposium (unpublished), 2 text books (1955, 1971), and 2 journal articles (1965, 1970). He never mentions Holmes,[80] Freer,[81] Mason,[82] Spielberg,[83] or House[84] because, in all likelihood, he was either indifferent or oblivious of the American literature. Below is the list of references by Hunter Fry in the journal: Aust N Z J Surg. 1973 Feb;42(3):291—4.

1. Cantor C. (1972), personal communication.
2. Caust, LJ. (1968), "The Surgical Relief of Nasal Obstruction" paper read at general scientific meeting of Royal Australasian College of Surgeons, Adelaide, but not published.
3. Caust LJ. (1972), personal communication.
4. Clarke G. (1972), in symposium on "Turbinectomy" at the University Department of Otolaryngology, Royal Victorian Eye and Ear Hospital
5. Duouek E. (1971) in Scott-Brown's "Diseases of the Nose," Butterworths, London: 220.
6. Ewert G. (1965), Acta oto-laryng. (Stockh.), Suppl.200 (Complete citation is added by authors as follows: Ewert G. On the mucus flow rate in the human nose. Acta Otolaryngol Suppl. 1965; 200:SUPPL 200:1—62. PMID: 14326391.)
7. Thomson ST C, Negus VE. (1955), "Diseases of the Nose and Throat" Cassell & Co., London: 195.
8. Watkins ABK. (1970), Med J Aust, 1: 382.
   (The complete citation is added by authors as follows: Watkins AB. Middle turbinate headache. Med J Aust. 1970 Feb 21; 1(8):382—4. doi: 10.5694/j.1326-5377.1970.tb77928.x. PMID: 5439147.)

Unfortunately, Fry, in his turbinectomy assertion, provides neither illustrations nor any data. He referred to rhinitis sicca as atrophic rhinitis, not making the distinction between primary and secondary atrophic rhinitis writing:

"To the writer's knowledge, there has been no hard evidence ever available that this (rhinitis sicca-atrophic rhinitis) is a sequel of turbinectomy." Furthermore, Fry adds: "Rhinitis sicca appears to be a constitutional disease rather than a surgically induced condition."

Alarming us the most is, how many young surgeons were likely influenced by this paper written in an esteemed medical journal? (Bold italics added highlighting our marvel as to which revered reviewers permitted publication of this paper.)

To understand how much has stayed the same in medicine, it benefits to hop on a proverbial "Time Machine" and voyage back over a century to September 1914 when Dr. Albert Mason of Waycross, Georgia, warned us in his plea for the conservation of the inferior turbinate as follows:

"…I have also seen a condition resembling atrophic rhinitis follow the removal of part of the turbinate."[82]

In his final remarks, Dr. Mason wrote:

*"In conclusion, **I plead with you**, both rhinologist and general practitioner, to **respect the function of the inferior turbinate and to save it when possible to do so."**[82]* (Bold italics added)

Obviously not every experienced surgeon was listening, reading, or grasping the medical and surgical literature of the day, or for that matter, approximately a complete *century* of pertinent medical literature.

In a wide-ranging historical review, spanning more than a century (actually over the past 130 years) of treating inferior turbinate pathology, with 13 various techniques, Hol and Huizing updated the profession in the millennial year of 2000 with their extensive bibliography (141 references) in the journal *Rhinology* outlining both borders of the debate immediate to the inferior turbinate.[25] Regarding the debated treatment disagreements, they thought that:

"Some authors consider turbinectomy as an appropriate method, while others condemn it as too aggressive and irreversibly destructive. In the light of these and other controversies, this article reviews and evaluates the literature on the surgical treatment of hypertrophied turbinates."[25]

And after their intensive and thoughtful critical analysis, Hol and Huizing declared:

*"Our review of the literature revealed a serious lack of qualified studies. Research meeting the criteria for a prospective comparative randomized surgical study is extremely rare. Studies that meet all the criteria of a prospective comparative surgical study do not exist, with the notable exception of the recently published study by Passali et al. In our opinion, the purpose of surgically reducing the inferior turbinates should be to diminish complaints while preserving function. From that perspective, it seems that electrocautery, chemocautery, (total and subtotal) turbinectomy, cryosurgery, and laser surface surgery **should not be used**, as these techniques are too destructive. Intraturbinal turbinate reduction (intraturbinal turbinoplasty) would seem to be the method of choice."[25]* (Bold italics added)

Their recommendation of intraturbinal turbinoplasty was based on both their literature review and extensive clinical experience in concert with understanding the importance of preserving the physiology of the inferior turbinate. Hol and Huizing synthesized and summarized the function of the inferior turbinates beyond the warming and humidification of the inspired air to include its significant inspiratory breathing (respiratory) function of providing inspiratory resistance as follows:

"First of all, they (inferior turbinates) contribute to inspiratory resistance, which is necessary for normal breathing. The greater the nasal resistance, the greater the negative intrathoracic pressure needed for inspiration. Greater negative pressure, in turn, enhances pulmonary ventilation and venous backflow to the lungs and the heart (Butler, 1960; Haight and Cole, 1983). This is what we would like to call the ,'**resistor function**' of the turbinates. Secondly, as part of the valve area, the inferior turbinate helps change the inspiratory lamellar airstream into a turbulent flow. Turbulence in the outer layers of air increases the interaction between air and nasal mucosa. Humidification, warming up, and cleansing of the air are thus enhanced. Thanks to their large mucosal surface and extensive blood supply, the inferior turbinates play a major role in this process. This role may be called the '**diffusor function**' of the inferior turbinates. Finally, they (inferior turbinates) are essential to the nasal defence system (mucociliary transport, humoral and cellular defence). All of these functions require a large amount of normally functioning mucosa, submucosa, and turbinate parenchyma."*[25] (Bold italics added)*

*References noted: Butler J (1960) The work of breathing through the nose. Clin Sci 19:55–62, Haight JSJ, Cole P (1983) The site and function of the nasal valve. Laryngoscope 93:49–55.

Hol and Huizing considered the anterior portion of the inferior turbinate head (the posterior portion of the internal nasal valve area) to be a frequent site of nasal airway obstruction.[25] We agree with these observations along with their thinking, which harmonizes with the pioneering landmark work of Haight and Cole previously referenced.[5]

Resection of the anterior portion of the inferior turbinate (anterior turbinectomy) was advocated by numerous other surgeons.[86–88] In the early 1980s, Richard Mabry from Dallas, Texas, introduced the term "turbinoplasty," aptly named, by reducing both the submucosal parenchyma and conchal bone of the inferior turbinate all the while preserving the overlying pseudostratified ciliated respiratory epithelium designed to preserve physiological nasal function.[89–91]

Turbinoplasty[92–94] fleetingly held sway until another dark age descended upon the rhinologic panorama with the reintroduction of turbinate trauma by a number of enthusiastic practitioners of total turbinectomy who we unashamedly term turbinate traumatologists. Turbinectomy after falling from grace was resurrected and recommended by these traumatologists, initiating a new reign of turbinate terror.[85,87,95-116] Claiming that adverse consequences of total turbinectomy had never been recognized or documented, Courtiss and Goldwyn (1984) stated that:

"Fears for dry nose syndromes are unfounded."[97]

Obviously, these authors were either indifferent or unaware of their American compatriots Holmes (1900),[80] Mason (1914),[82] Spielberg (1924),[83] House (1951),[84] and Mabry (1982).[91]

Ophir et al. after performing total turbinectomy in 150 patients followed for 1–7 years (mean 2.5 years) trumpeted that:

"Postoperative complications are minimal, and no patient complained of crusts, dryness, or foul odor."[100]

Seven years later in 1992, Ophir et al. affirmed that after interviewing and examining 186 inferior turbinectomy patients followed for 10 to 15 years (mean 12.3 years) that:

"Atrophic changes of the nasal mucosa and chronic purulent infection were not observed in any of the patients."[102]

These were the sorts of statements spread by some sides,[81,85,87,96,97,100-103,105,106] which were disputed by the other side who witnessed and described long-lasting signs and symptoms of persistent nasal airway obstruction, crusting, dryness, and postoperative posttraumatic pain syndromes in a multitude of other patients.[2-4,9,18,19-21,24,25,28,110,112,114-116,118] With the turbinate argument ablaze, Hol and Huizing, after examining the evidence, offered their cool and somewhat detached diktat:

"In our opinion, there is no justification for performing a total or subtotal turbinectomy in patients with a hypertrophic inferior turbinate. Turbinectomy is not compatible with the goal of 'preservation of function'. Turbinectomy is irreversible and deprives the nose of one of its important organs. There is thus no place for this technique in modern functional nasal surgery. There are more conservative surgical methods to achieve the desired effect."[25]

Hol and Huizing also noted that intraoperative and postoperative hemorrhage was a significant issue associated with total inferior turbinate resection that definitely required reporting.[25,85,95,115,116]

As it is impossible to be totally objective, so in the spirit of fair-mindedness, we have taken the liberty of presenting the contrary viewpoints using their own words. ***The tenor and tone of the turbinate debate*** is clearly conveyed with several examples from exceptionally influential surgeons, including some particularly persuasive plastic surgeons, charismatic and forceful in expressing their opinions abstracted from their papers.

Courtiss (1978) and colleagues stipulated that:

> *"We report a series of 88 patients in whom 119 obstructing inferior nasal turbinates were resected for airway obstruction, and who have been followed for 3 months to 3 years. The airways were consistently improved and,* **to date, there have been no undesirable sequelae***"*[95] (Bold italics added)

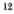

Eugene H. Courtiss

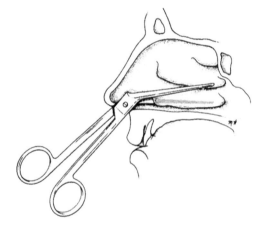

Figure 1. Placement of turbinate scissors with one blade on each side of the inferior turbinate. (*From* Courtiss EH, Goldwyn RM, O'Brien JJ: Resection of obstructing inferior nasal turbinates. Plast Reconstr Surg 62:249, 1978; with permission.)

In a follow-up paper, Courtiss and Goldwyn (1983) specifically stated:

> *"In 1977, we advocated partial resection of the inferior turbinates when turbine hypertrophy was the cause of nasal airway obstruction. The purpose of this communication is to present a follow-up of the 88 patients and, in particular, to assess any adverse effects that might have occurred."*[96]

Those authors determine as follows:

> *"On the basis of these findings, we conclude that our original recommendations and observations are correct:* **Partial resection of the inferior turbinate is proper treatment** *if that is the cause of airway obstruction."*[96] (Bold italics added)

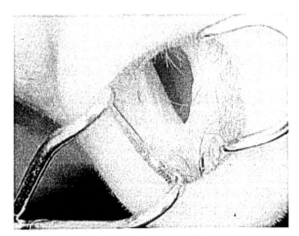

Fig 10. Left internal valve obstruction. (Photograph courtesy of Jack Sheen, M.D.)

From this 1984 "Nasal Physiology" paper by EH Courtiss, TJ Gargan, and GB Courtiss,[97] note that their Fig 10 announces a left internal nasal valve obstruction. We raise the following two issues. First, the left internal valve *obstruction is not observable* on this photograph. Second, the photograph is shown *upside down*, of course, adverse mishappenings may occur even after corrected galley proofs are submitted to a journal, otherwise knowledge and complete understanding of the anatomy involving the internal nasal valve may possibly be deficient. Their section on nasal reflexes contained a meager 5 sentences, which is certainly not an all-encompassing discussion of nasal physiology plus the paper lacked information regarding any of the extensive and critical defensive functions of the nose. Then in 1990, Courtiss and Goldwyn wrote:

> *"On the basis of our examination of these 25 patients, all of whom had bilateral inferior turbinate subtotal resection performed at least 10 years ago, **we believe that this kind of resection is the treatment of choice** for airway obstruction due to hypertrophy of the inferior turbinates and that **fears of dry nose syndromes are unfounded**."[98]* (Bold italics added)

It is astounding to us that this 1990, 10-year follow-up paper by Courtiss and Goldwyn seen in Table 5.1 on page 153 of their paper, *they recorded 2 of 23 patients with dry nose after* surgery and *5 of 20 patients with crusting after surgery*, that is a crusting complication rate of 25%. (Bold italics added) What's even more perplexing is that in the first line of their discussion these authors state:

> *"We have not observed a dry nose syndrome in any of these 25 patients, all of whom were followed for over 10 years."[98]* (Bold italics added)

That statement of certitude certainly conflicts with their printed table number II (our Table 5.1 below). We wonder how they define a dry nose after surgery versus a dry nose syndrome as there's nothing in their paper that makes the distinction or addresses these discrepancies.

Table 5.1 Patient assessment of symptoms before and after surgery.

	Before surgery		After surgery	
	Yes	**No**	**Yes**	**No**
Runny nose	4	21	6	19
Dry nose	4	21	2	23
Crusting	3	22	5	20
Postnasal drip	6	19	7	18
Nose bleeds	5	20	7	18

Table 5.1 from: Courtiss EH, Goldwyn RM. Resection of obstructing inferior nasal turbinates: a 10-year follow-up. *Plast Reconstr Surg.* 1990;86:152–4.[98]

Another formidable contributor leading the charge headlong into the turbinate debate was Dr. Dov Ophir who also championed and advocated aggressive turbinectomy that we find appallingly atrocious. He and his colleagues wrote in 1985:

"Eighty percent of the patients reported improvement in nasal breathing, and 14 (27%) of the 51 patients who suffered from nasal drainage preoperatively reported that it had stopped after the operation. Of the 39 patients who had anosmia preoperatively, 46% reported the restoration of their sense of smell. **Postoperative complications are minimal**, *and* **no patient complained of crusts, dryness, or foul odor.***"[100]* (Bold italics added)

Several years later in 1990, Dr. Ophir proclaimed that:

*"***Total inferior turbinectomy** *was carried out in 38 patients who complained of nasal obstruction following rhinoplasty or rhinoseptoplasty and in whom hypertrophied inferior turbinates were found to be the cause of obstruction." And he added: "***Atrophic changes of the nasal mucosa** *or chronic purulent infection* **were not observed in any of the patients**. *Because the results of partial procedures on the inferior turbinates are often unsatisfactory,* **I suggest performing total inferior turbinectomy in patients with obstructing inferior turbinates following rhinoplasty.***"[101]* (Bold italics added)

Apparently cognizant and sensitive to the reality that *secondary atrophic rhinitis* may require years to develop, Dr. Ophir and colleagues published (1992) a 10–15-year follow-up paper and quoted:

*"**The long-term** effectiveness and **safety of inferior turbinectomy** were assessed in 186 patients who were interviewed and examined 10 to 15 years after surgery (mean 12.3 years). Relief of nasal obstruction was reported by 82% of the patients; rhinoscopy showed wide, clean nasal airways in 88%. The authors continued: '**Atrophic changes of the nasal mucosa and chronic purulent infection were not observed in any of the patients'.**"[102]* (Bold italics added)

Talmon and colleagues,[105] published a paper in 2000, a portion which read:

*"Over a 6-year period, **357 total inferior bilateral turbinectomies were performed at our institution.** We present the results of these procedures and describe our surgical technique. We conclude that even in a hot and dusty climate, **total inferior turbinectomy is an effective and relatively safe procedure.**"* (Bold italics added)

The authors continued: **"Total removal of the inferior turbinate is an accepted surgical procedure for the relief of chronic nasal obstruction.** Surgeons hesitated to use it for two main reasons: (1) total turbinectomy is not "physiologic"; (2) the procedure is not "safe." As for the interference of the operation with the physiology of the nose, this might be true for healthy people. We, instead, operate on patients with nasal obstruction who are unable to use their noses for breathing. The term "physiologic" in this connection is inappropriate, and the term "pathological" should be considered. The results show clearly that the vast majority of patients who undergo this operation do enjoy its outcome and are better off after the operation."

They continued*:*

*"Ozena **(atrophic rhinitis)** is believed by some to be related to total inferior turbinectomy. This is a serious disease that may discourage surgeons from performing the operation. In our series, conducted in a hot, dusty climate, no such complication was observed, nor did we find any documented case in the literature. We therefore cannot regard ozena as a possible complication of this operation." They concluded: "We conclude that total inferior turbinectomy is an effective and relatively safe procedure, and using the described technique makes it even safer."[105]* (Bold italics added)

We emphasize the importance of agreed upon definition of the terms because *ozena* is an example of *primary atrophic rhinitis,* and we are discussing *secondary atrophic rhinitis.* By what standards of evidence-based medicine is total inferior turbinectomies an accepted and "relatively safe" surgical procedure as Talmon and colleagues claim?

What do they mean by **relatively safe** and **total inferior turbinectomy** is an accepted procedure, by whom? Have any of these practitioners performed a randomized control trial (RCT) to remove the possibility of bias and placebo effects?

In Letters to the Editor, Dr. Olawale Olarinde, FRCS(Oto) Department of Otorhinolaryngology Head and Neck Surgery Singleton Hospital Sketty, Swansea SA2 8QA, Wales, was critical of Talmon and colleagues as follows:

"It would have been more appropriate to analyze their results in patients who had turbinate surgery alone, as this was the procedure being studied. While it is clear

that the authors selected their patients for this procedure, it is unclear what the selection criteria were. They only state that all patients suffered from chronic nasal obstruction and failed to respond to local and systemic treatment. This diagnosis is unfortunately vague."[104]

So, Dr. Talmon responded to Dr. Olawale Olarinde in Letters to the Editor as follows:

"The article is about total inferior turbinectomy. The usual patient has more than one cause for his or her complaints and usually requires a combined procedure. Therefore, it is more appropriate to analyze reality rather than a theoretical model. Second, no operation has a 100% success rate, and inferior turbinectomy is no exception. Patients should be warned. Unsuccessful intervention is usually due to reasons other than the excised inferior turbinates: inferior turbinates do not regenerate after total trimming. I see patients who underwent total turbinectomy 20 years ago and still enjoy the results of the operation. A failure of the procedure might be due to reasons such as an abundant soft palate or lack of a nasal valve. Recurrent symptoms are due to conditions such as nasal polyps or hypertrophy of the medial turbinates." Yoav Talmon, MD Dept of Otolaryngology Head and Neck Surgery Western Galilee Hospital, Nahariya, Israel.[105]

Also commenting on the paper of Talmon et al. in Letters to the Editor, Ron Eliashar, MD Department of Otolaryngology Head and Neck Surgery Hadassah University Hospital, Jerusalem, Israel, stated:

*"I read the paper by Talmon et al. (Talmon Y, Samel A, Gilbey P. Total inferior turbinectomy: operative results and technique. Ann Otol Rhinol Laryngol 2000; 109:1117—9) with great interest. **We ourselves perform total (or subtotal) inferior turbinectomies routinely** in our department. Whenever we discuss this procedure with our American colleagues, they condemn it because of the risks of ozena or " empty nose syndrome." It seems that they often regard us almost as "criminals" when we mention inferior turbinectomy! The most serious complication encountered by us was massive epistaxis requiring anterior and posterior nasal packing. **There were only a few cases of atrophic rhinitis, and no cases of ozena or of empty nose syndrome**. Some patients developed crusting, but it was mostly temporary and was relieved by nasal irrigation and application of lubricating gel. The results of our very large series are therefore in line with the results published by Talmon et al. **Hence, I join in their conclusion that total inferior turbinectomy is effective and relatively safe, at least in our Israeli climate."* (Bold italics added)

Ron Eliashar, MD Department of Otolaryngology Head and Neck Surgery Hadassah University Hospital, Jerusalem, Israel.[106]

*So, Dr. Eliashar joins Talmon et al. by promulgating that "**total inferior turbinectomy is effective and relatively safe**," nevertheless Dr. Eliashar observed and reported that: "There were only a few cases of atrophic rhinitis, and no cases of ozena or of empty nose syndrome." (Bold italics added)*

We wonder if it is possible for Talmon et al. or Eliashar to find their previously operated patients and publish their present-day findings on these patients and concurrently consider enrolling and performing an important RCT on a new cohort of patients to remove the possibility of bias and placebo effects?

In a paper from East Africa, Oburra found atrophic rhinitis after bilateral inferior turbinectomy in 15% of patients, disputing assertions to the contrary.

*"Thirty-four patients undergoing bilateral inferior turbinectomy for obstruction of the upper airway are prospectively reviewed. The indication for the operation was persistent nasal obstruction interfering with sleep and speech. Their **ages ranged from seven years to 50 years**. The most common postoperative complications were synechiae **(15%), atrophic rhinitis (15%), persistent obstruction (12%), and abnormal nasal sensation (9%)."*[110] (Bold italics added)

We, the authors of this book, note: that the average annual relative humidity in Nairobi, Kenya, is 69.0% where the average annual relative humidity in Tel Aviv, Israel is 70.5%. The fact that **Dr. HO Oburra reported a 15% incidence of atrophic rhinitis (in 5 patients) after bilateral inferior turbinectomy** clangs and clashes with the claim by Dr. Dov Ophir that the relative humidity in Israel **prevent** the patients from experiencing atrophic rhinitis after bilateral inferior turbinectomy. (Bold italics added).

Table 5.2 Pattern of complications.

Complication	No. of patients	%
Synechiae	5	15
Atrophic rhinitis	5	15
Persistent obstruction	4	12
Abnormal sensation in the nose	3	9
Severe epistaxis	2	6
Rhinnorrhoea	2	6
Infection	1	3
Numbness of the left incisors	1	3

Table 5.2 "Pattern of complications" following bilateral turbinectomy in the paper by Oburra.[110] **Note the incidence of atrophic rhinitis 15% and** "severe" **epistaxis 6%.** (Bold italics added)

Others declared that patients who received partial or even full total turbinectomy experienced no "untoward sequelae." So, a debate, which flourished for more than a century was sustained and nourished by colleagues in Europe, the Middle East, and in our country was again in full bloom even after ample numbers of previous surgeons cautioned the profession that the nasal mucosa is "the organ of the nose" and that total resection *can result in disaster*, as we also have observed on hundreds of occasions.[18] In our country, other highly experienced and respected surgeons wrote:

> "***Full***-*thickness excision of the anterior third to half of the inferior turbinate (turbinectomy) became a favored procedure. Relief of nasal obstruction was obtained in greater than 90% of patients. Healing was satisfactory regardless of the method, and complications, including hemorrhage and infection, were few.* ***Long-term follow-up revealed no untoward sequelae, and no patient developed atrophic rhinitis.***"[87] (Bold italics added)

Wondering and questioning, what happened to the other 10% of their patients? In 1983, while at the University of Nebraska, Martinez et al. published in *The Laryngoscope*:

> "***Total inferior turbinectomies*** *have been performed on 40 patients over the past 5 years; 29 of these patients have been followed from 2 to 60 months postoperatively by clinical examination and by formal questionnaire." The authors continue: "The* ***inferior turbinates*** *play a role in humidification and temperature regulation of inspired air.* ***The removal of them, however, does not seem to be fraught with the morbidity which has heretofore been attributed to this procedure.***"[103] (Bold italics added)

George Drumheller, MD of Everett, Washington, wrote a letter to the editor of *The Laryngoscope* regarding the Martinez et al. paper: Martinez SA, Nissen AJ, Stock CR, Tesmer T. Nasal turbinate resection for relief of nasal obstruction. Laryngoscope 1983 Jul; 93 (7):871−5.

> "*The teachers of the American Rhinologic Society are frequently being asked by students and others regarding our treatment of malfunctions and pathologic situations which are manifested in the nasal turbinates. It is most incredible that the article shows a picture of 'normal regenerated respiratory epithelium with mucous and serous glands.' In order to be normal, the nasal cycle must be present, and certainly this is not the case after turbinectomy. In addition, many other nasopulmonary reflexes are disturbed, and certainly pre- and postoperative case studies should be included in any article addressing this subject. It is regrettable that many of our young surgeons will take the easy route of resecting a turbinate which nobody can reconstruct, and the morbidity rate will be markedly increased as a result of this very poorly worked up article.*"

In the same edition of *The Laryngoscope,* Pat Barelli, MD, a rhinologist from Kansas City, Missouri, said:

"I have in my practice many people who have had turbinectomies with disastrous results. The treatment of these postoperative turbinectomies is extremely unsatisfactory as one cannot reconstruct a turbinate which is not present."

*Editorial Note (from The Laryngoscope): "This paper (Martinez et al.)[103] is a Southern Section meeting paper. Triological Society papers are not usually reviewed. They are accepted, for the most part, for publication when the author is accepted as a speaker for a Triological meeting. Publication does not necessarily mean approval, but rather indicates what is going on in the profession."

Moore et al. also at the University of Nebraska followed the identical patients initially reported by Martinez et al. With the additional follow-up of several years, Moore and colleagues ***emphatically contradicted*** the initial findings by Martinez et al.[103] concluding that:

*"Total inferior turbinectomy has been proposed as a treatment for chronic nasal airway obstruction refractory to other, more conservative, methods of treatment. Traditionally, it has been criticized because of its adverse effects on nasophysiology. In this study, patients who had previously undergone total inferior turbinectomy were evaluated with the use of an extensive questionnaire. **It confirms that total inferior turbinectomy carries significant morbidity and should be condemned.**"[2]* (Bold italics added)

Segal and colleagues from Tel Aviv University Israel operated on 227 children under the age of 10 followed one year after surgery and to our dismay and disappointment concluded:

*"Conclusions: A **complete inferior turbinectomy** should be considered in children <10 years of age who have hypertrophied inferior turbinates that cause major interference with nasal breathing."[113]* (Bold italics added)

At this moment, we ask Dr. Segal or one of his colleagues (Eviatar, Berenholz, Kessler, or Shlamkovitch), can you please present to the profession, an update regarding the "long-term results" of your 227 children after your "complete inferior turbinectomy" published 18 years ago in your paper of 2003?[113]

Admittedly, we are not reluctant reticent envoys but ferocious opponents of the brazen ideology of total inferior turbinectomy along with others[2–4,18–28] including, arguably the greatest, 20th century American rhinologist and pedagogue Maurice H. Cottle, MD of Chicago, who once told me, and to the best of my recollection, and most assuredly the word "criminal" remains in mind:

"...aggressive resection of the inferior turbinate for nonmalignant disease can be considered a criminal act." Personal communication (EBK).

In present-day state-of-the-art of nasal surgery, it would be vastly valuable to understand how much nasal mucosal tissue, with its critical breathing (respiratory) and defensive functions can be safely removed, damaged or impaired, without producing nasal functional failure resulting in empty nose syndrome (ENS). How often does the contemporary nasal surgeon consider the conjectural functional residual capacity of the nose (FRCn) before or after surgical intervention, especially with total inferior turbinectomy in mind?

Another confounding reality is that in the current state of nasal functional testing, it appears an estimate of nasal function is often based on observation or the patient's subjective assessment, using a visual analog scale. Several other pertinent quotations from Lord Kelvin's scientific perspicacious pen include:

"To measure is to know." "If you cannot measure it, you cannot improve it."*

*PLA, Volume 1, "Electrical Units of Measurement", 1883-05-03 PLA- Popular Lectures and Addresses (1891–1894, 3 volumes)

Concluding this overworked and well-worn section of the historical perspective of the turbinate debate, the work of Jackson and Koch from the Division of Otolaryngology Head and Neck Surgery, Stanford University Medical Center published in the journal *Plastic and Reconstructive Surgery* in 1999 summarized the advantages and disadvantages of inferior turbinate treatment as follows:

"After correcting septal and nasal valve pathology persistent nasal airway obstruction may be the result inferior turbinate enlargement (hypertrophy) for which a graduated "staged" approach is recommended all the while minimizing hemorrhage and postoperative atrophy (nasal drying)."[119]

1. **Injections:** Intraturbinate steroid injections although minimally invasive improvement is not long-lasting and the potential for blindness exists, but it is not as common as was once thought.[120–122]
2. **Out-fracture (lateralization):** Minimally invasive with a low risk of complications; however, turbinate mucosal pathology is not addressed.
3. Non-surgical **T**urbinate **R**eduction **A**djunctive **P**rocedure (n-s TRAP):
   (a) Electrocautery... routine and not technically difficult; delayed hemorrhage may occur.
   (b) Cryosurgery... routine and not technically difficult; brief relief of symptoms.
   (c) Laser surgery ... routine and not technically difficult; brief relief of symptoms, postoperative crusting unable to change the bony (concha).
4. **Surgical procedures:**
   (a) Partial turbinectomy... routine and not technically difficult; severe hemorrhage can occur, nasal airway relief can last for years; however, synechia, prolong crusting, and *ENS* can develop.
   (b) Total turbinectomy... routine and not technically difficult; severe hemorrhage can occur, nasal airway relief can last for years; however, synechia, protracted crusting, and *ENS* may develop along with a disturbance in physiological function, resection is irrevocable.
   (c) Turbinoplasty... pseudostratified ciliated respiratory epithelium is preserved, reduction of cases of hemorrhage, high incidence of relief of nasal

airway obstruction, incidence of nasal atrophy, and ***ENS is exceedingly low*** and can be combined with out-fracture (lateralization).

There are three options for turbinoplasty while still maintaining preservation of the pseudostratified ciliated respiratory epithelium.

1. Submucosal (parenchymal) resection alone, WITHOUT conchal bone resection
2. Conchal bone resection alone, WITHOUT submucosal (parenchymal) resection
3. Combined submucosal (parenchymal) resection combined WITH conchal bone resection

Jackson and Koch concluded that nasal airway obstruction secondary to turbinate hypertrophy must first receive medical therapy before contemplating any surgical intervention. They clearly recognized that surgical treatment should be conservative, with minimal morbidity. As a consequence of that reality, they favored "increasingly invasive interventions" after a failure of medical management, first with laser application as an initial office procedure followed by partial inferior turbinectomy or submucosal resection, "and rarely total turbinectomy or vidian neurectomy" if other treatments are unsuccessful. They unambiguously acknowledged that definitive guidelines for rational therapeutic decisions regarding the inferior turbinate were lacking; therefore, they favored continued studies as a necessary requirement for sensible therapeutic choices.[119]

2. Turbinate anatomy

Customarily, the general term turbinate is understood to mean the nasal structure composed of an overlying pseudostratified ciliated respiratory epithelium with a subepithelial layer (synonyms include submucosa, lamina propria, stroma); this submucosa (lamina propria, stroma) is composed of neurovascular bundles, especially large capacitance vessels. This submucosa (lamina propria, stroma) together with the conchal bone and the overlying epithelium form the entire turbinate. Anatomically, the turbinates are often divided into the anterior portion (head), a midportion (body), and posterior portion (tail), which has utility allowing thinking about which portion of a turbinate to modify.

2.1 Anatomy of the *middle turbinate*

The middle turbinate is part of the ethmoid bone; superiorly, it connects to the cribriform region receiving its blood supply posteriorly by the sphenopalatine artery and anteriorly from the anterior ethmoid artery, a branch off the ophthalmic artery supplied by the internal carotid arterial system. The osseous skeleton can be structured as lamellar or bullous bone (concha bullosa). The concha bullosa is lined with pseudostratified ciliated respiratory epithelium, which drains into the ethmoid infundibulum, which on occasion may expand significantly to obstruct the nasal airway.

As pointed out by Scheithaurer,[28] there are numerous middle turbinate anatomic variations which may be classified as follows:

1. Bulbous form (concha bullosa) with pneumatization in the horizontal plane
2. Lamellar form with pneumatization in the vertical plane
3. Combined bulbous and lamellar forms
4. Paradoxical curve
5. Extra concha

The most common form of middle turbinate anatomic variant is the concha bullosa, while the most common pathologic form is the polypoid change, which is commonly associated with chronic rhinosinusitis. Since the mucosa of the middle turbinate is highly vascularized, it plays an important role in humidification of the inspired air.

2.2 Anatomy of the *inferior turbinate*

The inferior turbinate is the largest of the turbinates and slightly larger in males than in females being approximately 4.9 cm in men and 4.7 cm in women. The outer mucosal layer is pseudostratified ciliated respiratory epithelium, while the subepithelial layer (submucosa, lamina propria, stroma) contains an extensive network of venous capacitance vessels (sinusoids). Figs. 5.1–5.3.

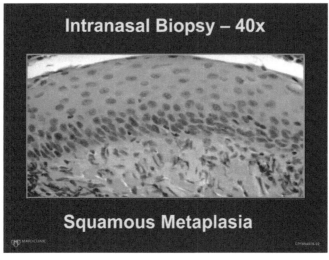

FIGURE 5.1

An intranasal mucosal biopsy of a patient with the *"Empty Nose Syndrome."* The normal ciliated columnar respiratory epithelium is frequently replaced by squamous metaplasia seen in these patients with the *"Empty Nose Syndrome."*

(Kern and Friedman. By permission of Mayo Foundation for Medical Education and Research. All Rights Reserved).

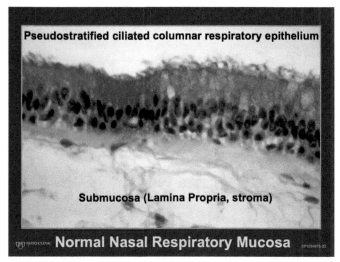

FIGURE 5.2

The normal nasal mucus membrane is composed of an outer epithelial layer with four different cell types and a deeper submucosal layer. The outer epithelial layer contains the *ciliated columnar* cells (approximately 100 to 250 cilia/cell with microvilli) and *nonciliated columnar* cells (with microvilli, increasing their functional surface area), *mucus-secreting goblet cells* and *basal cells,* which are diminutive in size and rest upon a basement membrane. Submucosa (lamina propria, stroma). The submucosa contains neurovascular fenestrated capillaries, mixed glandular elements, and an extensive zone of venous cavernous plexuses.

(Kern and Friedman. By permission of Mayo Foundation for Medical Education and Research. All Rights Reserved).

It is the subepithelial layer that is involved in the "*nasal cycle,*" defined as the alternating episodic congestion and decongestion of the nasal turbinates. Figs. 5.4−5.7. The physiologic reality of the "*nasal cycle*" has to be taken into consideration when examining the patient; therefore, the internal nose requires examination *before* and *after decongestion.*[123,124]

This fluctuation induced by the submucosal venous sinuses results in a variation of nasal airflow from one nasal chamber to the other side, which occurs over several hours throughout the day. This cycle occurs in approximately 80% of healthy adults.[125,126] Flanagan and Eccles observed the nasal cycle in 20%−40% of (*n* = 52) healthy volunteer adults. They went on to say:

> *"The cycle is adrenergic-stimulated. It is suspected that the activity of the sympathetic nerve is subject to changes which are regulated via the respiratory center in the brain stem and which are closely associated with breathing activity."*[12,127]

According to Williams and Eccles, the *nasal cycle* slows with age and the reciprocal changes in nasal airflow may be organized and controlled from the

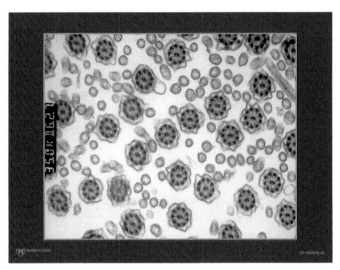

FIGURE 5.3

Electron microscopic view of nasal respiratory cilia. The central strand of a cilium is composed of two single centrally located microtubules surrounded by an array of nine pairs of peripheral microtubules with both inner and outer dynein arms. The dynein arms are absent in patients suffering from primary ciliary dyskinesia.

(Kern and Friedman. By permission of Mayo Foundation for Medical Education and Research. All Rights Reserved).

hypothalamus and brainstem.[128,129] The answer to the question, what is the function of the *nasal cycle* was proposed by Eccles who stated:

> *"It is proposed that the periodic congestion and decongestion of nasal venous sinusoids may provide a pump mechanism for the generation of plasma exudate, and that this mechanism is an important component of respiratory defence."[130,131]*

These venous capacitance vessels (sinusoids) in the submucosa (lamina propria, stroma) exist in the middle turbinate but are more numerous in the inferior turbinate. These vessels can dilate to the point of totally obstructing the nasal airway. The blood supply is controlled by sympathetic innervation to the arterial resistance vessels. The mucous membrane is decongested when both the venous capacitance vessels (sinusoids) and the resistance vessels receive sympathetic stimulation as both are surrounded by adrenergic nerve fibers.[132,133]

Fundamentally, the nasal autonomic nervous system maintains the ability to control systems:

> System 1 controls nasal secretion with parasympathetic innervation, and system 2 controls nasal airflow with sympathetic innervation.

In addition to controlling nasal secretions, the parasympathetic system influences the vascular system by the neurotransmitter acetylcholine and the potent vasodilator, vasoactive intestinal polypeptide. The sympathetic nerves are distributed to both the

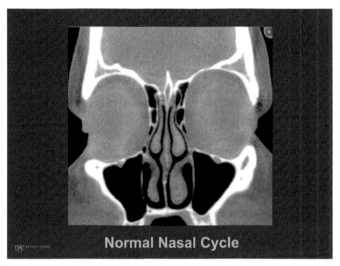

FIGURE 5.4

The Nasal Cycle is described as the normal physiologic alternating *congestion* and *decongestion* of the nasal turbinates. This alternating *congestion decongestion* cycle produces rotating changes of the nasal resistance on each side (uninasal resistance alterations) of the nasal airway. As a consequence of this nasal cycling, the side congested (obstructed) rotates or "cycles" to become decongested (unobstructed), while the opposite side becomes congested (obstructed). This nasal cycling occurs between 20% and 80% of the adult population.[126–130] On this CT scan above, source Wikipedia, https://en.wikipedia.org/wiki/Nasal cycle, at that specific time, the left inferior turbinate is congested while the right inferior turbinate is decongested by comparison.

blood vessels and nasal glands.[134] The venous capacitance vessels (sinusoids) in the submucosa have a dense adrenergic sympathetic innervation, and sympathetic nerve stimulation produces vasoconstriction with a mucosal blood volume reduction.[135,136] Noradrenaline is the primary sympathetic neurotransmitter along with neuropeptide Y, both are vigorous vasoconstrictors.[137]

The role of the nasal venous sinuses in the control of nasal airflow is now well recognized, and their ability to swell and completely obstruct the nasal passage has been observed and reported.[5,131,134] The location of the nasal venous sinuses at the anterior tip of the inferior turbinate and nasal septum is critical for controlling nasal airflow, and this area of the nose is often referred to as the "nasal valve." The nasal valve area is the narrowest point of the nasal passage, which determines the nasal resistance to airflow.[5,25,138,139] However, there is some dispute in the literature as to whether the nasal valve lies in the nasal vestibule or more posteriorly within the bony cavum of the nose. The anatomical and physiological evidence indicates that the nasal valve occurs at the entrance of the piriform aperture, with the major site of nasal resistance just anterior to the tip of the inferior turbinate.[140,141]

The inferior turbinate is inserted into the lateral wall of the nose at approximately the mid-maxillary wall location. This insertion is located at varying angles, ranging from approximately 20° to 90° from the mid-maxillary wall. This anatomic fact has surgical implications when performing out-fracture (lateralization) of the inferior

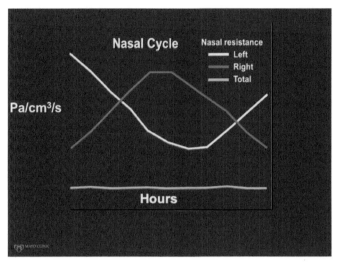

FIGURE 5.5

Composite graph demonstrating the presence of a nasal cycle, which occurs in 20% to 80% of the adult population. The values were obtained over a five-hour study period using active anterior rhinomanometric techniques. Using rhinomanometry, transnasal pressure and transnasal airflow during active breathing (inspiration and expiration) can be measured when breathing only through the right side, breathing only through the left side, and when breathing through both sides (both nostrils) at the same time. The Nasal Cycle is described as the normal physiologic alternating *congestion* and *decongestion* of the nasal turbinates. This alternating *congestion decongestion* cycle produces alternating changes of the nasal resistance on each side (uninasal resistance alterations). After the passage of time, the opposite side "cycles" becomes congested (obstructed), while the opposite side becomes decongested. Nasal resistance in Pa/cm^3/s is measured at 150 Pa (Pascals) pressure. The nasal resistance can be *calculated* by measuring transnasal pressure divided by transnasal nasal air flow. The nasal resistance for either right or left side is an "uninasal" resistance that can be calculated from the pressure and flow measurements. The total nasal resistance is calculated from the transnasal pressure divided by the transnasal airflow when breathing through both nostrils at the same time. When breathing through both sides, the patient feels unobstructed as the **total nasal resistance** is lower (less) than either one of the individual's right-sided resistance or left-sided resistance of the nose as depicted in the graph of *the nasal cycle* above. Most people are simply unaware of the presence of the alternating *congestion decongestion* phases of the nasal cycle.

(Kern and Friedman. By permission of Mayo Foundation for Medical Education and Research. All Rights Reserved).

turbinate as the optimal point of out-fracture (lateralization) should be as close to the actual insertion to the lateral wall as possible, thereby producing a comminuted fracture of the conchal bone, allowing repositioning of the inferior turbinate in a more lateral position, thereby opening (widening) the internal nasal valve area.

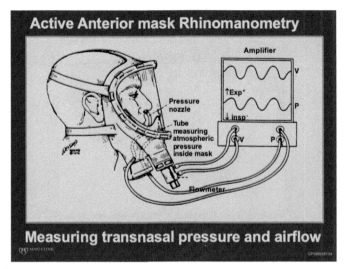

FIGURE 5.6

With this schematic drawing of active anterior mask rhinomanometry, as used at the Mayo laboratory, the investigator is able to objectively measure the pressure difference between the nostril and the nasopharynx while simultaneously measuring the airflow through the side under study. Each nasal cavity, right and left side, is measured separately. The measurements of transnasal airflow and pressure changes during breathing (inspiration and expiration) can be reordered and visualized. From these measurements, nasal resistance can be calculated using the formula: Nasal resistance equals transnasal pressure *divided* by transnasal air flow.

(Kern and Friedman. By permission of Mayo Foundation for Medical Education and Research. All Rights Reserved).

3. Physical examination

Recollect that effective medical management of turbinate enlargement involves accurate diagnosis and eliminating medical iatrogenic causes of turbinate swelling. Infection (by viral, bacterial, rickettsia, fungal, or other infectious agents), allergic rhinitis, nonallergic rhinitis (NARES syndrome), pregnancy, hypothyroidism, and medications such as beta-blockers, antihypertensives, antidepressants, some certain oral contraceptives can induce nasal mucosal engorgement. Abuse of topical decongestants may result in "rhinitis medicamentosa" that can be reversed with medication. Environmental irritants such as cigarette smoke can be responsible and eliminated by smoking cessation and/or air filtration. Turbinate swelling is regularly caused by venous congestion, capable of producing both the *nasal cycle* and a well-known gravitational and physiological response, especially when a person assumes a lateral or supine position. These gravitational and physiological responses can be mitigated with positional changes and elevation of the head with pillows or elevating the head of a bed with blocks. The examining physician needs to be mindful of the assorted sources of turbinate enlargement so that accurate diagnosis is reached.

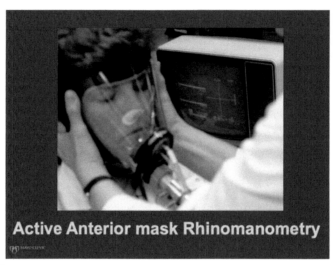

Active Anterior mask Rhinomanometry

FIGURE 5.7

With active anterior mask rhinomanometry, as used in our clinical laboratory at Mayo, the individual is studied while seated during quiet breathing. The pressure changes between the nostril opening and the posterior nasopharynx are measured through an airtight fitted tube, on the one side, measuring the transnasal pressure changes on the opposite side, in this example, the left side. A pneumotachograph is connected to the mask which measures the nasal airflow on the tested side, in this example, the left side. From these reordered and visualized measurements of transnasal pressure and transnasal airflow during breathing (inspiration and expiration), nasal resistance can be calculated and the existence of a *nasal cycle* confirmed.

(Kern and Friedman. By permission of Mayo Foundation for Medical Education and Research. All Rights Reserved).

Preoperative evaluation includes complete medical, surgical history, and physical examination including anterior rhinoscopy of the internal nasal structures including the internal and external nasal valves, the septum, all mucosal surfaces, including evaluation of the turbinates, the cribriform region, and choana before and after topical sympathomimetic decongestion (and 4% xylocaine when instrumentation, palpation, or biopsy is indicated). Subsequent to anterior rhinoscopy, endoscopic (rigid and flexible telescopes) examination is performed studying all nasal structures including the nasopharynx to evaluate the nasopharyngeal space and the posterior portion (tails) of the turbinates.

Farmer and Eccles found no evidence for cellular hypertrophy despite the common use of the term "turbinate hypertrophy" arguing that the term "turbinate hypertrophy" should be replaced with a more correct term, "turbinate enlargement."[142]

The precise definition of **hypertrophy** is an **increase in cell size** while **hyperplasia** is an **increase in cell number**. Farmer and Eccles found that turbinate enlargement is largely the result of, "cellular hyperplasia, tissue edema, and vascular congestion" and **not** the result of an increase in cell size. Continuing with definitions, **metaplasia** is the conversion of one type of cell to another, for example, cellular change from pseudostratified ciliated columnar epithelial cells to squamous cells, **squamous metaplasia**. Fig. 5.1. Any normal cell may become a cancer cell by changing to an abnormal cell first by hyperplasia (increase in the number of cells) and then dysplasia (increase in the number of abnormal cells).

4. Rhinologic evaluation with assessment tests and biopsy

The diagnostic assessment tests are summarized in Table 5.3.

Table 5.3 Assessment tests and biopsy.

1. Saccharine test of mucociliary transport[143,144]
2. Schirmer test[145,146]
3. Olfaction testing[147,148]
4. Acoustic rhinometry (AR)[149]
5. Rhinomanometry (RM)[150,151]

   Note: Rhinomanometry is generally accepted as the standard technique of measuring nasal airway resistance and assessing the patency of the nose.
6. Peak nasal inspiratory flow (PNIF)[152,153]

   Note: The peak nasal inspiratory flow (PNIF), acoustic rhinometry (AR), and rhinomanometry (RM) assess different aspects of nasal obstruction. These methods "generally" relate to each other and can be alternatively *applied to research and clinical practice* (Bold italics added).
7. Computational fluid dynamics (CFD)[154]
8. Nasal secretions[155,156]
   a. Secretory IgG, IgA, IgM, IgE, IgD
   b. CSF fluid
9. Nasal smear cytology[157]
   a. Lymphocytes
   b. Eosinophils

   Note: *"A significant correlation was obtained between secretion eosinophilia and allergy. Nasal provocation tests correlated with skin tests in 87%, whereas the correlation between nasal provocation tests and IgE determinations in the serum was poorer."* [157]
10. Allergy testing
    a. Skin prick testing
    b. Blood immunoassay testing

    Note: Enzyme-linked immunosorbent assay (ELISA or EIA) is obtained for allergen-specific antibodies
    c. Elimination diet
    d. Provocation testing
11. Imaging studies
12. Nasal biopsy
    a. Light microscopy
    b. Electron microscopy

Results from these tests are combined with clinical findings to reach a reasoned conclusion in the decision-making process. Therefore, it is the blending and correlation of the patient's symptoms, findings of the diagnostic studies integrated with the pathology found on physical nasal examination that allows accurate diagnosis. Currently, because of the immense improvements made in measurement technology, the objective assessment of the minimal cross-sectional area (acoustic rhinometry)[149] along with the investigation of the transnasal airflow and transnasal pressure changes (rhinomanometry)[150] have now attained a very high standard. Nevertheless, the data collected do not always correspond to the subjective experience of the patient. Cole has previously acknowledged this drawback as early as 1989 with the finding that approximately 20% of patients experiencing nasal airway obstruction when measured rhinomanometrically had either a normal or reduced nasal resistance when compared to controls (general population).[158,159] Nonetheless, in the context of the preoperative assessment, these two procedures, acoustic rhinometry and rhinomanometry have been established, by the leader of the University of Toronto group, Professor Philip Cole, MD, as important tools in the *routine* diagnostic assessment of the rhinologic patient with nasal airway obstruction.[158,159]

Brief history of evidence-based medicine —David Sackett, MD

According to Thoma and Eaves, *The British Medical Journal* conducted an online poll of its readers in January 2007 finding that evidence-based medicine (EBM) was ranked seventh among the 15 most momentous milestones molding modern medicine. Some of these major milestones included sanitation (germ theory of disease), immunization (vaccines), antibiotics, and anesthesia along with imaging (radiology) noting that a Google search today (in 2015) regarding anything to do with EBM would be in the millions.[160]

Who was behind the concept of EBM, simply, what is EBM, how did it all come about, and why is it pertinent to our conversation in this book?

The imaginative original unifying ideas behind EBM comes from David Sackett, MD considered the "father" of EBM. We reason that EBM is primarily about discovery. Discovery of the "best evidence," optimistically "proof positive"; using that proof of the best medical **"scientific evidence,"** as opposed to the best **"expert opinion,"** for crafting clinical choices, judgments, and rational therapeutic decisions in the best interest of the patient.

In their tribute to Dr. Sackett, authors Thoma and Eaves[160] defined EBM essentially as the combination of:

1. Finding, from the literature, the supreme scientific research evidence coupled
2. With a given physician's clinical expertise
3. Integrated with an understanding of an individual patient's unique situation, values, and wishes.

In other words, EBM is defined as the combination of the best research evidence integrated with a given clinicians expertise and blended with the individual patient's needs and values.[161–163]

Dr. David Sackett, born in Chicago in 1934, obtained his medical degree at the University of Illinois, trained in internal medicine with a subspecialty in nephrology. He attended Harvard University earning a Master's degree in epidemiology practicing clinical medicine in Chicago, Buffalo, and Boston in the United States. At age 33 (1967), he left the United States and founded the first Department of Clinical Epidemiology at McMaster University Medical School in Hamilton, Ontario, Canada, which was the first department of epidemiology in the world.[160]

EBM effectively began when a group of McMaster University epidemiologists, guided by Dr. Sackett, published their 1979 article in *The Canadian Medical*

Empty Nose Syndrome. https://doi.org/10.1016/B978-0-443-10715-3.00006-8

Association Journal counseling physicians as to how to evaluate the medical literature. The precise term "evidence-based medicine" was actually conceived and publicized by internist Dr. Gordon Guyatt, who was one of Dr. Sackett's students.[160,163–165]

The bedrock of EBM is the tiered system of organizing evidence known as levels of evidence (LOEs). The concept of "LOEs" was initially presented and explained in the report by the Canadian Task Force on the Periodic Health Examination in 1979.[165] The Task Force's purpose was to provide recommendations for the periodic health examination based on evidence obtained from the medical literature. The authors established a system of rating the evidence from the published literature determining the value of that particular evidence. For example, a high-level value was assigned to exceptional evidence supporting a recommendation for a specific medical condition which was to be included in the health examination.

In a 2011 paper by Burns et al., a clear summary of the history of LOEs was succinctly presented and described in tables below (Tables 6.1 and 6.2).[166]

Both systems place randomized controlled trials (RCTs) at the highest level and case series or expert opinions at the lowest level. The hierarchies rank studies according to the probability of bias. RCTs are given the highest level because they are designed to be unbiased having less risk of systematic errors.

A case series or expert opinion is often biased by the author's experience or opinions, without controlling for confounding factors. In order to answer any clinical question, the highest LOE should always be applied. In other words, a major goal of EBM practice is finding the highest LOE to solve a clinical problem. It is important to understand the history behind the levels and how they should be interpreted since not all level I evidence even from an RCT is perfect.[169] Since the introduction of LOEs, numerous organizations and journals have adopted variations of the classification system. Diverse specialties are often asking different questions, and it was

Table 6.1 Canadian task force on the periodic health examination's levels of evidence[a].

Level	Type of evidence
I	At least one RCT* with proper randomization
II.1	Well-designed cohort or case-control study
II.2	Time series comparisons or dramatic results from uncontrolled studies
III	Expert opinions

*RCT, *randomized controlled trial.*
[a] *Adapted from Canadian Task Force on the Periodic Health Examination. The periodic health examination. Can Med Assoc J 1979;121:1193–1254.[165]*
Table 6.1 amended from Burns et al.[166]

Table 6.2 Levels of evidence from Sackett[a].

Level	Type of evidence
I	Large RCTs* with clear-cut results
II	Small RCTs with unclear results
III	Cohort and case-control studies
IV	Historical cohort or case-control studies
V	Case series, studies with no controls

*RCTs, randomized controlled trials.
[a] Adapted from Sackett DL. Rules of evidence and clinical recommendations on the use of antithrombotic agents. Chest. 1989;95:2S–4S.[169]
Table 6.2 amended from Burns et al.[166]

recognized that the type of evidence and LOE needed modification accordingly. Research questions are divided into the following four categories:

1. Treatment (Therapeutic)
2. Prognosis
3. Diagnosis
4. Economic/decision analysis.

For example, Table 6.3 shows the LOEs developed by the American Society of Plastic Surgeons for *prognosis*[167], and Table 6.4 shows the levels developed by the Centre for Evidence-Based Medicine for *treatment (therapeutic studies)*.[168] These two tables feature the types of studies that are appropriate for the question of *prognosis* versus questions of *treatment*. This very important distinction is made because RCTs are *not appropriate* when looking at the *prognosis* of a disease.

Table 6.3 Levels of evidence for prognostic studies[a].

Level	Type of evidence
I	High-quality prospective cohort study with adequate power or systematic review of these studies
II	Lesser quality prospective cohort, retrospective cohort study, untreated controls from an RCT*, or systematic review of these studies
III	Case-control study or systematic review of these studies
IV	Case series
V	Expert opinion; case report or clinical example; or evidence based on physiology, bench research, or "first principles"

*RCT, randomized controlled trial.
[a] Adapted from the American Society of Plastic Surgeons. Available at: http://www.plasticsurgery.org/For_Medical-Professionals/Legislation-and-Advocacy/Health-Policy-Resources/Evidence-based-GuidelinesPracticeParameters/Description-and-Development-of-Evidence-based Practice-Guidelines/ASPS-Evidence-Rating-Scales.html. Accessed December 17, 2010.[167]
Table 6.3 amended from Burns et al. for questions of prognosis.[166]

Table 6.4 Levels of evidence for therapeutic studies[a].

Level	Type of evidence
1a	Systematic review (with homogeneity) of RCTs*
1b	Individual RCT (with narrow confidence intervals)
1c	All-or-none study
2a	Systematic review (with homogeneity) of cohort studies
2b	Individual cohort study, including low-quality RCTs; (e.g., <80% follow-up)
2c	"Outcomes" research; ecological studies
3a	Systematic review (with homogeneity) of case-control studies
3b	Individual case-control study
4	Case series (and poor-quality cohort and case-control study)
5	Expert opinion without explicit critical appraisal or based on physiology, bench research, or "first principles"

RCTs, randomized controlled trials.
[a] *From the Centre for Evidence-Based Medicine (Web site). Available at: http://www.ccbm.net. Accessed December 17, 2010.[168]*

Table 6.4 amended from Burns et al. for questions of treatment.[166]

A prognosis does not compare treatments; therefore, the highest LOE comes from a cohort study and not from an RCT for questions of prognosis. Obviously, the physician must consider the quality of the data, since a poorly designed RCT has little merit; consequently, it may be at the same LOE as a cohort study. The question in this instance is, "What will happen to the patient if we do nothing at all?" Because a prognosis question does not involve comparing treatments, the highest evidence would come from a cohort study or a systematic review of cohort studies and again not from an RCT.

The LOEs must also consider the quality of the data. For example, in Table 6.4 from the Centre for Evidence-Based Medicine, a poorly designed RCT has the same LOE as a cohort study. A grading system that provides strength of recommendations based on evidence has also changed over time.

Table 6.5 shows the Grade Practice Recommendations developed by the American Society of Plastic Surgeons. The grading system provides an important component in EBM and assists in formulating clinical decisions. For example, a strong recommendation is given when there is level I evidence in concert with consistent evidence from level II, III, and IV studies available. The grading system does not degrade lower-level evidence when deciding recommendations if the results are consistent. Although RCTs are often assigned the highest LOE, not all RCTs are conducted properly, and it is our responsibility to scrutinize the results carefully.[167,168]

Sackett[169] stressed the importance of estimating types of errors and the power of studies when interpreting results from RCTs. For example, a poorly conducted RCT may report a negative result because of low power when in fact a real difference exists between treatment groups. The Jadad scale has been developed to judge the

Table 6.5 Grade practice recommendations.*

Grade	Descriptor	Qualifying evidence	Implications for practice
A	Strong recommendation	Level I evidence or consistent findings from multiple studies of levels II, III, or IV	Clinicians should follow a strong recommendation unless a clear and compelling rationale for an alternative approach is present
B	Recommendation	Levels II, III, or IV evidence, and findings are generally consistent	Generally, clinicians should follow a recommendation but should remain alert to new information and sensitive to patient preferences
C	Option	Levels II, III, or IV evidence, but findings are inconsistent	Clinicians should be flexible in their decision-making regarding appropriate practice, although they may set bounds on alternatives; patient preference should have a substantial influencing role
D	Option	Level V evidence: little or no systematic empirical evidence	Clinicians should consider all options in their decision-making and be alert to new published evidence that clarifies the balance of benefit versus harm; patient preference should have a substantial influencing role

From the American Society of Plastic Surgeons. Evidence-based clinical practice guidelines. Available at: http://www.plasticsurgery.org/MedicalProfessionals/HealthPolicyandAdvocacy/HealthPolicyResources/Evidence-basedGuidelinesPracticeParameters/DescriptionandDevelopmentofEvidence-basedPracticeGuidelines/ASPSGradeRecommendationScale.html. Accessed 3 March 2011.

quality of RCTs.[170] Remember, do not assume that all level 1 studies are of higher quality than level 2 studies. Although the goal is to improve the overall LOE in medicine and surgery, this does not mean that all lower-level evidence should be discarded. Case series reports are important for **hypothesis** generation, which leads to more questions and further controlled studies. In addition, in the face of overwhelming evidence to support a treatment, such as the use of antibiotics for wound infections, there is no need for an RCT.

Some basic items that should be considered for assessing RCTs include a description of the randomization and blinding process, a description of the number of subjects who withdrew or dropped out of the study, the confidence intervals around study estimates, and a description of the power analysis. Although RCTs may not be appropriate for many surgical questions, well-designed and well-conducted cohort or case-control studies could boost the LOE.

Clearly, LOEs are an important component of EBM. Understanding the levels and why they are assigned to publications and abstracts helps the reader to prioritize information. This is not to say that all level IV evidence should be ignored and all level I evidence accepted as fact. The LOEs provide a guide, and the reader needs to be cautious when interpreting these results.[166]

Many of the current studies in the literature tend to be descriptive and lack a control group. The way forward seems clear. Surgery researchers need to consider using a cohort or case-control design whenever an RCT is not possible. If designed properly, the LOE for observational studies can approach or surpass those from a RCT. In some instances, observational studies and RCTs have yielded similar results.[171] If enough cohort or case-control studies become available, the prospect of systematic reviews of these studies will increase, which will increase overall evidence levels in surgery.

So, it is the understanding of the LOE, also titled the hierarchy of evidence, and how studies are assigned specific levels are purely based on the methodological quality of their design, validity, and applicability to a specific patient care situation. These decisions are assigned levels of strength or hierarchies of recommendation.

Table 6.6. Level of evidence.

Level of evidence (LOE)	Description
Level I	Evidence from a systematic review or metaanalysis of all relevant andomized controlled trial (RCTs) or evidence-based clinical practice guidelines based on systematic reviews of RCTs or three or more RCTs of good quality that have similar results.
Level II	Evidence obtained from at least one well-designed RCT (e.g., large multisite RCT).
Level III	Evidence obtained from well-designed controlled trials without randomization (i.e., quasiexperimental).
Level IV	Evidence from well-designed case-control or cohort studies.
Level V	Evidence from systematic reviews of descriptive and qualitative studies (metasynthesis).
Level VI	Evidence from a single descriptive or qualitative study.
Level VII	Evidence from the opinion of authorities and/or reports of expert committees.

Adapted from Ackley BJ, Swan BA, Ladwig G, Tucker S. Evidence-based nursing care guidelines: medical-surgical interventions. *St. Louis, MO: Mosby Elsevier; 2008:7.[172]*

Diverse clinical questions are best answered by different varieties of research findings. Realize that the answer to your clinical question might not be found at the highest LOE, that is with a systematic review or metaanalysis. If this occurs, choose the next highest LOE. This table below suggests study designs best suited to answer specific clinical questions.[172]

Table 6.7. This is a "best research design approach" to answer a specific clinical question using a particular research design.

Clinical question	Suggested research Design(s)
All clinical questions	Systematic review, metaanalysis
Therapy	Randomized controlled trial (RCT), metaanalysis
	Also: cohort study, case-control study, case series
Etiology	RCT, metaanalysis, cohort study
	Also: case-control study, case series

Adapted from: Ackley BJ, Swan BA, Ladwig G, Tucker S. Evidence-based nursing care guidelines: medical-surgical interventions. *St. Louis, MO: Mosby Elsevier; 2008:7.*[172]

Ultimately, as per Straus and Sackett *"Firstly, practicing EBM begins and ends with clinical expertise."*[173] EBM is seen as a way to improve medical practice by limiting errors even when there is no evidence to identify the gold standard of treatment. By asking questions and searching for the best alternative among all the various alternatives available, thousands of authors working with the **Cochrane Collaboration** worldwide have fashioned systematic reviews to lower ambiguity in medical decision-making. The conclusions and deductions from the Cochrane reviews of RCTs influence their recommendations for clinical practice and research.[174] About 10 years ago, a rigorous system of evaluating data was introduced by the Oxford Centre for Evidence-Based Medicine specifying the quality of the methodology.[168]

"Evidence-based medicine has not been universally accepted in all quarters of medicine and surgery."

In a letter to the editor published in 2018 entitled:

"Rethinking Evidence-Based Medicine (EBM) in Plastic and Reconstructive *Surgery,"* N.F. Al Deek[175] argued against EBM as follows:

"Evidence-based medicine is not without weakness; it is inherently restrained by the quality of evidence in the literature, affected by the timing of proposal of the technique, experience of the operator, instruments used, anatomical understanding, and volume, and the list goes on."

Near the close of the editorial, he continued as follows: "If comparison must be made, let it be among experts, not among a pool of data."[175]

While advancing, in our opinion, a contrary and a most rational view, Dr. Eric Swanson of Leawood, Kansas, said:

*"**Evidence-based medicine is our true North Star. It ranks data over institutional authority, consensus of experts, mainstream views, and the tyranny of conventional wisdom .... Evidence-based medicine empowers the pioneer to challenge the** status quo **on an even playing field, where only the facts matter. Let us not abandon but rather recommit to our scientific roots ... surgeons attend medical school—not a fine arts academy or business school for a reason. If we turn our backs on evidence-based medicine now, not only will we fail, but we will deserve to fail."*[176] (Bold italics added)

On the other hand, arthritis researchers Peter Croft et al.[177] in the United Kingdom, while discussing the pros and cons of EBM thought that criticism of EBM needed to be openly expressed and freely discussed. They thought that the proponents of EBM needed to accept clinical expertise especially in the area of innovation. They believed that inventiveness and new ideas could be rationally resolved… "by allowing the use of the new, innovative interventions at an early stage within the setting of RCTs, or observational, monitoring, or audit studies." The alternative is to define characteristics of interventions or situations that would be acceptable as exceptions to EBM.[177]

Others saw EBM primarily as a guide to excellence in the clinical decision process by integrating expertise with patient preferences thereby improving medical practice especially avoiding errors when a specific gold standard is not available. But these authors were also concerned about the implied suppression of innovation, pointing out that the most deleterious aspect of EBM is when it operates as an excuse to:

> "…block the access of the innovation to patients certainly not the best way to maximize the benefits of EBM"[178]

Colleagues from McGill University, Montréal, Québec, Canada, division of cardiology, department of medicine, clearly recognized the aim of EBM was to facilitate the physician's ability to make rational clinical decisions based on superior knowledge from RCTs and metaanalysis. However, the reality is, as they pointed out, evidence from RCTs is frequently imperfect, incongruous, contradictory, or evidence is nonexistent, even for clinical questions which have been scrupulously studied. They reminded us that the likelihood of therapeutic success or failure of a given therapy is not identical in all the individuals treated in any specific trial because results from any trial cannot be assuredly applied to every other individual patient. This is true even if that patient matches all the entry benchmarks for the particular trial in question. They went on to say that important sources of knowledge come from guidelines; however, there are limits to the quality and the transferability of evidence, so physicians and surgeons nevertheless require rational thought, "clinical reasoning" to select the "best choices," especially in the absence of complete knowledge, decisions must be made. So, Sniderman and colleagues recognized that we are ultimately left with:

> "Clinical reasoning is the pragmatic, tried-and-true process of expert clinical problem solving that does value mechanistic reasoning and clinical experience as well as RCTs and observational studies. Clinicians must continue to value clinical reasoning if our aim is the best clinical care for all the individuals we treat."[179]

In the middle of last century, Dr. Harry Bakwin of New York City wrote an interesting inquiry into some of the then contemporary pediatric errors exploring the various reasons for their perseverance. He adroitly referred back to Sir Thomas Brown's huge 17th century treatise entitled *Pseudodoxia Epidemica,* which is illuminated as the *"Enquiries into very many received Tenents and commonly Presumed Truths."*[180] Bakwin observed that Sir Thomas investigated the abundant fallacies then acknowledged as truths of the day all the while authenticating their absurdity.[180] As we now know so well, science, in general, has debunked the magical, the mystical, and the reigning superstitions that prospered during the 1600s. But even today, in our "modern scientific era," there are practices and delusions that endure in the practice of medicine despite their patent fallaciousness. Think complete and total turbinectomy as a treatment for benign nasal airway obstruction or that turbinate hypertrophy is a serious complication of deafness. *Pseudodoxia Epidemica* could be rewritten today, in modern times of the 21st century, as *Pseudodoxia Rhinologica.*

Recall the citation of T. Carmalt Jones* at a meeting of the British Medical Association chronicled in *The Lancet* in 1895 as follows:

> *"**Removal of hypertrophied inferior turbinals** and moriform growths **should be practiced** in cases of **deafness and** tinnitus where the auditory nerve was in a healthy condition."*[78] *(Bold italics added)*

*Jones T. Carmalt. "Turbinotomy in cases of Deafness and Tinnitus Aurinm": The Lancet 2. The British Medical Association. August 24, 1895 p.496.

Generally, the medical profession acknowledges the adverse effects of flawed teachings by experts, even professors who practice predominantly without any scientific objective evidence, mainly possessing a wealth of "experience" enjoying to be greeted by colleagues and christened by the exhalated term, "expert" or at medical conferences as "esteemed professor." Just as authorities once proclaimed the healing power of leaches or bloodletting, major errors in contemporary medical rhinologic education appear to be the failure to properly educate the student in the fundamentals of nasal physiology. For example, the ideas and opinions regarding upper airway surgery were often based on observation alone while scientific knowledge regarding the upper airway must of necessity be based on objective testing and comprehension of the fundamental principles of physics incorporating and accepting the aerodynamics of nasal airflow during both inspiration and expiration. The salient concepts regarding the influence and physiologic realities of aerometry of both the internal or external nasal valve are both fundamental and crucial knowledge for the coherent cogent practice of upper airway nasal surgery.

Diagnosis and treatment concepts require evolution in scientific thinking, which in our field seems to be painfully sluggish, inevitably accompanied by errors delaying and at times derailing progress. No doubt, despite errors, progress requires identification and confirmation with substantiation of those identified miscalculations to be reduced, for a steady arc of improvement, regrettably we must accept missteps. We proclaim that progress is two steps forward and one step back. Dr. Bakwin[180] perspicaciously noted that error-prone medical progress was already shrewdly detected and reflected upon by the French critical essayist and author Marcel Proust (1871−1922) who observed:

"For, medicine being a compendium of the successive and contradictory mistakes of medical practitioners, when we summon the wisest of them to our aid, the chances are that we may be relying on a scientific truth the error of which will be recognized in a few years' time. So that's to believing medicine would be the height of folly, if not to believe in Medicine were not greater folly still, for from this mass of errors there have emerged in the course of time many truths."[181]

Dr. David L. Sackett died in May 2015, leaving behind a major philosophical influence on the clinical practice of medicine with his commanding concepts of EBM. As a concluding statement on the matter, according to Dr. Sackett, EBM is really all about the prudent use of contemporary "best evidence" from the literature to be used in formulating rational decisions about the care of a particular patient. Practicing EBM means incorporating three fundamental requirements:

1. Primarily, harvesting the "best scientific" research from the literature
2. That best research evidence must be combined with the physician's unique clinical expertise
3. Integrating the patient's values, desires, and specific situation into the decision-making process

In summary, for Dr. Sackett before a final therapeutic decision can be made, those three requirements needed to be considered and integrated into the decision process. Primarily and most prominent was the necessary fundamental research evidence from the literature. Although research evidence was supreme, it required coupling with the individual specific clinical circumstances (conditions) of a given patient and eventually integrated with the unique individual patient's preferences before reaching a concluding clinical decision apropos of future action.

Recognize, moreover that the practice of EBM requires a physician's lifetime commitment to education and remaining abreast of the contemporary literature regarding diagnosis, treatment, and prognosis for any given medical and surgical condition.[173]

Ultimately, those of us in rhinology must accept the remaining reality that as of March 2023, there were no studies listed for inferior turbinate reduction, turbinate surgery, or turbinoplasty at the Oxford Centre's database.[168] Therefore, we need to continue utilizing our rational clinical reasoning to manage the problem of nasal airway obstruction secondary to inferior turbinate enlargement ("hypertrophy"); cautious clinical reasoning, while minimalizing turbinate trauma in the absence of definitive RCTs, is the order of the day, avoiding a catastrophic result for an innocent trusting patient.

In answer to the question, why is EBM pertinent to our conversation in this text, it's because understandably, the most reliable treatment information, the best evidence, comes from well-conceived and well performed RCTs; however, that is not to say that all level IV evidence should be ignored and all level I evidence accepted as fact. The LOEs provide a guide for us the reader, and we are required to be cautious when interpreting these results.[166]

The turbinates—management

1. Middle turbinate management

The debate regarding middle turbinate preservation has a heated history of disagreement raging for more than a century, the rhinologic equivalent of the Hundred Years' War, 1337−1453, in the blossom of the Middle Ages. Middle turbinate "resectors" are surgeons who remorselessly rationalize resection of the middle turbinate to forestall formation of synechia in the region of the middle meatus.[182−184] Proponents on the other side of the divide champion ***respecting not resecting*** the middle turbinate for its importance as a critical anatomical landmark and as an independent functional organ system.[185−187]

Among all the brother and sister surgeons, there are effectively two schools of thought regarding managing the middle turbinate. Without wavering, all agree that the middle turbinate dispassionately represents an important landmark in nasal sinus surgery since the olfactory cribriform region is superior and medial to the middle turbinate. Lateral to the middle turbinate is a plethora, a surplus of important structures including the frontal recess, the floor of the anterior cranial fossa, the middle meatus, semilunar hiatus, the uncinate process, the infundibulum, the maxillary sinus ostium, the ethmoidal bulla, and the orbital contents. The medical literature both favors and criticizes middle turbinate resection.[182−187] So, what are we left with?

For the historical record, the practice of middle turbinate resection was condemned by Professor Walter Messerklinger, MD, (1920−2001)[185] the "father" of modern endoscopic sinus surgery (ESS) and mentor to the incomparable surgeon and educator, Professor Heinz Stammberger, MD, (1946−2018) of Graz, Austria,[187] both *favoring middle turbinate preservation* whenever possible. They accepted a *"conservative"* approach that embodied preserving a maximum aggregate of normal tissue, whereas *partial* middle turbinate resection was tolerated only in cases of concha bullosa and paradoxical middle turbinate.

Other surgeons promoted "routine" total or partial middle turbinate resection as a fundamental step in essentially every endoscopic sinus operation. We think that "routine" total or partial middle turbinate resection as a prelude to every sinus surgery is "unreasonable"; we display computerized tomography (CT) scans from patients having had, in all "likelihood," *essential middle turbinate resections,* who developed "empty nose syndrome (ENS)." These middle turbinectomies were performed elsewhere, not at the Mayo Clinic; seen in Figs. 7.1–7.4.

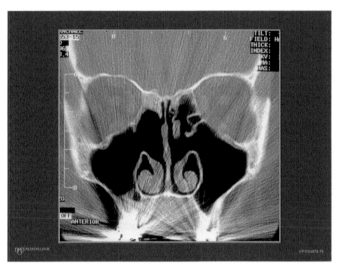

FIGURE 7.1

Coronal CT scan of a patient exhibiting the common findings of bilateral *middle turbinectomy* seen in patients with the **"empty nose syndrome,"** performed elsewhere, not at the Mayo Clinic. This procedure is not supported by authors.

(Kern and Friedman. By permission of Mayo Foundation for Medical Education and Research. All Rights Reserved).

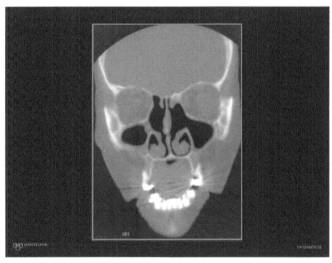

FIGURE 7.2

Coronal CT scan of a patient exhibiting the common findings of *middle turbinectomy* seen in patients with the **"empty nose syndrome,"** performed elsewhere, not at the Mayo Clinic. This procedure is not supported by authors.

(Kern and Friedman. By permission of Mayo Foundation for Medical Education and Research. All Rights Reserved).

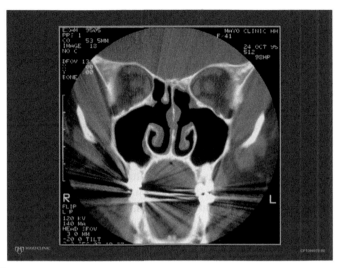

FIGURE 7.3

Coronal CT scan of a patient exhibiting the common findings of *middle turbinectomy* seen in patients with the **"empty nose syndrome,"** performed elsewhere, not at the Mayo Clinic. This procedure is not supported by authors.

(Kern and Friedman. By permission of Mayo Foundation for Medical Education and Research. All Rights Reserved).

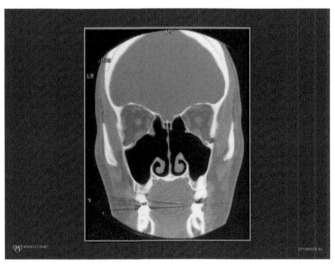

FIGURE 7.4

Coronal CT scan of a patient exhibiting the common findings of *middle turbinectomy* seen in patients with the **"empty nose syndrome,"** performed elsewhere, not at the Mayo Clinic. This procedure is not supported by authors.

(Kern and Friedman. By permission of Mayo Foundation for Medical Education and Research. All Rights Reserved).

In addition, we assessed and treated a patient for **"ENS"** after septectomy (squamous cell carcinoma) and subtotal resection of a portion of the left lateral wall of the nose who developed symptoms several years after the initial tumor surgery. Both middle turbinates were resected with a partial reduction (subtotal resection) of the left inferior turbinate. Note: the surgery was not performed at the Mayo Clinic, by a Mayo Clinic surgeon. Fig. 7.5

Both approaches, *preservation* and *resection* of the middle turbinate have produced "successful" outcomes; nonetheless, there are various variables that have not been controlled, so practically every study in the literature has their conclusions based on nonrandomized retrospective assessments. Many, if not all, of these studies probably have dubious conclusions and associated problematic prejudices.

The argument even included possible potential peril to the frontal recess resulting in an increased incidence of frontal sinusitis subsequent to partial resection of the middle turbinate. In 1995, Swanson et al. at the University of Pennsylvania observed a statistically significant rise in *secondary frontal sinus* disease when a portion or the entire middle turbinate was surgically removed.[188]

Figs. 7.6 and 7.7 are examples of patients, seen at the Mayo practice, who developed *secondary frontal sinusitis* after previous middle turbinectomies, performed elsewhere, not at the Mayo Clinic.

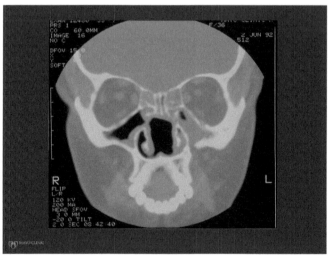

FIGURE 7.5

Coronal CT scan of a patient who developed symptoms of the **_"empty nose syndrome"_** after septectomy and subtotal resection of a portion of the left lateral wall for squamous cell carcinoma of the nasal septum. Both middle turbinates have been resected with a partial reduction (subtotal resection) of the left inferior turbthee. Note: the primary surgery was not performed at the Mayo Clinic or by a Mayo surgeon.

(Kern and Friedman. By permission of Mayo Foundation for Medical Education and Research. All Rights Reserved).

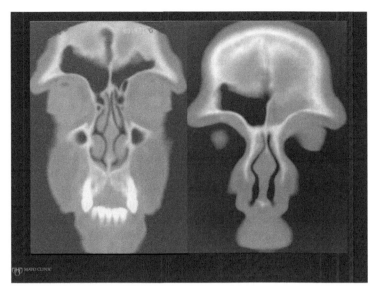

FIGURE 7.6

Coronal CT scans of a patient who developed frontal sinusitis subsequent to a *middle turbinectomy*. The CT scan on the left is prior to the *middle turbinectomy*, while the CT scan on the right is taken some time after a bilateral *middle turbinectomy,* performed elsewhere, not at the Mayo Clinic. This procedure is not supported by authors.

(Kern and Friedman. By permission of Mayo Foundation for Medical Education and Research. All Rights Reserved).

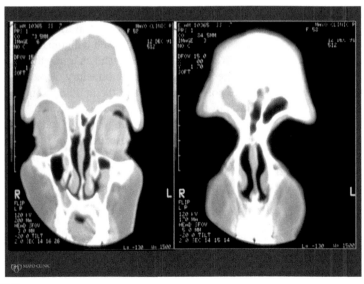

FIGURE 7.7

Coronal CT scan of a patient who developed frontal sinusitis sometime after a bilateral *middle turbinectomy,* performed elsewhere, not at the Mayo Clinic. This procedure is not supported by authors.

(Kern and Friedman. By permission of Mayo Foundation for Medical Education and Research. All Rights Reserved).

Zhou and Li in a retrospective analysis ($n = 87$) investigated the effect of partial middle turbinectomy on the frontal sinus and concluded that partial middle turbinectomy has no effect on the incidence of frontal sinusitis.[189]

In control a review of 155 consecutive patients, utilizing the "Duncavage technique" for partial middle turbinectomy, Fortune and Duncavage found a 10% incidence of frontal sinusitis subsequent to partial middle turbinate resection.[190]

Havas and Lowinger attempted to resolve the debate by studying a population composed of ($n = 1106$) patients, some patients **with** ($n = 509$) middle turbinate surgery, and ($n = 597$) patients **without** middle turbinate surgery. Their team recorded few complications while lauding the benefits of thoughtful partial middle turbinate resection in patients with extensive sinus disease.[191] In a study from New York University involving ethmoidectomy operations in 100 patients, conservative partial middle turbinate resection was performed in 50 patients with preservation of the middle turbinate in the other 50 patients. After a two-year follow-up, the:

> *"…clinical and endoscopic findings revealed no difference in the incidence of frontal sinusitis or frontal recess stenosis between groups."[192]*

In a prospective study, ($n = 31$) patients in 2003 from the University of California Los Angeles found that:

> *"…middle turbinate resection has no deleterious effects on the results of endoscopic sinus surgery."[193]*

So, if the middle turbinate is significantly involved with an inflammatory process as with extensive polypoid disease and associated exposed bone, then resection is advisable, since leaving a large "raw surface" has the potential for developing postoperative adhesions. Remember, the turbinates are involved with the nasal cycle, the maintenance of a proper airflow, in addition to warming and charging the inspired air with moisture, the middle turbinate also contains some olfactory elements. Overall, authorities agree that if extensive polypoid changes of the middle turbinate mucosa are present, then partial resection of the damaged mucosa is indicated.[194,195]

Stewart in 1998 found that *partial* middle turbinate resection had a lower adhesion rate when compared with *total* middle turbinate resection.[196] In other words, the presence of extensive polypoid degeneration with the destruction of a major portion of the middle turbinate, concomitant with chronic rhinosinusitis (CRS), obviously turbinate preservation is virtually impossible; therefore, cautious resection is almost statutory.

As pointedly observed by Nurse and Duncavage,[197] the kerfuffle and brouhaha surrounding middle turbinate resection centers around any specific surgeon's actual approach or philosophy regarding nasal physiology and those opinions are currently widely diverse, distinct, and disparate.

Fundamentally, we completely agree with Kennedy's assertion that in the presence of a normal middle turbinate, then surgical resection is not necessary to access either the ethmoid labyrinth or the frontal recess.[194]

Kennedy, Rice, and other experienced surgeons agree that the middle turbinate should be partially resected removing extensive polypoid changes of that particular middle turbinate when existent.[193-198]

In the presence of an airway obstructing middle turbinate concha bullosa, it is universally agreed that some type of surgical intervention is indicated to reduce the obstruction. For a concha bullosa, we favor incision into the body of the concha bullosa with instrument collapse; thereby, minimizing the airway obstruction while maintaining both the medial and lateral mucosal surfaces of the middle turbinate structure since mucocele is rare Figs. 7.8–7.13.

So, what are we left with?

Remarkably after the searing perspicacious 2001 paper by Clement and White who unequivocally specified that after judging 283 papers over a 35-year period of both middle and inferior turbinate surgery that since there were no randomized controlled trials (RCTs), not a one, specifying:

> *"The evidence supporting the efficacy of these procedures remains debatable."[199] (Bold italics added)*

As of 2010, Scheithauer[28] astutely noted while supporting Clement and White unfortunately it was virtually impossible to make a clear recommendation regarding middle turbinate preservation or excision due to the lack of controlled, long-term randomized studies in the literature.

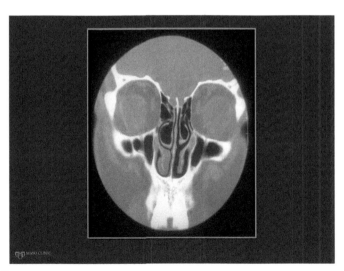

FIGURE 7.8

Coronal CT scan of a patient (from our practice) exhibiting the typical findings seen with *bilateral concha bullosa* (both middle turbinates), right larger than the left.

(Kern and Friedman. By permission of Mayo Foundation for Medical Education and Research. All Rights Reserved).

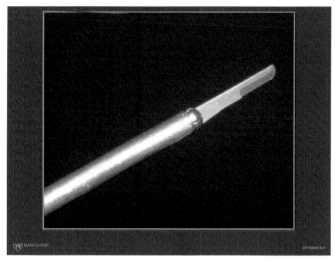

FIGURE 7.9

Photograph of a #64 Beaver knife blade for incision into the anterior portion of the middle turbinate in the process of reducing a concha bullosa.

(Kern and Friedman. By permission of Mayo Foundation for Medical Education and Research. All Rights Reserved).

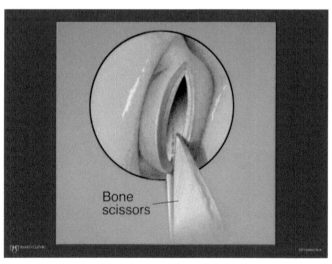

FIGURE 7.10

Illustration of a bone scissor cut into the body of the middle turbinate to reduce the concha bullosa after the #64 Beaver knife blade incised the anterior portion of the middle turbinate allowing for the introduction of the bone scissors.

(Kern and Friedman. By permission of Mayo Foundation for Medical Education and Research. All Rights Reserved).

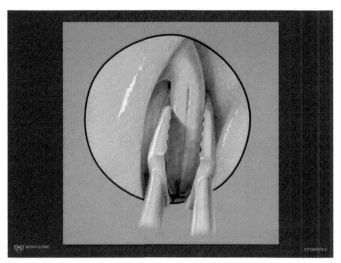

FIGURE 7.11

Illustration of a collapse of the middle turbinate, reducing the concha bullosa, with a modified Ferris Smith forceps.

(Kern and Friedman. By permission of Mayo Foundation for Medical Education and Research. All Rights Reserved).

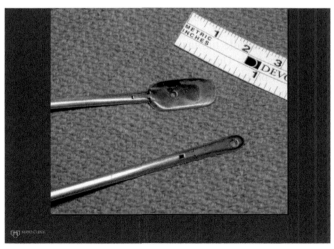

FIGURE 7.12

Photograph of a Ferris Smith forceps (below) with the modified Ferris Smith forceps (above) used specifically to collapse an incised concha bullosa of the middle turbinate.

(Kern and Friedman. By permission of Mayo Foundation for Medical Education and Research. All Rights Reserved).

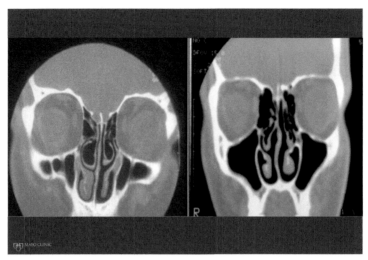

FIGURE 7.13

Coronal CT scan of a patient (from our practice) exhibiting the typical findings seen with *bilateral concha bullosa,* on the ***left,*** note the inferior turbinates exhibiting evidence of the nasal cycle on the right side is congested while the left is the decongested side. On the ***right*** is a CT scan of the same patient one year after bilateral reduction (collapse, **without** resection) of the concha bullosa of middle turbinates, preserving the nasal turbinate mucosa.

(Kern and Friedman. By permission of Mayo Foundation for Medical Education and Research. All Rights Reserved).

Fortunately, for the middle turbinate debate, we have a recent, 2018 RCT by Hudon and colleagues from Université de Sherbrooke, Sherbrooke, Canada, who looked at the effect of preservation versus resection of the middle turbinate (middle turbinectomy) on surgical outcomes after ESS for CRS[200]. In 16 patients, 15 males (15 initial and primary cases), the nasal cavities were randomized:

> *"…so that middle turbinectomy was performed on one side while the middle turbinate was preserved on the other. Each participant acted as their own control." After 6 months follow-up, they concluded that there was: "…**no sustained objective endoscopic benefit of routine middle turbinectomy**" in their 16 CRS patients with polyposis after ESS.[200] (Bold italics added)*

Finally, for the moment, of ***"approximate temporary truth"*** in the absence of certainty from RCTs, we champion saving the middle turbinate for both its physiological function and as a critical anatomical landmark, especially for potentially revision surgery in patients with CRS with recurrent polyps; therefore, unless reduced or destroyed by polypoid disease concomitant to CRS, or a paradoxical middle turbinate, or a concha bullosa, for our crowd, preservation of the middle turbinate is the word of the day. We favor discrete resection of middle turbinate polypoid disease and conservative surgical treatment of a concha bullosa as summarized and presented in Figs. 7.8–7.13.

2. Inferior turbinate management

2.1 Classification: inferior turbinate enlargement ("hypertrophy")

There are a number of published systems for classifying enlargement ("hypertrophy") of the inferior turbinate.

Three are based on the clinical physical examination and one on CT. [201−204] The nasoendoscopic system proposed by Camacho et al. is the most recent, 2015, from the Stanford Outpatient Medical Center in Redwood City, California. It is a validated grading system based on a study of 100 consecutive patients (200 inferior turbinates) that were prospectively graded by two different individuals on two separate occasions. Grading of the 200 inferior turbinates was as follows:

> *"…classified as a **grade 1** when the inferior turbinate occupies 0% to 25% of the total airway, **grade 2** is 26% to 50%, **grade 3** is 51% to 75%, and **grade 4** is when the inferior turbinate occupies 76% to 100%."[201] (Bold italics added)*

Over 20 years ago, Friedman et al. proposed a *simplified system* using a three-part grading system where:

Grade 1 is "normal" or slight enlargement of the inferior turbinate *without* airway obstruction,
Grade 2 is *partial* airway obstruction, and
Grade 3 is *complete* obstruction of the nasal airway at the level of the inferior turbinate.[202]

A study correlating the nasal anatomy to the severity of obstructive sleep apnea classified inferior turbinate enlargement ("hypertrophy") as: 0—normal, 1—mild, 2—moderate, or 3—severe.[203]

By studying the inferior turbinate (concha) bone using CT, Uzun et al. rated the inferior turbinate size as:

Type 1 (lamellar),
Type 2 (compact bone),
Type 3 (combined), and
Type 4 (bullous).[204]

Whichever classification of turbinate enlargement ("hypertrophy") is your favorite, we suggest using it during your clinical evaluations.

2.2 Turbinate reduction: surgical and nonsurgical procedures

Since the mid-1980s, during the evidence-based medicine (EBM) milieu, the optimal study design for comparing therapeutic interventions is the unrivaled RCT. In 2001, colleagues Clement and White from the Department of Otolaryngology, University of Dundee, Ninewells Hospital and Medical School, Dundee, United Kingdom, reviewed more than 500 papers covering 35 years identifying

283 papers detailing turbinate surgery and noted a recent increase in the number of endoscopic and laser turbinate procedures. Astoundingly, as previously mentioned, there was a total absence of any RCTs among those papers for both middle and inferior turbinate surgery.[199] They concluded, somewhat sardonically, that this field of clinical research is *"driven by technological advancement rather than by establishment of patient benefit."*

Since the introduction of EBM about 30 years ago, the righteous clamor in otorhinolaryngologic practice and academic circles has been for RCTs to determine rational guidelines for achievable goals vis-à-vis the turbinates designed for a predictable benefit for our patients. Unfortunately, *a dearth* describes the *quantity* of RCTs in both otorhinolaryngology and in the plastic surgery literature; however, auspicious trends may be promising. [205–209] In 2009, Cleveland Clinic authors Batra, Seiden, and Smith presented an exhaustive review of the current evidence from 96 studies of inferior turbinate surgery containing a prodigious list of references.[210] They cited 93 (97%) of the 96 studies as level 4 or 5 with two level 2[211,212] and only one of the highest order, level 1 study.[26]

Recently, in 2015, Peters et al. from University Medical Center Utrecht, Utrecht, the Netherlands, went as far as to sneeringly brand the *quality* of the RCTs in our ENT literature as **"suboptimal."**[213] (Bold italics added)

As of 2023, we ask, what are the comprehensive choices, evidence-based or otherwise, available for the management of the inferior turbinate following a medical treatment failure?

Based on the all-inclusive reviews of Hol and Huizing, (2000),[25] Scheithauer, (2010),[28] Abdullah and Singh, (2021),[214] we have integrated and modified their inferior turbinate management framework with ours as: Inferior Turbinate Reduction: Surgical and Nonsurgical Procedures 2022 Table 7.1.

Within our ecosphere, we hold that the triad of principal objectives or goals for inferior turbinate treatment are:

1. Relief of nasal airway obstruction secondary to inferior turbinate enlargement ("hypertrophy")
2. Preservation of physiologic turbinate function
3. Avoidance of complications, immediate and delayed (hours, days, weeks, months, and years into the future)

To grasp the entirety of turbinate management techniques utilized over the years, there are principally two types of turbinate procedures: streamlined and simplified as follows:

(a) Epithelial mucosal *destruction: Transmucosal* approach (including partial and complete-total turbinectomy)
(b) Epithelial mucosal *preservation: Submucosal* approach

For a brief anatomy lesson, recall that the nasal mucosa (epithelium and submucosa) itself is basically composed of two distinctive layers, the epithelium and the submucosa (lamina propria, stroma) Fig. 5.2:

Table 7.1 Inferior turbinate reduction: Surgical and non-surgical procedures.[a]

  A. Epithelial mucosal *destruction* (transmucosal approach)
    1. Surgical resection-turbinectomy (partial or complete-total)
    2. Electrocautery
    3. Laser therapy
    4. Cryotherapy
  B. Epithelial mucosal *preservation* (submucosal approach)
    1. Submucosal soft tissue surgical reduction (turbinoplasty)
      a. Submucosal soft tissue reduction only
      b. Conchal bone reduction only
      c. Combined: soft tissue and conchal bone reduction
    2. Microdebrider
    3. Radiofrequency
    4. Coblation
    5. Ultrasound
    6. Electrocautery
  C. Complimentary: out-fracture (lateralization)
    1. Solitary-isolated intervention
    2. Combined with other procedures

---

[a] *Specifically, as previously written, surgery is: the medical practice of managing diseases, deformities, and injuries by actually "cutting" into a part of the body, while, on the other hand, electrocautery, chemocautery, lasers, radiofrequency, coblation, or ultrasound are not surgery in the traditional sense of cold knife "cutting," but nonetheless they are currently considered "surgery" by some authors; however, we choose to call these practices the **n**on-**s**urgical **T**urbinate **R**eduction **A**djunctive **P**rocedures (n-s TRAPs).*

1. Epithelium—The outer most epithelial layer composed of pseudostratified ciliated columnar respiratory epithelium consisting of ciliated columnar cells, goblet cells, intermediate cells, and basal cells, resting on a basement membrane.
2. Submucosa—The second deeper layer is the submucosa (lamina propria, stroma), which is composed of a loose connective tissue with a rich complex vascular erectile venous sinusoid system along with seromucous glands and mesenchymal cells.

Although "usually" effective in relieving nasal airway obstruction, the epithelial mucosal *destruction* (including resection-partial and complete-total turbinectomy) procedures have been associated with postoperative complications such as profuse bleeding, pain, crusting, and ENS (paradoxically the procedure to relieve nasal airway obstruction has been associated with exacerbating nasal airway obstruction) with a protracted period for recovery.

Because untoward complications are largely avoided in the epithelial mucosal *preservation* approach, epithelial mucosal *preservation* is our preference. Currently, since numerous and various inferior turbinate reduction practices are utilized worldwide, a comprehensive review and commentary regarding each surgical and **n**on-surgical **T**urbinate **R**eduction Adjunctive **P**rocedure (n-s TRAP)* intervention is presented for completeness.

* Specifically, as previously written, surgery is: the medical practice of managing diseases, deformities, and injuries by actually "cutting" into a part of the body, while, on the other hand, electrocautery, chemocautery, lasers, radiofrequency, coblation, or ultrasound are not surgery in the traditional sense of cold knife "cutting," but nonetheless they are currently considered "surgery" by some authors, but we choose to call these practices the **n**on-surgical **T**urbinate **R**eduction **A**djunctive **P**rocedures (n-s TRAP).

Different techniques, surgical and nonsurgical, have been used to increase the cross-sectional diameter of the nasal airway by reducing the inferior turbinate size, thereby enlarging (opening) the internal nasal valve area.[25,28,211,214,216] These techniques include conventional surgical turbinectomy (partial or complete-total) or turbinate reduction using nonsurgical modalities such as electrocautery, lasers, and cryotherapy. In addition, conventional (cold knife) turbinoplasty, microdebrider turbinoplasty, radiofrequency turbinoplasty, coblation turbinoplasty, ultrasound turbinoplasty, and submucosal electrocautery have all been ***introduced submucosally*** reducing the turbinate size, thereby enlarging (opening) the internal nasal valve area to improve nasal breathing.

Overall, these surgical and nonsurgical techniques are classified into two broad categories:

First, the epithelial mucosal ***destruction***
Second, the epithelial mucosal ***preservation***

These techniques are based on the destructive damage or preservation of the nasal epithelial mucosal surface of the inferior turbinate summarized in Table 7.1.

External surgical resection (turbinectomy-partial and complete) resects (excises and removes) the entire epithelial mucosa (pseudostratified ciliated columnar respiratory epithelium), including the submucosal (lamina propria, stroma) erectile tissue, the neurovascular bundles, and conchal (turbinate) bone.

Turbinoplasty is an epithelial mucosal *preservation* technique that reduces the submucosal soft tissue (lamina propria, stroma) with or without conchal (turbinate bone) removal.

According to Silkoff et al. in Philip Cole's unimpeachable impeccable nasal airway laboratory at the University of Toronto, Canada, nasal obstruction secondary to inferior turbinate enlargement ("hypertrophy") can be objectively and accurately quantitated with both active anterior rhinomanometry and acoustic rhinometry.[215] These twin techniques have become the *first-line routine standard methods* to objectively confirm nasal airway obstruction.[214]

In general, indications for surgical or nonsurgical reduction of the inferior turbinate are considered sensible after 3 months of medical therapy that is unable to resolve the nasal airway obstruction secondary to usually bilateral turbinate enlargement ("hypertrophy") regardless of etiology.[28]

2.2.1 *Epithelial mucosal* destruction: *Transmucosal approach (including partial and complete total turbinectomy)*

1. Surgical resection-turbinectomy (partial or complete-total)
2. Electrocautery
3. Laser therapy
4. Cryotherapy

For precision, turbinectomy is defined as the removal of a portion of the turbinate (partial turbinectomy) or the entire turbinate, complete (total turbinectomy) and may be performed with or without endoscopic visualization. Elwany and Harrison compared partial turbinectomy against three other types for inferior turbinate reduction evaluating subjective and objective outcomes for comparison.[117] They found both partial turbinectomy and laser turbinectomy superior to inferior turbinoplasty and cryoturbinectomy for relieving nasal airway obstruction, by reducing resistance to nasal airflow and improving olfaction. Muco-ciliary clearance was unchanged postoperatively. Those patients with partial turbinectomy despite an "improved" nasal airway developed postoperative nasal pain, headache, mucosal atrophic changes, and postoperative bleeding more frequently than the patients in the other three randomly assigned study groups who were evaluated one year posttreatment.

In two important papers, 1999 and 2003, Passali et al. reported on long-term (four and six years) outcomes in ($n = 382$) patients randomly assigned to six different treatment groups:[211,216]

1. Electrocautery (62 patients)
2. Cryosurgery (58 patients)
3. Laser surgery (54 patients)
4. Submucous resection *without* lateral displacement (69 patients)
5. Submucous resection *with* lateral displacement (94 patients)
6. Turbinectomy (45 patients)

After data collection ($n = 382$) and analysis, Passali et al. concluded that:

"After six years, only submucosal resection resulted in optimal long-term normalization of nasal patency and in restoration of mucociliary clearance and local secretory IgA production to a physiological level with few postoperative complications ($p < .001$). The addition of lateral displacement of the inferior turbinate improved the long-term results. We recommend, in spite of the greater surgical skill required, submucosal resection combined with lateral displacement as the first-choice technique for the treatment of nasal obstruction due to hypertrophy of the inferior turbinates."[211]

They found that while inferior turbinectomy reduced nasal airway obstruction, it was associated and coupled with additional complications including, remarkable pain, nasal crusting, and excessive bleeding. As was plainly pointed out by Abdullah and Singh[214] referencing Chhabra and Houser[21] declaring:

"… that atrophic rhinitis and the empty nose syndrome are now acknowledged as delayed sequalae following total turbinectomy."[214] (Bold italics added)

Numerous authors[2–4,18–28,214] have made these observations that significant nasal turbinate trauma may lead to dryness and nasal crusting, which can develop after disrupting the normal mucociliary activity, shredded raw mucosal edges along with exposed bare bone all leading to secondary atrophic rhinitis and the ENS years into the future. ENS may result from surgical excision or from other traumatic turbinate injuries effected by electrocautery, laser, or cryosurgery. These observations of significant nasal turbinate trauma leading to delayed nasal atrophy and ENS may appear years after the inciting trauma has been appreciated and has been reported by various and abundant eyewitnesses.[2–4,18–28]

Passali et al. also noted that while turbinectomy had its major favorable effect on nasal breathing (objective test results from rhinomanometry and acoustic rhinometry), the functional effect was unfavorable with a parade of findings involving: abnormal mucociliary transit times, abnormal secretory IgA testing, and an increased incidence of secondary hemorrhage, which ultimately hinders the utility of total turbinectomy, banishing its station as a rational therapeutic preference.[211,216] Their data strongly supported submucosal resection (turbinoplasty) plus outfracture (lateralization) of the inferior turbinate as the treatment of choice, since this results in excellent nasal airflow while maintaining nasal functional integrity with the slightest probability of future complications.

Electrocautery when applied as electrical current induces unpredictable damage to the epithelium and submucosa depending on the duration and voltage of the current and is the least effective mode of improving nasal airway resistance; additionally, there is an increased rate of crusting and synechiae.[211]

As named by Abdullah and Singh[214] for inferior turbinate reduction, the lasers regularly used are diode and CO_2 lasers such as neodymium-doped: yttrium aluminum garnet (Nd-YAG), holmium: YAG, potassium titanyl phosphate, and argon plasma lasers which are cited in the literature.[214,217]

Essentially the laser varieties are centered on their manner and method of application, for example: *"…contact or noncontact mode, pulsed or continuous wave emission, emitted wavelength, and output power."*[218] According to the literature, the preferred choice is the diode laser as it allows accurate cutting of the inferior turbinate tissue coupled with excellent hemostatic control.[218] A RCT comparing radiofrequency with the diode laser reduction of airway obstruction found that the patients had a significant improvement of nasal breathing for both diode laser and radiofrequency application 3 months after treatment. Although there were no major complications observed, patients in the radiofrequency arm complained of significant discomfort.[219] With a colossal patient population ($n = 3219$), Prokopakis et al. compared three study arms including CO_2 lasers, radiofrequency, and electrocautery turbinate reduction treatments with a subjective (visual analog scale, VAS) and objective (rhinomanometry) measurements. Mucociliary transport disturbances and difficulties in manipulating the device were the only significant drawbacks of using the CO_2 lasers, but all three groups had outstanding postoperative breathing results, without statistical differences, reported at one month and one year posttreatment.[220]

Cryotherapy is considered minimally invasive, using either liquid nitrogen or nitrous oxide as the thermal freezing agent initiating necrosis with extensive damage of surface epithelium of both the nasal mucosa and submucosal stromal tissue. Since the quantity of tissue reduction was unpredictable and the beneficial results where unsustainable cryosurgery was eventually discarded.[211]

2.2.2 Epithelial mucosal preservation: Submucosal "turbinoplasty" approach

1. Submucosal soft tissue surgical reduction (conventional "cold knife" "turbinoplasty")
   (a) Submucosal soft tissue reduction only
   (b) Combined: soft tissue and conchal bone reduction
   (c) Conchal bone reduction only
2. Microdebrider
3. Radiofrequency
4. Coblation
5. Ultrasound
6. Electrocautery

Principally, all the epithelial mucosal *preservation* (submucosal "Turbinoplasty") treatments are directed toward the submucosal stroma containing erectile neurovascular bundles.

2.2.2.1 Submucosal soft tissue surgical reduction (conventional "cold knife" "turbinoplasty")

2.2.2.1.1 *Submucosal soft tissue reduction only* All these procedures are intended to remove the obstructive submucosal stromal portion of the inferior turbinate, largely at the anterior head, which is the posterior portion of the internal nasal valve area. The goal is reduction of the submucosal stromal tissue thereby reducing obstruction of the critical internal nasal valve area, improving breathing all the while preserving as much of the stromal tissue as possible so as not to interfere with physiologic functions. All these treatments are basically termed "turbinoplasty" approaches. Only the submucosa is removed claiming the advantage over the other turbinate procedures by preserving sufficient overlying mucosa, while removing adequate amounts of obstructing tissue to improve the airway sufficiently and significantly to improve breathing without reducing nasal function.

Another term labels this technique a "submucosal" resection or treatment, referring to the submucosal stromal location of the reduction treatment procedure. It was Mabry[91] who used the term "inferior turbinoplasty" that involved directing the treating modality below the epithelial mucosal surface within the inferior turbinate, affecting only the submucosal stromal tissues with or without removing part of the conchal (turbinate) bone.

*2.2.2.1.2 **Combined: soft tissue and conchal bone reduction*** Occasionally, the inferior conchal (turbinate) bone is remarkably thickened and obstructing requiring reduction of the bone *in addition* to reduction of the submucosal stromal soft tissues. Mabry said that he utilized the procedure for more than nine years, and he did not observe any of the formally dreaded complications such as bleeding, foul odor, discharge, crusting, and by extension *secondary atrophic rhinitis* in any of his study population ($n = 40$). His histologic studies of "inferior turbinoplasty" patients, observed five years postoperatively, as expected, revealed normal epithelial mucosal surfaces with submucosal stromal fibrosis along with a decreased mucous gland population.[91]

*2.2.2.1.3 **Conchal bone reduction only*** On very rare occasion, the conchal bone may be extremely thick and readily seen on direct CT scan. In this situation, the thicken conchal bone can be successfully reduced with a dental drill without complication as has been experienced by the Mayo team (EBK) on one occasion.

Many modalities can be utilized for performing the "inferior turbinoplasty." Methods and instruments used to accomplish a turbinoplasty may include any one of a host of options: "cold knife," microdebrider, radiofrequency, coblation, ultrasound, and even electrocautery; something, anything to reduce the subepithelial submucosal stromal tissues for the relief of nasal airway obstruction. Some of the submucosal techniques are, of course, blind with obvious limitations as the tissue removal is inexact; therefore, tissue reduction is frequently imprecise.

Various designs and methods of "inferior turbinoplasty" compared to other therapeutic modalities have been offered to the profession. From our literature review and subsequent to Abdullah and Singh's comprehensive paper in 2021, we located the pertinent literature supporting the physiologic and therapeutic logic of the "inferior turbinoplasty," which has happily and overwhelmingly captured the data-driven class of rhinologists.[214,221–229]

2.2.2.2 Microdebrider

The microdebrider deserves special mention as a significant advancement coupled with the endoscope, which allows aspiration of the hematogenous dissemination (blood) permitting precise tissue removal sparing the overlying epithelium, entirely, with minimal thermal damage to the surrounding tissues.[221,225]

Subjective and objective evaluations are currently common practice including symptom questionnaires, endoscopic scoring, and acoustic rhinometry which revealed microdebrider turbinoplasty as a superior method for accomplishing nasal airway relief lasting beyond a year.[221–225] In another outcome study, objectively using anterior rhinomanometry, patient's nasal breathing resistance calculations were substantially reduced after endoscopic microdebrider inferior turbinoplasty.[226] Other authors presented a matched study comparing conventional turbinoplasty with microdebrider turbinoplasty which exhibited ($n = 46$) substantial reduction in both blood loss and operative times compared to conventional turbinoplasty.[228]

In a study by Cingi et al., microdebrider turbinoplasty ($n = 124$) was compared with radiofrequency turbinoplasty ($n = 144$), while symptom improvement was statistically significant in the microdebrider group and the objective rhinomanometric measurements demonstrated increased nasal airflow, improved breathing, in the microdebrider group when compared to the radiofrequency group; nonetheless, using the power instrument microdebrider still has the inherent risk of intraoperative and or postoperative bleeding.[230]

2.2.2.3 Radiofrequency

Radiofrequency turbinoplasty is a minimally invasive method that accomplishes precise and pointed turbinate volume reduction using radiofrequency energy at an estimated temperature range of 60°C (140°F) to 90°C (194°F), while electrocautery temperatures reach a range of 400°C (752°F) to 600°C (1112°F). Radiofrequency lessens tissue injury, minimizing surrounding tissue trauma, and reducing posttreatment pain.[214] In addition to pain reduction, there is a reduction in turbinate tissue bulk, reducing nasal airway obstruction, thus improving nasal breathing.[230–235] Rhinomanometric measurements were markedly improved validating an increased nasal airway breathing. The few sequalae noted included negligible epistaxis, some dryness, little crusting, or inconsequential adhesions.[234,235] In two separate studies comparing microdebrider turbinoplasty with radiofrequency turbinoplasty, the investigators found markedly improved nasal airflow with objectively improved rhinomanometry scores similarly improved VAS showing that both techniques are treatment successes. As expected, the only noted downside was impaired mucociliary transport function with the conventional turbinectomy.[236,237]

In 2012, Garzaro et al. compared radiofrequency turbinate reduction ($n = 26$) with partial turbinectomy ($n = 22$) finding that while both techniques improved breathing, radiofrequency turbinoplasty preserved nasal physiology more efficiently, as anticipated, than partial turbinectomy and was deemed the superior method of choice for reducing inferior turbinate enlargement (hypertrophy).[238]

Interestingly, in another study using the Nasal Obstruction Symptom Evaluation scale, developed by the American Academy of Otolaryngology Head and Neck Surgery, as a validated way for comparing different treatments of patients with nasal airway obstruction. Although the patient follow-up was merely 6 months, both patient groups had septal deviations and inferior turbinate hypertrophy and those treated by radiofrequency turbinoplasty alone had similar results with those who were treated by a combined radiofrequency turbinoplasty and septoplasty. Of course, the explicit surgical details and the passage of adequate time, measured in years, are required before uttering any definitive statements with any legitimacy.[239]

2.2.2.4 Coblation

Coblation ("controlled ablation" meaning tissue reduction in a precise "controlled" manner or "cold ablation" meaning tissue reduction by a lower or "colder" temperature) is radiofrequency energy supplied in a saline or lactated Ringer's solution that energizes the sodium and chloride ions producing a plasma field which decreases the thermal tissue trauma, thereby reducing postoperative pain, accelerating recovery.[214] By vaporizing and destroying the submucosal neurovascular erectile tissues, the turbinate volume is reduced by the contracting fibrosis of the healing process, which is maintainable well into the future. Passali et al. accomplished coblation turbinoplasty in ($n = 40$) patients collecting preoperative data repeated at one and three years postoperatively. Using a VAS for *subjective data* and active anterior rhinomanometry and acoustic rhinometry for *objective data*, they noted that both coblation and radiofrequency provided an improvement in nasal airflow. Complications were reduced to just trivial bleeding and minor crusting. Notably, together coblation and radiofrequency were less painful, especially in the immediate postoperative period compared to other procedures; however, while both methods reduced nasal airway obstruction, improving breathing, the ***effectiveness decreased*** through time, over their three-year study interval.[240]

The outcome of both radiofrequency and coblation was better than conventional turbinoplasty with fewer and less severe complications than conventional turbinectomy.[214] The short-term excellent coblation effects seen at 3 months by Farmer et al. were objectively and subjectively recorded by rhinomanometry and by a VAS score.[241] In a longer study of 32 months, Leong et al. studied the effect of coblation in a limited population, starting with 18 patients reduced to 13 patients using objective posterior rhinomanometry and subjective VAS. The nasal breathing was statistically significantly improved objectively ($p = .033$), but the subjective calculations did not attain statistical significance.[242]

Most recently, in 2020, Singh et al.[243] compared coblation-assisted turbinoplasty (CAT) with microdebrider-assisted turbinoplasty (MAT) in a prospective comparative trial. Patients ($n = 33$) were randomized for coblation CAT ($n = 16$) and microdebrider treatment MAT ($n = 17$). Evaluation was by a VAS for nasal obstruction, sneezing, rhinorrhea, headache, and hyposmia. Turbinate size, edema, and secretions were assessed by endoscopic examination. The assessments were done preoperatively, at the first postoperative week, second and third postoperative months. Their recorded postoperative sequalae included pain, bleeding, crusting, and synechiae. The authors concluded that both procedures were able to improve symptoms equally by effectively eliminating the enlarged submucosal neurovascular erectile soft tissues jointly with the conchal bone exclusive of complications.[243]

2.2.2.5 Ultrasound

Ultrasound technology, with its destructive capability, was somewhat new to the rhinology community in 2010. So, it was most intriguing and very refreshing to read the paper by Gindros et al. who gifted the profession with a prospective RCT using ultrasound for inferior turbinate treatment.[27] They presented ($n = 60$) patients diagnosed with nonallergic chronic hypertrophic rhinitis; separated into two groups:

Group 1: 30 patients, using *ultrasound* treatment on the *left* side and monopolar *electrocautery* on the *right*.

Group 2: 30 patients, using *radiofrequency coblation* treatment on the *left* side and *ultrasound* on the *right.*

Subjective evaluation for nasal breathing and pain was attained using a VAS. Objective evaluation was achieved by both active anterior rhinomanometry and acoustic rhinometry. Data collected before treatment and 1, 3, and 6 months post-treatment documented both subjective and objective improvement in all cases. The best results were obtained with the ultrasound procedure, secondly with the radiofrequency technique. They decided, after data assessment, that the ultrasound treatment was safe, secure, and superior to both the radiofrequency and electrocautery group as the electrocautery group demonstrated the smallest improvement.[27]

2.2.2.6 Electrocautery

As is well known, when electrocautery is performed submucosally, blindly into the inferior turbinate, the amount of tissue destruction is impossible to estimate and there is considerable risk of soft tissue and conchal bone thermal damage that may ultimately result in a secondary osteomyelitis. Doubtless, it is not difficult to grasp that adverse and significant thermal trauma may result from a "prolonged" or "elevated" voltage applied to the surrounding submucosal neurovascular erectile stromal tissues and to the conchal bone of the inferior turbinate. Remember that the electrocautery temperatures reach a range of 400°C (752°F) to 600°C (1112°F). As a consequence of imprecision and the chance of significant thermal damage, **we do not recommend** using electrocautery for a submucosal approach for treating turbinate enlargement.

2.2.3 Complimentary out-fracture (lateralization) techniques

1. Solitary-isolated and sole intervention: out-fracture (lateralization)
2. Combined with other procedures

Out-fracture (lateralization) of the inferior turbinate may be performed as a solitary-isolated and sole intervention or alongside all the other turbinate reduction techniques, except of course when the turbinate is appallingly and dreadfully deleted, expunged, as in the case of total turbinectomy.

Out-fracture (lateralization) involves lateral displacement of the inferior turbinate usually first by an initial in-fracture, moving it medially toward the midline septum from its normal connection to the lateral wall of the nose. The mechanical anatomical concept for this procedure is creating added space when the inferior turbinate is lateralized away from the midline which permits opening (enlarging) the region of the head of the inferior turbinate, which is the posterior portion of the internal nasal valve area.[5] Many surgeons believe that inferior turbinate's out-fracture (lateralization) efficacy is variable, causing criticism over its long-term utility as there is a propensity for the inferior turbinate to return to its original position after out-fracture (laterization), so some surgeons do not recommended it as a single procedure, but it may be used to supplement the other techniques.[211,214,216]

2.2.3.1 Solitary-isolated and sole intervention: out-fracture (laterization)

According to Hol and Huizing,[25] Killian introduced out-fracture (laterization-lateropexia-conchopexy) because of the adverse effects of total inferior turbinectomy and Kressner, in 1930, introduced crushing of the inferior turbinate with specific forceps followed by trimming and his method has since been recycled and reused by several surgeons including usual use at their own institution in The Netherlands.[2] For the record, as has been pointed out previously by Farmer and Eccles[142] although the inferior turbinate thickening results from submucosal vascular congestion, interstitial tissue edema, and at times conchal bony thickening or even undisputable genuine microscopic cellular hyperplasia, but most often there is no proof of cellular hypertrophy despite the common use of the term "turbinate hypertrophy."[142] They suggest that the term "turbinate hypertrophy" is imprecise and should be changed to "turbinate enlargement." Naturally, the primary pathology producing the inferior turbinate enlargement needs accurate diagnosis for appropriate management.

Hol and Huizing also pointed out that out-fracture (laterization) is relatively risk-free, preserves function, is technically simple although they thought that it tends to resume its original position concluding that out-fracture (laterization) may best serve as complementary when combined with other procedures[25,86]

Moss et al.[244] from Division of OtolaryngologyHead and Neck Surgery University of California, San Diego San Diego, California, performed a systematic literature review in 2015 writing in Viewpoints in *Plastic and Reconstructive Surgery* thought the superbly designed studies for inferior turbinate out-fracture (laterization) came from the authors, Aksoy et al. in 2010,[245] Marquez et al. in 1996,[246] and Passàli el al. 2003.[211,216] It was Aksoy et al. who studied out-fracture (laterization) alone in a prospective study ($n = 40$), 80 turbinates which showed convincing evidence that out-fracture was *durable* at 1 and 6 months postseptal and turbinate surgery with CT evidence of fixed bony change. According to Moss et al., in another prospective study ($n = 21$), the out-fractures were *durable* supported by statistically significant rhinometric data presented by Marquez et al.[246] Buyuklu et al., including one of our former visiting surgeons to Mayo Clinic, Dr. Ozcan Cakmak from the Departments of Otorhinolaryngology and Radiology, Baskent University Faculty of Medicine, Ankara, Turkey, studied CT scans of out-fractures (laterization) as a solitary-isolated turbinate intervention in septal surgical patients ($n = 10$), 20 turbinates. Based on their persuasively documented CT scans, they concluded, as did Moss et al., that out-fracture (laterization) can be effortlessly performed, effective in improving the nasal airway, and what's more, it's a *reliably durable* procedure for inferior turbinate surgery.[247]

2.2.3.2 Combined with other procedures

It was Passali et al. in 1999 and 2003, respectively, ($n = 382$) who confirmed (at four and six **years** follow-up) that turbinoplasty accompanied **with** an out-fracture (laterization) is an effective approach to inferior turbinate enlargement ("hypertrophy") when compared to electrocautery, cryotherapy, laser cautery, turbinectomy, and sub-mucosal resection ***without*** an out-fracture (lateral displacement).[211,216]

In their most compelling randomly assigned prospective study, Passali et al. used subjective and objective measures (acoustic rhinometry, anterior rhinomanometry, mucociliary transport time, and secretory immunoglobulin A levels) to confirm the superiority of turbinoplasty ***with*** an out-fracture (lateralization) over all other methods studied.[11,216]

English authors found that by adding the uniquely *multiple submucosal* out-fractures (lateralization) of the inferior turbinates to turbinoplasty, results were improved, although not statistically significant the trend was "improvement," arguing that the additional steps appeared to improve the outcomes without additional risk of complications.[248]

On the other hand, other English authors added to the dilemma by their anterior rhinomanometry findings, ($n = 28$), that out-fracture (lateralization) with amputation of the posterior ends (tips) of the inferior turbinates failed to demonstrate any improvement in the nasal airway.[249] Though just over half the patients had an objective improvement in nasal airflow, only half of this group reported a subjective improvement in their symptoms.

The Chinese added to the out-fracture (lateralization) discussion with a paper in 2013 in which the inferior turbinate "hypertrophy" was documented by both endos-copy and CT scan in a total of ($n = 50$) patients.[250] Supporting the out-fracture (lateralization) debate with statistical data assessments (t-test and correlation tests) of the subjective VAS and the objective studies (acoustic rhinometry and rhinoman-ometry), these authors concluded that out-fracture (lateralization) was an "*ideal sur-gical method*" to improve nasal airway function secondary to an expanded nasal cavity.

A few years later, in 2016, Sinno and colleagues presented conflicting data chal-lenging the notion that out-fracture (lateralization) was an "ideal surgical method."[251] Publishing in *Plastic and Reconstructive Surgery*, they performed a sys-tematic review of 58 surgical papers involving surgical treatments for inferior turbi-nate "hypertrophy" covering total turbinectomy, partial turbinectomy, submucosal resection, "turbinoplasty," laser surgery, cryotherapy, electrocautery, radiofrequency ablation, and turbinate out-fracture (lateralization).[251] After their careful systematic review of operative results and complications, they concluded that submucous resec-tion (turbinoplasty) with radiofrequency ablation was the superior method of treat-ing turbinate "hypertrophy" and that out-fracture (lateralization) should only be used in combination with tissue-reduction procedures ... They also noted that:

> "...turbinectomy (partial/total) and submucosal resection showed crusting and epistaxis at comparatively higher rates, whereas more conservative treatments such as cryotherapy and submucous diathermy failed to provide long-term results."[251]

A year later, in a very shrewd retrospective study in transnasal transsphenoidal brain tumor patients ($n = 55$), Lee and colleagues questioned whether out-fracture (lateralization) was permanent or not.[252] They were especially interested in these practices since inferior turbinate out-fracture (lateralization) was practiced alone or in concert with other procedures in rhinoplasty patents. Using coronal CT images scans for conchal bone objective measurements, they answered their question, yes, *"inferior turbinate out-fracture is preserved for at least 6 months."*

In addition, they noted that subsequent to out-fracture (lateralization), the thickness of the medial mucosa increased, which supports the idea that turbinoplasty plus out-fracture (laterization) is perhaps the treatment of choice for inferior turbinate enlargement ("hypertrophy"). This is yet another study supporting the idea that inferior turbinate out-fracture (lateralization) is possible to be maintained (durable) contrary to finding of other surgeons. Obviously, the exact and specific details of any out-fracture (lateralization) technique make a meaningful difference and probably answers the question of discrepancy.

For a comprehensive coverage of the turbinate subject, Hol and Huizing[25] also presented the out-fracture (lateralization) *"discarded"* techniques of Fateen and Legler using the terms lateropexia (or conchopexy). Conchopexy is the procedure where the inferior turbinate is displaced (out-fractured) into the maxillary sinus through a large inferior meatal antrostomy. This technique was generally unpopular; therefore, eventually abandoned.

Additionally, Golding-Wood's vidian neurectomy of the 1980s was also *"discarded"* since it only controlled the nasal secretions but did not alter the nasal airway obstruction (breathing difficulty).[25]

The work of Salam and Wengraf[114] was fascinating as ($n = 25$) patients were randomly chosen as to which side would receive a total inferior turbinectomy, while the other side received a conchoantropexy. At 6 months after surgery, as expected, there was no statistically significant differences in relief of nasal airway obstruction between the two sides. However, 16% of the patients experienced ***dryness and crusting on the side of the total turbinectomy*($p < .05$)**, which was statistically significant; yet separately and strikingly, there was a higher incidence of postoperative pain ($p < .05$) on the total inferior turbinectomy side, whereas these findings ***did not occur on the conchoantropexy side*** since the turbinate mucosa was preserved intact on that side.[252]

Out-fracture (lateralization) is fundamentally free of peril; however, some questions did arise regarding the effect of out-fracture (lateralization) on the ostiomeatal unit complex and a possible "silent sinus syndrome." These intriguing questions were answered by Lee and colleagues who demonstrated in a number ($n = 23$) of patients that out-fracture *does not* adversely affect the ostiomeatal unit complex in anyway.[253] In 2011, Jung and Gray presented a case of a *unilateral silent sinus syndrome* in a 41-year-old man attributed to a prior (6 months previously) bilateral out-fracture (lateralization) procedure concomitant to a septorhinoplasty.[254] Fracture of the orbital floor is the usual cause of silent sinus syndrome, which is characterized by enophthalmos and hypoglobus secondary to a prolapse of the orbital contents into the maxillary sinus.

Another interesting question was answered by measuring the nasolacrimal transit time after inferior turbinate out-fracture (lateralization) and radiofrequency ablation. Twenty patients with septal surgery and unilateral out-fracture (lateralization) had *nasolacrimal* transit times measured by the saccharine test, which was totally normal at 2 months postsurgery in all 20 patients.[255]

We close this section citing studies celebrated above, Passali et al.,[11,216] Moss et al.,[244] Aksoy et al.,[245] Marquez et al.,[246] Buyuklu et al.,[247] Zhang et al.,[250] and Lee et al.[252] that inferior turbinate out-fracture (lateralization) *is possible to be maintained (durable)* for a prolonged period of time and may be safely combined with other turbinoplasty procedures on the inferior turbinate.

One of us (EBK) has performed *multiple closed comminuted fractures* of the inferior turbinate (conchal bone) on multiple occasions over many years that has been sustained (durable) over a prolonged period of time, measured in years (anecdotal).

It is technically possible to create *multiple closed comminuted fractures,* especially when the out-fracturing (lateralization) begins in close proximity to the origin of the inferior turbinate, at the lateral maxillary wall. In this instance of *multiple comminuted fractures* of the inferior turbinate (conchal bone), internal nasal dressings ("packs" of various lengths of ½ inch gauze soaked in antibiotic and steroid solution) are introduced after intranasal septal stents are sewn in place. Both "packs" and stents are removed after approximately 7 days. This practice supports the findings of Passali et al.,[216] Moss et al.,[244] Aksoy et al.,[245] Marquez et al.,[246] Buyuklu et al.,[247] Zhang et al.,[250] and Lee et al.[252] that an inferior turbinate out-fracture (lateralization) *is possible to be maintained (durable)* for a prolonged period of time.

In order to accurately assess and evaluate any specific surgical technique, the exact and defined details of any operative procedure, specifically the out-fracture (lateralization) technique, must be clearly presented in an unambiguous and explicit meaningful manner, so it can be precisely visualized and duplicated, then for bias reduction and efficacy, a well-designed and well-performed RCT is vital and authoritative.

2.2.4 Histopathology

Lately, in 2016, an elegant and sophisticated ultrastructural histopathologic study was presented by the Italian academic investigators Neri et al.[256] They examined the ultrastructural features (scanning electron microscope for cell surfaces and transmission electron microscope for intracellular and extracellular spaces) of the nasal mucosa after Microdebrider-Assisted Turbinoplasty (**MAT**) in seven patients with two normal controls.[256] The tissues were obtained preoperatively then at 4 months and again at four years after surgery and processed for transmission electron microscopy.[256] At 4 months, the nasal mucosa appeared normal with normal pseudostratified ciliated columnar respiratory epithelium with normal cellular morphology. The submucosa was also normal as the interstitial edema disappeared. At four years, tissue was again acquired, observed, and confirmed that the normal cellular architecture was restored. Neri and colleagues specified that after "cold knife" excision mucosal basal cells can proliferate and repair the injury. They noted:

> "…that p63 gene plays a central role in the epithelial stem cell self-renewal although critical information on the properties of nasal epithelial stem cells is lacking."[256]

These authors explicitly reminded us that the nasal mucosa is physiologically involved with two equally important and distinct functions: the defensive immune response function and the breathing (respiratory) function of providing airway resistance (**'resistor function'**—**the internal nasal valve area** for breathing, lung expansion, and enhancing venous return) and of air conditioning (**'diffusor function'**—**turbulent air flow**) of charging the inspired air with warmth and humidification by the mucus from the seromucous glands and goblet cells.[256] Furthermore, the nasal mucosal cells have the defensive power to fuel IgE production and liberate immunoglobulins IgA and IgG, leukotrienes, histamine, prostaglandins along with interleukin (Il) cytokines including the all-important Il-4, Il-5, Il-8, and Il-13.

The nasal epithelium (pseudostratified ciliated columnar respiratory epithelium) is the physical barricade against pathologic organisms and particulate matter gaining entrance to the lower airway. The submucosa (lamina propria, stroma) also has a meaningful functional contribution through the venous sinusoid vascular system and a vibrant cellular defensive system including the dendritic cells which present foreign proteins to T and B lymphocytes to initiate immune responses. Other specific defensive cells include eosinophils, mast cells, basophils, plasma cells, and the antimicrobial proteins all proceeding and presiding in the submucosal vascular system.[15–17,256]

Because the nasal mucosa (epithelium and submucosa) has a multitude of significant functional commitments, many surgeons side with those of us who campaign for the preservation of the nasal mucosa, as much as possible, during any type of inferior turbinate surgery saving nasal functioning tissue avoiding the possible unfavorable unsavory sequalae, from a radical turbinate terminator, resulting in the ENS.[256] So, they strongly favor cold knife reduction of an enlarged "hypertrophic" inferior turbinate avoiding any thermal injury to the epithelium and the submucosa since:

> "Thermal techniques cause coagulation of venous sinuses resulting in fibrosis and scarring of the submucosal tissue. Gindros et al. found loss of cilia after submucous diathermy. Ultrastructural changes after radiofrequency include squamous metaplastic epithelium with basal cells and lack of ciliated, brush cells and columnar cells, fibrosis of the lamina propria, intense inflammatory infiltration, and reduction of seromucous glands. It was demonstrated also that thermal techniques cause nerve fibers devitalization resulting in reduced sensation of nasal airflow."[256]

The paper of Gindros et al.[257] cited by Neri et al.[256] is significant since they also examined all specimens by electron microscopy comparing monopolar diathermy, radiofrequency coblation, and ultrasound in 60 patients, divided into two groups of 30 with a diagnosis of airway obstruction secondary to chronic nonallergic inferior turbinate "hypertrophy." Gindros et al. studied these tissues before and at 1, 3, and 6 months after treatment. In the pretreatment study of "hypertrophic" tissue, they observed a global degeneration of epithelial cells, ciliary loss, disrupted and disordered intercellular connections, edema, nasal mucus overproduction, and inflammatory cell infiltration. After intervention with monopolar diathermy and radiofrequency coblation, the histopathologic findings included a reduction of both intercellular edema and reduced mucus production with a degenerated disorientated epithelium, yet an exuberant assembly of collagen, by another name, vigorous submucosal fibrosis. On the other hand, after ultrasound treatment in some patients, they observed islets of normally organized ciliated columnar cells appearing in the epithelium. They concluded that in several cases treated with ultrasound, epithelial regeneration occurred:

> *"... resulting to anatomical and functional restoration of the nasal physiology"*[257]

In an earlier histopathologic paper, Berger and colleagues noticed that when the inferior turbinate mucosa is hypertrophied, histological examination reveals a generalized increase of the submucosal width (of the lamina propria, stroma) with venous sinusoid vascular engorgement, with the associated gross external thickening of the mucosa overlying the medial portion of the turbinate accounting for the gross increased turbinate size.[258] The submucosal glandular elements and vessels in the surrounding connective tissue in the submucosa (lamina propria, stroma) basically remain unchanged. It is imperative that after turbinate treatment, the mucociliary transport blanket be preserved by protecting the mucosal surface epithelium, the pseudostratified ciliated columnar respiratory epithelium, so normal ciliary clearances are maintained. In another histopathologic study, Berger et al. looked at two groups or patients specifically examining the epithelium and the submucosal tissues:[259]

Group 1: Coblation treatment $n = 16$ (22 samples)
Group 2: Control inferior turbinectomy treatment $n = 14$ (18 samples)

After coblation, qualitative analysis displayed marked fibrosis with the depletion of submucosal glands and venous sinusoids in the lamina propria. The coblation group exhibited an increased connective tissue and a significantly ($p < .001$) decreased fraction of both the submucosal glands and venous sinusoids. A significantly decreased proportion of intact epithelium and a significantly increased relative proportion of partial epithelial shedding ($p = .03$ and $p = .04$, respectively). The long-term histological effects of coblation of the inferior turbinate resulted in partial epithelial shedding, probably due to the thermal submucosal vascular damage of the lamina propria stroma, with significant fibrosis generating glandular and venous sinusoid depletion.[259]

With our physiological thinking, any practitioner pursuing inferior turbinate reduction has the duty, responsibility, and obligation to preserve the pseudostratified epithelial mucociliary transport system, minimize damage to the submucosal (lamina propria, stroma) neurovascular morphologic structures avoiding adverse physiologic consequences and the resultant sequalae all the while improving the nasal airway breathing function.

Consequently, "cold knife" techniques appear to have the edge for now, avoiding thermal trauma as submucosal vascular choking fibrosis also deprives the overlying epithelium with the necessary nutrition to maintain a healthy mucociliary transport system, and the secretory deprivation robs the requisite moisture needed to charge the inspired air with heat and moisture allowing optimal exchange of oxygen and carbon dioxide at the alveolar level.

All studies need the great equalizer, the final arbitrator, "Father Time," to "weigh in" before making a "final" adjudication regarding our interventions. Duration after treatment matters before a "final" therapeutic result can be determined and "final" promulgation for therapeutic recommendation. With duration in mind, the 2016 work of Pelen and associates while laudable and praiseworthy comparing the "cold knife" microdebrider reduction with radiofrequency ablation concluded that both techniques were minimally invasive and could reliably provide an improved nasal airway subjectively and objectively assessed as statistically significant without any disruption of nasal physiology.[260] The only issue of concern and disquiet was one of duration. Their posttreatment follow-up was, in their own words:

> *"Nasal obstruction, the grade of turbinate hypertrophy, and other symptoms were evaluated with subjective nasal obstruction scale and anterior rhinoscopy **before the operation, and 3 days, 7 days, 4 weeks, and 8 weeks after the surgical intervention**."*[260] *(Bold italics added)*

Certainly, projecting the long-term effects of a given procedure based on after 8 weeks of treatment results is a startling speculative leap of faith, for "who knows" where that leap will land you?

How do you find the "Best Reduction Method" for inferior turbinate enlargement ("hypertrophy") reduction?

1. A Context with discussion of some specific critical confounding questions

As we all know too well, when medical therapy fails to reduce an enlarged inferior turbinate, a "surgical" reduction is advocated.

Is there clear agreement, any unanimity of unswerving direction, a signposting as to the "best method" the "gold standard," that one shining technique from the literature, for inferior turbinate reduction? The answer to the that question is a resounding "possible perhaps."

And that's because of all the five superior level 1 papers reviewed by Larrabee and Kacker[264] they thought that the findings of the randomized trial ($n = 382$) of Passali et al.[211,216]

> *"…was the most effective at decreasing nasal obstruction caused by inferior turbinate hypertrophy."[264]*

Therefore, to strictly and decisively answer the question of what is the "best method," a well-designed and well-performed randomized controlled trial (RCT) is needed to *confirm or contradict* the randomized trial of Passali et al.[211,216]

So, in the meantime, what's a rhinologist to do?

In 2001, as previously cited, the doctors from the United Kingdom, Clement and White did not find any RCTs in their MEDLINE literature review of 35 years of inferior and middle turbinate surgery, declaring that properly conducted RCTs were essential to establish long-term benefits from turbinate treatment.[199] After the challenge issued by Clement and White in this new era of evidence-based medicine (EBM) for "properly" conducted RCTs, Batra et al. in 2009 did an evidence-based review focusing on the inferior turbinate in adults finding only one level 1 and two level 2 reports in their PubMed database search assessing 143 abstracts and included 96 articles in their report.[210] They thought that, in the future, all studies should include control groups and must be prospective in design. In discussing EBM's emphasis on levels of evidence, they designated the hierarchy of levels of evidence (level 1 the highest) from the literature as:

Level 1: RCTs
Level 2: prospective cohort study or low-quality randomized trials
Level 3: retrospective case-control studies
Level 4: case series or retrospective chart review
Level 5: case reports or expert opinion

They reviewed 143 international studies including turbinectomy, lasers, thermal techniques, and turbinoplasty. They commented that although level 1 evidence from RCTs is the highest level of evidence, that an RCT may not be necessary since all inferior turbinate interventions gave an overwhelming initial positive response for airway reduction, improved breathing, citing the parachute paper of Smith and Pell demanding common sense when considering risk and benefits from various procedures and that an RCT may not be required for every study to be valid when the result is obvious, an RCT is **not** required to realize that parachutes are effective in reducing injury following jumping from airplanes.[261]

A year later, Leong and Eccles clearly recognized, for the moment, that no clear directive for patient selection for inferior turbinate surgery existed because inferior turbinate treatment was still evolving and definitive evidence regarding the "best" treatment technique remained unresolved; therefore, prospective studies, RCTs, with validated objective and subjective outcome measures appropriately controlled were mandatory to answer the question, what is the best method for reducing an inferior turbinate to improve nasal airway breathing?[262]

Over the next decade, some astute authors repeatedly reviewed the literature in the leading ear, nose and throat (ENT) journals evaluating the level of evidence of RCTs and concluded that essentially the quantity and quality of all the RCTs in the ENT literature could be improved.[205,207,263]

1.1 Randomized controlled trials searching for the "Best Reduction Method" from the literature

In 2014, Larrabee and Kacker from the Department of Otolaryngology New York-Presbyterian/Weill Cornell Medical College, New York asked the question: Which inferior turbinate reduction technique best decreases nasal airway obstruction?[264]

They reviewed and presented the results of five superior papers they thought had the most convincing level 1 data for effective reduction of nasal airway obstruction secondary to enlargement ("hypertrophy") of the inferior turbinate. All their level 1 presented papers are listed below falling into the category of "possible perhaps" as to a "Best Reduction Method" for inferior turbinate enlargement ("hypertrophy"):

1. Passali F, Passali G, Damiani V, Bellussi L. Treatment of inferior turbinate hypertrophy: a randomized clinical trial. *Ann Otol Rhinol Laryngol*. 2003;112: 683−688.[211]
2. Nease C, Krempl G. Radiofrequency treatment of turbinate hypertrophy: a randomized, blinded, placebo-controlled clinical trial. *Otolaryngol Head Neck Surg*. 2004;130:291−299.[26]
3. Liu CM, Tan CD, Lee FP, Lin KN, Huang HM. Microdebrider-assisted versus radiofrequency assisted-inferior turbinoplasty. *Laryngoscope*. 2009;119: 414−418. https://doi.org/10.1002/lary.20088.[235]
4. Cingi C, Ure B, Cakli E, Ozudogru E. Microdebrider-assisted versus radiofrequency-assisted inferior turbinoplasty: a prospective study with objective and subjective outcome measures. *Acta Otorhinolaryngol Ital*. 2010;30: 138−143.[230]
5. Gindros G, Kantas I, Balatsouras D, Kaidoglou A, Kandiloros D. Comparison of ultrasound turbinate reduction, radiofrequency tissue ablation and submucosal cauterization in inferior turbinate hypertrophy. *Eur Arch Otorhinolaryngol*. 2010;267:1727−1733.[27]

After reviewing those level 1 papers, Larrabee and Kacker concluded with the best practice:

> *"Of conventional inferior turbinate reduction techniques,* **submucosal resection combined with lateral displacement is the most effective at decreasing nasal obstruction caused by inferior turbinate hypertrophy.** *In the turbinoplasty group, based on the current evidence, microdebrider-assisted and ultrasound turbinate reduction have been shown to be the most effective. A prospective randomized trial comparing the microdebrider-assisted and ultrasound turbinate reduction has not yet been performed. Little research exists on the ultrasound procedure; thus, the microdebrider-assisted turbinate reduction technique has the advantage of more widespread familiarity."[264]* (Bold italics added)

Since Larrabee and Kacker challenged the profession to perform a RCT comparing ultrasound turbinate reduction with microdebrider-assisted turbinoplasty, we searched the literature for that study to no avail. To our knowledge, such a study has yet to be published, last searched for on the first of March 2023.

1.2 Future studies—designing the "Best Study" for finding the "Best Reduction Method"

The constructive challenge commanded by numerous authors asserted that all future turbinate studies should be randomized with control groups, RCTs, which must be prospective in design following the philosophic principles of EBM.[199,205,207,210,262,263,265]

So, what are the essential elements necessary to design the "Best Study" for determining the "Best Method" for inferior turbinate reduction?

Taking the lead from Hol and Huizing,[25] Batra et al.,[210] Leong and Eccles,[262] Agha et al.,[266] and Peters et al.,[215] we added some thoughts to their suggestions concerning creating the criteria for an "ideal" or a "Best Study," which includes the following for clarity, consistency, and transparency in crafting an RCT that will definitively answer the question as to the "best method" for inferior turbinate reduction.

1.3 Thoughts for designing a "Best Study" for finding the "Best Reduction Method" for treating patients with inferior turbinate enlargement ("hypertrophy")

1. Funding source(s)—transparency with a conflict of interest (COI) statement
2. Ethical considerations—institutional review board approval (when appropriate) and compliance with principles included in the Belmont Report,* NIH guidelines,* AMA's Code of Medical Ethics guidelines, and the World Medical Association-Declaration of Helsinki Ethical Principles for Medical Research Involving Human Subjects
3. Informed written consent
4. Prospective study with clearly written and available "approved" protocol
5. Careful selection of primary and secondary endpoints to determine efficacy
6. Clear and easy to use case report form(s)
7. Protocol deviations (notated if and when they occur)
8. Randomly assigned treatment groups
9. Baseline demographics and clinical characteristics of each group
10. Blinding when feasible (***note: blinding is possible in surgical and procedural studies when the operator remains "silent" as to his/her specific involvement with subjective and objective outcome studies performed by blinded evaluators-coded study***)
11. Matched control group—medical therapy group (blinding) and surgical and/or procedural group(s)
12. Eligibility: inclusion and exclusion criteria
13. Adequate sample size—prestudy power analysis
14. Statistical analysis with statistician involved—P values and confidence intervals
15. Drop-out rate and cause(s)
16. Adverse events—data details and specifically mentioning if adverse events did not occur
17. Histology—light and electron microscopy (scanning and transmission electron microscope)
    Coded samples—blinding pathologist to study purpose
18. Follow-up period minimum one year extending to 10 years with retrospective study evaluation at a later date

19. Pretreatment and posttreatment evaluation of:
   (a) Endoscopic classification of turbinate enlargement ("hypertrophy")
   (b) Validated scores: Coded samples or study-blinding technician as to study methods and purpose
      1. Subjective visual analog score (VAS)
      2. Subjective Snot-25 score or NOSE scale
      3. Objective measurement of nasal airway pressure/flow change—rhinomanometry-coded study
      4. Objective measurement of nasal airway dimensions—acoustic rhinometry-coded study
   (c) Mucociliary transport times measurement-coded study
   (d) Secretory IgA measurements-coded study
   (e). Olfaction evaluation (subjective and objective)-coded study
20. Interpretation of results with primary and secondary outcomes within context of "current" evidence
21. Study weaknesses freely and clearly presented
22. Blinding of all third-party evaluators-coded

   *Ethical principles in research with human participants:
   1. Belmont report (1979) entitled: Ethical Principles and Guidelines for the Protection of Human Subjects of Research. The National Commission for the Protection of Human Subjects of Biomedical and Behavioral Research.
   2. The National Institute of Health (NIH) Clinical Center researchers published seven main principles to guide the conduct of ethical research:
   Social and clinical value.
   Scientific validity.
   Fair subject selection.
   Favorable risk—benefit ratio.
   Independent review.
   Informed consent.
   Respect for potential and enrolled subjects.

1.4 When are randomized controlled trials NOT needed?

With the rigor of the "Best Study" design for finding the "Best Method for treating, we, the authors of this book, totally support: How to design the "Best Study" for finding the "Best Method" for treating patients with enlarged inferior turbinates? Allowing physicians to make intelligent treatment decisions based on the best data of the day has been the history of medicine "evidence first" is the way to progress.

Although "evidence first" is the way to progress and EBM is the sacred "holy grail" of modern medicine with the RCT the epitome of study design, there are many clinical situations where *common sense* reigns and RCTs are *not required* as pointed out by Smith and Pell[261] and Paul Glasziou with coauthors[267] who noted some stark examples in medicine where **RCTs were not needed** calling them "historical examples of treatments with dramatic effects" with a "Top 10" list listed below alphabetically:

1. Blood transfusion for severe hemorrhagic shock
2. Closed reduction and splinting for fracture of displaced long bones
3. Defibrillation for ventricular fibrillation
4. Drainage for pain associated with abscesses
5. Ether for anesthesia
6. Insulin for diabetes
7. Neostigmine for myasthenia gravis
8. One-way valve or underwater seal drainage for pneumothorax and hemothorax
9. Suturing for arresting hemorrhage
10. Tracheostomy for tracheal obstruction

These are our "Top 10" examples of such dramatic effects, as Glasziou et al. reasoned, that biases can be unambiguously ruled out *without the need* for RCTs. They defined the dramatic effects by "the size of the treatment effect (signal) relative to the expected prognosis (noise)."[267]

Nonetheless, we think that for a definitive answer to the question, what is the best method for treating inferior turbinate enlargement ("hypertrophy")? a well-designed and well-performed RCT is needed to confirm or contradict the randomized trial ($n = 382$) of Passali et al.[211,216]

1.5 Asking answerable questions: empiricism versus rationalism

Practicing intelligent EBM, according to Kenny et al.[268] revolves around asking answerable clinical questions; the soul of EBM by:

(a) Framing a specific and clear-cut clinical question
(b) Searching for the best evidence in the literature
(c) Critically evaluating the evidence
(d) Integrating the evidence with clinician's clinical capability coupled with the unique features of the patient and their situation, expectations, and rights
(e) Evaluation of the clinician's performance

The now former chief editor of the *Mayo Clinic Proceedings* Bill Lanier, MD and his colleague S. Vincent Rajkumar discussed the medical applications of the two major competing philosophies of *empiricism* and *rationalism*.[269] *Empiricism* is based on observational experimentation, research evidence in the Western tradition of Francis Bacon, John Locke, David Hume, and others, while *rationalism* is that method of gaining knowledge through intellectual reasoning, in medicine (clinical judgment).

Empiricism is knowledge, from facts, *evidence* from *experimentation*, while rationalism is knowledge, from *intellectual reasoning*, from experience, it's *clinical judgment*.

EBM rationally favors *empiricism,* but what happens when new information reaches the clinician and before deciding what action is demanded and defensible, the clinician needs time for reflection with decision modulated by rational thought. As in the case when clinical decisions require action, but evidence is limited, incomplete, inconclusive, conflicting, or starkly nonexistent. What about inconclusive conflicting poorly performed RCTs? What to do then? Rationalism to the rescue. The reasonable belief approach employs the good "clinical judgment" idea and the aphorism from Canadian physician Kerr Lachlan White, MD (1917−2014) "Good judgment comes from experience; experience comes from bad judgment."[270]

Bad judgment, well-known and lamentable, has occurred in medicine often without maliciousness of forethought. Once conventional and notable treatments promulgated by experts have been overturned, invalidated, and abolished by employing the scientific method, medical progress ensues. In an astounding 2013 article, Vinay Prasad and colleagues from the NIH reviewed over 2000 articles with the intent of determining which medical practices have no benefit for the patients.[271] We quoted from their abstract because of the authority of their findings; provides pause for reflection:

"We reviewed 2044 original articles, 1344 of which concerned a medical practice. Of these, 981 articles (73.0%) examined a new medical practice, whereas 363 (27.0%) tested an established practice. A total of 947 studies (70.5%) had positive findings, whereas 397 (29.5%) reached a negative conclusion. A total of 756 articles addressing a medical practice constituted replacement, 165 were back to the drawing board, 146 were medical reversals, 138 were reaffirmations, and 139 were inconclusive. Of the 363 articles testing standard of care, **146 (40.2%) reversed** that practice, whereas 138 (38.0%) reaffirmed it." And they concluded: "**The reversal of established medical practice is common** and occurs across all classes of medical practice. This investigation sheds light on low-value practices and patterns of medical research." [271](Bold italics added)

With this powerful paper, it is understandable that Prasad favors the rigor of science since so many medical practices have been reversed (40.2%) over the years of their study. EBM and RCTs are the orders of the day, *empiricism* over *rationalism.* Agreed.

Wait, not so fast. What about uncertainty? How do we manage our patients then? Prasad in Letters to the Editor of the *Mayo Clinic Proceeding* conceded but:

"There will always be a place for the thoughtful deliberation of physicians in medicine; however, I continue to believe that given the pressures of the modern marketplace and university promotions, most decisions should be firmly grounded in RCTs powered for hard end points."[272]

In the same issue, Donald G. Ross, MD wrote a response to Prasad in Letters to the Editor; the debate is a foot:

"Medical research cannot be held to the same standard as basic science, but we must remain aware of the (relative) weakness of the evidence we rely on in applying 'evidence-based' principles. There must always be a place for rational decision making based on experience and the situation of the individual patient. Survival curves for 2 different therapies that appear nearly identical to the eye are in fact nearly identical, even if complex statistics show a 'significant' difference between them. I find that this line of reasoning is upsetting to some of my colleagues; they are looking for certainty where there are only probabilities. However, the diagnosis and treatment of the individual patient will always involve making choices with some degree of uncertainty, and one must make one's peace with that."[273]

1.6 Are controlled trials (RCTs) really needed? Can they actually be accomplished in a surgical setting?

What about the role of EBM especially RCTs in the clinical practice of surgery especially when evaluating new procedures? The thoughtful approach addressing these questions was tackled in a comprehensive manner, about 30 years ago, by Professor of Obstetrics and Gynecology Gordon M. Stirrat and his colleagues from the United Kingdom.[274] They understood that all new surgical procedures must, for ethical reasons, be assessed comparing the new to the contemporarily accepted method(s). Not to make the comparison between the new procedure and the currently accepted method was clearly unethical. They noted examples, from the surgical literature, where less scrupulously evaluated procedures were eventually found to be *ineffective*. Gastric freezing for bleeding was eventually found to be harmful. Of course, they recognized that the optimum comparison method was by an RCT, which is ideal for a medication trial because drug trials could be an RCT that is double-blinded and placebo-controlled. However, for evaluating a new surgical technique or for the reevaluation of any surgical technique, there are major issues to consider for ***randomization in surgical practice:***

(a) Factually, a truly placebo operation is the unethical "sham operation," which must ***never*** be performed. Although this position is debated by Franklin G. Miller, PhD on page 149. Surgical trials are rarely ever fully placebo-controlled.

(b) Blinding the surgeon for the procedure can ***never*** be achieved.

(c) In trials comparing new methods with established techniques, the surgeon's experience strongly determines results, inevitably results will be "better" for the standard method and not directly comparable to the new method especially with "learning curve" concerns. Further bias accrues because new surgical techniques are often originated by fervently skilled surgeons, while the standard technique is performed by the balance of the surgeons in that specialty.

Stirrat et al. concluded by accepting the reality that the ideal double-blind placebo-controlled trial cannot easily be applied for surgical comparisons. But the optimal design of RCTs for surgery must be attempted, nonetheless with input from epidemiologists and/or statisticians.[274]

They presented a table listing suggested **absolute** and **relative** criteria for a valid RCT.[274]

(a) Absolute criteria for a valid RCT
   1. Random allocation mandatory
   2. Trial size large enough to avoid erroneously false-positives or false-negative outcomes
   3. The number of patients required in each study arm must be large enough to demonstrate a treatment effect and must be determined in advance of the study starting
   4. No alteration of the protocol is permitted without justification and documentation
   5. Approval of an ethics committee
   6. Informed consent from patients before randomization
   7. Analysis of results on the basis of "intention to treat"

As long as the absolute criteria are met, other questions may be asked.

(b) Relative criteria for a valid RCT
   1. Although not always possible, every effort must be made to create the RCT
   2. The "first patient" should be randomized
   3. For large or controversial trials, an "independent data monitoring committee" can be useful

Dr. Stirrat noted that traditionally, surgical practice was formulated on the fundamental concepts and understanding of anatomy and pathophysiology of disease.[275] In essence, surgery was rational and technical, scientific and artistic, so with the emergence of the new paradigm of EBM and its reliance on RCTs, it was soon recognized that the data from these scientific studies did not possess generalizability. By definition, generalizability is a measure of how useful the results of a study are for a broader group of people or situations.

At the dawn of the innovative movement of EBM with RCTs, about 25 years ago, the critique, by the eminent Sir Nick Black, MD who served as the first Chair of the UK Health Services Research Network at the Department *of* Health Services Research and Policy at the London School of Hygiene and Tropical Medicine, was that the scientific evidence from an RCT was not generalizable. In other words, because the study results data were not widely transferable from the broad study population to a specific unique individual surgical patient, surgeons lost their enthusiasm, excitement, and zeal for the essence of EBM, the RCT.[276] Sir Nick Black thought that:

"although EBM clearly has a place, it does not have all the answers."[276]

Stirrat makes the distinction and reason for the inevitable tension between the "clinical surgeon" dedicated to a unique specific patient in the present, in the here and now, and the "clinical researcher" dedicated to the benefit of some patient somewhere and sometime in foreseeable future.[275] Writing in the *Journal of Medical Ethics*, Dr. Stirrat, in 2002, emphasized that medical intervention and new surgical procedures still require justification by the "best available evidence."[275] Therefore, RCTs are nevertheless needed and quite possible in surgery by well-designed and well-performed RCTs.

1.7 Evidence first, but what to do when RCT data are limited, incomplete, inconclusive, conflicting, or starkly nonexistent?

In the "evidence first" approach argued by Prasad,[272] that despite its acknowledged limitations, the "evidence first" worldview is the patented prescription designed for progress in medicine. Prasad continues the argument by asserting that physicians must *not remain neutral*, that choice is required, its either "evidence first" or "clinical judgment."[272] Sniderman et al. contended that in the hurly-burly of everyday clinical practice, in the atmosphere of uncertainty, when data from an RCT are either not available or limited, incomplete, inconclusive, conflicting, or starkly nonexistent, then "clinical judgment" ("clinical reasoning") is compulsory to save the day.[180] Prasad and Sniderman et al. agree that when comparing the two worldviews, *empiricism* versus *rationalism*, there is no substitute for "clinical judgment" ("clinical reasoning") to "fill in the gaps" while waiting for "the answers" in the current EBM era.[180] Is there a middle ground between *empiricism* versus *rationalism* regarding optimal patient care? Our view of optimal patient care, especially in an atmosphere of uncertainty, centers around a nonpolarized position, a sort of "bicameral" duality approach, we suggest; employ *empiricism* when results of RCT trials are available and use the *rationalism* of "clinical judgment" when trial data of an RCT is just not available or limited, incomplete, inconclusive, conflicting, or starkly nonexistent. In our opinion, *empiricism* and *rationalism* should cohabit in the same physician, with the pendulum swinging "to and fro," depending on the unique clinical condition calling for decisions.

As suggested by Prasad et al.,[271]

> *of the 146 verified and validated medical practices that were reversed (discontinued), no doubt, at first, those practices seemed logical and exquisitely rational when in fact they were ultimately flawed.*

As recently, in 2021, Tim Darsaut, MD a university neurosurgeon in Edmonton, Canada, and Jean Raymond, MD a university interventional neuroradiologist in Montréal, Canada, pointed out, reiterating the ethical medical care credo that care must be empirical, that ethical care is based on reliable, repeatable, established interventions with proven patient outcomes, essentially EBM, yet what to do in an atmosphere of uncertainty, when unproven interventions may either be useless or even harmful.

What is the ethical approach in those cases of comparing validated care and unvalidated care with its atmosphere of uncertainty? Of course, still guided by medical ethics, how to approach a patient or subject of a trial of a promising test or unproven intervention until they are validated as valuable and helpful and not the reverse? In the case of uncertainty, Darsaut and Raymond persuasively argued that medical ethics demands that a clear distinction be made between "research" and "care." That a "separation" between the two to protect patients from "research" studies designed to aid future patients.

Ethically, unvalidated care must be offered in the context of a "care research" trial protocol to optimize the potential benefits while minimizing possible adverse effects.[277] They propose pragmatic "care research" trials integrated into clinical practice to fulfill this need. Practicing good ethical medicine within the context of uncertainty was their main concern; therefore, the distinction was made between validated care and promising unvalidated care offered within the clearly announced pragmatic "care research" design which is proposed to: "act in the best medical interest of the patient." So, they concluded that any new or unvalidated care must be restricted to a "care research" trial and *never* practiced or offered as validated care to the unsuspecting patient.[277]

1.8 What are the influences of "placebo effects" in research and practice outcomes?

What, if any, are the influences of "placebo effects" in research and practice outcomes? In an erudite exploration from *The Lancet,* Finniss and colleagues surveyed the history and practice of placebo effects in medicine.[278] Dating back to the Canterbury Tales in the late 14th century, Chaucer named the flattering courtier character Placebo. Placebo controls, false or fake procedures began in the 16th century designed to discredit exorcisms and then applied to experimentations in medicine when Ben Franklin's commission, in 1784 debunked the "invisible natural force" of animal and vegetable magnetism (mesmerism) after the German doctor Franz Mesmer.[278] Placebo effects became a mainstream medical interest with the widespread acceptance of placebo-controlled RCTs.

Startling to the investigators was the finding that people improved; sometimes dramatically, in placebo-controlled arms of various studies.

Henry Beecher, MD, of Boston, Massachusetts, in 1955, popularized the idea of "placebo effects" claiming that about 35% ($35.2 \pm 2.2\%$) of patients responded positively to placebo treatments.[279] While Beecher boasted with an inflated impression of a "powerful placebo," he failed to distinguish the indisputable placebo response from other confounding factors.[279] Since then, especially in the last 10 years, there is increasing interest in investigating placebo effects by rigorous research methods. Finniss and colleagues are expansive in their thinking and offer compelling evidence of complexity regarding the "placebo effect" as they delved into and dissected the subject noting that evidence has emerged that "placebo effects" can exist in clinical practice, even if no placebo is given. Yes, a "placebo effect" can exist even if none is given. To highlight their thinking, they point to a shift in the emerging mechanistic understanding of "placebo effects" recognizing there is not one "placebo effect" but many. Succinctly, there are two overarching mechanisms: psychological and neurobiological with numerous other mechanisms involved in the "placebo effect."[278] Psychological mechanisms contributing to "placebo effects" include:

> "…expectations, conditioning, learning, memory, motivation, somatic focus, reward, anxiety reduction and meaning."[278]

Multiple studies have shown that *clinicians' beliefs* can also affect "placebo effects."[278] Accordingly, conditioning and expectancy are certainly entangled in the occurrence of "placebo effects" in clinical practice. The most reasonable interpretation of the recent literature is that expectancy is first, conditioning follows and is dependent on the success of the first encounter. That first encounter could be critical for the development of a subsequent robust placebo response.

> "There are also numerous neurobiological mechanisms contributing to 'placebo effects' involving different physiological systems in healthy volunteers and in patients with a host of different clinical conditions"[278]

This especially involves neurochemical mediators in the central nervous system. Research is ongoing.

Blease and colleagues pointed out that recent research has established that "placebo effects" are authentic psychobiological phenomenon attributable to a total therapeutic context, and the "placebo effect" can be influential in both research and clinical situations.[280] The "placebo effect" blinds many physicians to the reality that various treatments perceived as beneficial may in fact be merely a "placebo effect." Various flawed treatments have been retained merely because of a "placebo effect."[280]

> "This was emphasized recently in the study in which patients with irritable bowel syndrome were assigned to receive either an open-label placebo pill or no treatment. A large proportion of patients may perceive benefit from a placebo, and this perception may be influenced by patients' motivation or preconceived expectations of benefit. These scenarios cloud the thinking and judgment of all concerned and lead clinicians to reach faulty 'clinical impressions'. These aforementioned concerns including 'placebo effect' argue for treatment efficacy to be adjudicated primarily by randomized trials. In some situations, we need to recognize that no amount of expertise may substitute for data from randomized trials."[280]

It is fully understood that without evidence from RCTs, there is no choice but to rely on clinical reasoning, yet awareness of a possible flawed conclusion because of a "placebo effects" must *always* be kept in mind.

Understanding the seriousness of the "placebo question" appraisals defining the limits of placebos in both medicine and surgery is needed for authority and utility as both disciplines, medicine and surgery, stress the need for open discussions since as much unadulterated empirical data as possible are obligatory to make wise clinical decisions.

1.9 What are the ethics of using placebos in *medicine*?

The American Medical Association (AMA) has explicit guidelines on clinical use of placebos and supplies an ethical policy: Placebo Use in Clinical Practice (2007) advises:

> *"Physicians may use placebos for diagnosis or treatment only if the patient is informed and agrees to its use. A placebo may still be effective if the patient knows it will be used but cannot identify it and does not know the precise timing of its use. A physician should enlist the patient's cooperation by explaining that a better understanding of the medical condition could be achieved by evaluating the effects of different medications, including the placebo. The physician need neither identify the placebo nor seek specific consent before its administration. In this way, the physician respects the patient's autonomy and fosters a trusting relationship, while the patient may still benefit from the placebo effect."[280]*

1.10 What are the ethics of using placebos in *surgery*?

As specified repeatedly, placebo-controlled trials in both surgery and medicine are each respectively recognized as the "gold standard" way to test the efficacy of a *medical* therapy or a *surgical* procedure. Three recent papers, 2016[281,282] and 2021[283] from the United Kingdom, Germany, and Australia, respectively, tackled the issue of randomized placebo-controlled surgical trials head on. And one paper from an ethicist at the NIH discussing the landscape of "*sham surgery*" *approved* in **research surgical trials** but *forbidden* in **clinical surgical care**.[284]

Writing in the *Journal of Medical Ethics,* Julian Savulescu from the Faculty of Philosophy, Oxford Centre for Practical Ethics, Oxford, United Kingdom, along with doctors Karolina Wartolowska and Andy Carr from the Nuffield Department of Orthopaedics Rheumatology and Musculoskeletal Sciences University of Oxford, Oxford, United Kingdom, recognized that "surgical trial is a divisive issue," yet argued that just as in medicine, placebo controls for surgery are also necessary to reduce bias and control for "placebo effects."[281] They presented their defense, justification, and protocol for *surgical trials* as these trials are needed to acquire accurate unbiased data even more so than medical trials as medications can be suspended, but surgery can lead to *useless* surgery or *irretrievable harm* from a specific surgery. Doubtless, harmful procedures have no place in our ethical practice; therefore, these authors reason that surgical trials are inescapable to discover and avoid harmful surgical procedures. How to conduct such surgical trials has been considered by the AMA with a written position on both medical[280] and surgical trials.[281]

The most important document of ethical conduct in medical research is the Declaration of Helsinki which sanctions placebo-controlled trials in surgery when there is no proven treatment, and the importance of the study objectives offsets the risks for the human subjects. The AMA in their effort to provide guidance for placebo-controlled surgery followed the instruction and conditions of the Declaration of Helsinki highlighting the indispensable informed consent advocating standard nonsurgical treatment as a part of randomized placebo-controlled design. The AMA has adopted these tenants as their policy incorporated into the AMA's Code of Medical Ethics.[281]

From the University of Heidelberg, Germany, Probst et al.[282] performed a systematic review of *Central, MEDLINE, and EMBASE* researching randomized placebo-controlled trials, comparing placebo with a surgical procedure.

> "The ethical justification for the use of a placebo control remained unclear in two trials. Placebo-controlled surgical trials are feasible and provide high-quality data on efficacy of surgical treatments. The surgical placebo entails a considerable risk for study participants. Consequently, a placebo should be used **only** if justified by the clinical question and by methodological necessity. Based on the current evidence, a pragmatic proposal for the use of placebo controls in future randomized controlled surgical trials is made."[282] (Bold italics added)

Nelson and coworkers were interested in raising recruitment rates in placebo-controlled *surgical* trials, specifically in orthopedic arthroscopic surgery.[283] They presented four placebo-controlled surgical trials that demonstrated arthroscopic knee debridement with procedural lavage confirmed no benefit over the "placebo effect," which translated into a clinical guideline recommendation *against* further use of that arthroscopic surgical procedural lavage. Certainly, a big and important score for *surgical* RCTs. Nelson et al. also studied the issue of low recruitment rates in placebo-controlled *surgical* trials acknowledging that patients are often unwilling to accept a surgical procedure knowing the possibility of surgery without benefit. They listed those patient reluctance issues related to patient confusion, hesitancy, and unwillingness to participate because of:

> "Difficulties understanding concepts such as equipoise, placebo effects, randomization, and blinding may also leave many patients confused and unwilling to participate in a placebo-controlled surgical trial."[283]

Equipoise is the term meaning that the assumption is that neither the control nor experimental group is the "better" intervention and that is the reason for the RCT design to answer the question in the first place.

The most important influences for improving study enrollment for a *surgical* RCT are two specific topics:

1. The question to be answered must be considered important by the patient.
2. There must be a simplified method for providing the patient the important information and study details *before* obtaining consent.

One such strategy for improving informed consent and enhancing enrollment was the use of *video animation*, while two previous studies have demonstrated that "educational videos" *alone does not* improve enrollment. There is some evidence of the positive impact of *video animation* on enhancing patients' understandability of the research and fostering an affirmative attitude about participation in the research. This method of *video animation* should be explored further.[283]

1.11 *"Sham"* surgery, is there an ethical place for research surgical trials or is it forbidden?

The esteemed and lettered bioethicist Franklin G. Miller, PhD in philosophy from Columbia University is a senior faculty member at the National Institutes of Health (NIH), USA, and Professor of Medical Ethics in Medicine (Courtesy) Weill Cornell Medical College in New York City. Previously, in 2003, writing in the *American Journal of Bioethics* Miller presented an ethical analysis of "sham" surgery (placebo-controlled) in *surgical* clinical trials.[284] Although he mentions other commentators who think "sham" surgery unethical, he argues that:

> *"...there are no sound ethical reasons for an absolute prohibition of sham surgery in clinical trials."*

He goes on to make the distinction between clinical medical/surgical *research* and clinical medical/surgical *care*.

> *"This moral stance, which makes sham surgery appear inherently or presumptively unethical, confuses the ethics of clinical research with the ethics of clinical medicine (Horng and Miller 2002; Miller and Brody 2002). The randomized clinical trial is not a form of personal medical therapy. Rather, it is a scientific tool for evaluating treatments in groups of research participants, with the ultimate aim of improving medical care. Clinical trials routinely administer interventions whose risks to patients are not compensated by medical benefits but are justified by the anticipated value of the scientific knowledge that might be gained."[284]*

He cites internal mammary artery ligation for treating angina as a case where two sham-controlled trials *proved* that ligation of the internal mammary artery:

> *"... was no better than a sham operation involving skin incision under local anesthesia without ligation of the internal mammary artery (Cobb et al. 1959; Dimond, Kittle, and Crockett 1960)".[284]*

"The ethical analysis of the sham control in the arthroscopic surgery trial will examine six key ethical questions (Horng and Miller 2002):[284]

1. *"Was there scientific and clinical value in conducting this study?*
2. *Was the use of sham surgery methodologically necessary or desirable to achieve valid results?*
3. *Were the risks minimized for those randomized to sham surgery?*
4. *Were the risks of the sham surgery that were not balanced by the prospect of medical benefit within a reasonable threshold of acceptable research risk?*
5. *Were the risks justified by the potential value of the scientific knowledge to be gained from the research?*
6. *Did the subjects give informed consent?"*

He cites a number of arthroscopic knee surgery reports for arthritis to present his ethical examination of a procedural rationale for "*sham*" surgery with its risk-benefit calculation along with the associated promise to the patient, with the informed consent covenant.[284]

Miller concludes with a summation of his thinking regarding the ethics of "*sham*" surgery in research trials:

> "*Sham surgery is not inherently unethical. To criticize this research practice as a violation of the therapeutic obligation of physicians erroneously conflates the ethics of **clinical research** with the ethics of **medical care**. Nor is sham surgery necessarily contrary to the requirement of research ethics to minimize risks. In sum, there are no good reasons for an absolute prohibition of sham surgery in clinical trials. Ethical judgments should be case specific, depending on the strength of the methodological rationale for use of sham surgery and the level of risks posed to subjects.*"[284] *(Bold italics added)*

Lately, in 2019, Cotton et al. from the Medical University of South Carolina reported on their designed study of endoscopic treatment of patients with suspected sphincter of Oddi dysfunction. They were able to develop and effect a system of blinding in a "*sham-controlled*" study which they considered a viable and an effective "blueprint," a design, for future endoscopy trials. Regarding the issues of randomization and blinding, they wrote:

> "*Randomization and blinding are acceptable only if approved by Institutional Review Boards, and applicable only if patients understand and consent.*"[285]

Placebo control in surgical studies is not a capricious call but a vitally important demand because, "… ***a review of 53 placebo-controlled surgical studies found that half of them showed no benefit for surgery over the sham procedure.***"[285] (Bold italics added). That quotation was from Cotton et al. referencing a 2002 paper in the *Annals of Surgery* by Robert Tenery, MD and his colleagues.[286]

In a most important authoritative paper by the same Robert Tenery, MD and colleagues, mentioned above, from the Council on Ethical and Judicial Affairs of the AMA, following the ethical guidelines in the AMA's Code of Medical Ethics, they wrote in the *Annals of Surgery* the details of how blinding is not only possible but achievable in surgical evaluation studies. They clearly asserted the reasons for randomized, double-blind studies in the first place were because this design, the "gold standard," reduces the risk of random errors all the while eliminating overall bias as it diminishes the probability of eventual erroneous deductions and conclusions.[286]

> "*Studies of new operations that contain a surgical placebo control can be single or double blind (the patient only or the patient and the investigator blind to the patient's group). Double-blind studies are preferable and are possible even though the surgeon will always know what was done in the operating room. The group of investigators can be blind to the study groups if the surgeon, in*

follow-up, closely follows a prepared script with each patient, and if all of the follow-up measurements are done at an outside institution by investigators otherwise unconnected to the study. In this way, double-blind investigations can be achieved in the setting of surgical placebo-controlled studies."[286]

This is a vital consideration and an eminently ethically valuable design strategy because procedures that are ineffective or harmful must be eliminated from all surgical practices, and the most utilitarian study design to avoid ineffective or harmful procedures is the randomized, double-blind surgical placebo-controlled study. An important concept forwarded by Tenery et al. is that research is:

"... ethically acceptable only when there is 'equipoise', or a belief within the general medical community that the experimental intervention will provide at least equal or greater benefit than the standard therapy."[286]

1.12 What are the limitations, if any, to the doctrine of randomized controlled trials?

As we have repeatedly reported, the powerfully persuasive voice of EBM with the unimpeachable "gold standard" of RCTs rules the contemporary court of medical opinion, yet despite its dominance, there are voices of disquiet regarding limitations and concerns of the RCT especially in surgical design.[287] If the design employs multiple surgeons, of course, technical skill is a patient's fickle fate for even if the same "standardized" operative procedure is performed, just as master chefs using the "identical matching recipe" results can be disturbingly dissimilar, and so the same fortune for surgeons. Even extrapolation of the results from RCTs may be additionally hazardous for the same reason; not all surgeons enjoy similar technical mastery or the wisdom to apply that specific "procedure" for the "exact" same "type" of patient. This harkens back to the observations of Sir Nick Black[276] that the evidence from RCTs is a collection of representative data lacking specificity for that unique individual patient; therefore, results from the RCT are not widely transferable, generalizable, as it were, from the trial population to a specific unique surgical patient; it was for that reason that many surgeons lost interest in the total application of the RCT. The assumption that results from RCTs are transferable from the study population to other patients in other situations and that the proposed intervention to be performed is similar for the "same type" of patient by another surgeon is open to serious question.

Peter Rothwell from the Department of Clinical Neurology in the Stroke Prevention Research Unit writing a very extensive, complete, and well referenced article in *The Lancet* in 2005 also questioning generalizability, asking can the results of RCTs be rationally applied from a study population to a specific group of patients in another but "similar" clinical setting?[288] He points out that often the physician's concern is that poor external validity (generalizability) in that the results from RCTs has meager application to the specific patient population in question.

Quoting Archie L. Cochrane, *"Between measurements based on RCTs and benefit … in the community there is a gulf which has been much underestimated"*[288,289] Rothwell then deliberately declares, referring to RCTs:

*"They must be **internally valid** (i.e., design and conduct must keep to a minimum the possibility of bias), but to be clinically useful the result must also be relevant to a definable group of patients in a particular clinical setting; this is generally termed **external validity**, applicability, or generalizability. The beneficial effects of some interventions, such as blood pressure lowering in chronic uncontrolled hypertension, are generalizable to most patients and settings, but the effects of other interventions can be very dependent on factors such as the characteristics of the patient, the method of application of the intervention, and the setting of treatment. How these factors are taken into account in the design and performance of an RCT and in the reporting of the results can have a major effect on **external validity**."[288] (Bold italics added)*

He continues asking why there is clinician criticism and ubiquitous underuse by physicians of RCTs:

*"Lack of consideration of **external validity** is the most frequent criticism by clinicians of RCTs, systematic reviews, and guidelines, and is one explanation for the widespread underuse in routine practice of treatments that were beneficial in trials and that are recommended in guidelines."[288] (Bold italics added)*

This situation is even more troubling for our surgical sisters and brethren. Another very significant issue according to Rothwell is the reality that:

*"…researchers, funding agencies, ethics committees, the pharmaceutical industry, medical journals, and governmental regulators alike all **neglect external validity**…" (Bold italics added)*

External validity refers to generalizability, and generalizability is defined as a measure of the usefulness of the study results from a broad group of people to specific clinical situations. If the results of a **study** are broadly applicable to many different types of people or situations, then the **study** is said to have good **generalizability**. On the other hand, if an RCT study does not have applicability of their results to specific patients, then it has poor external validity. Most RCTs have poor external validity.

Now, despite the limitations of RCTs, Rothwell reassures us about the results of RCTs with:

"These inevitable limitations do not invalidate the results of RCTs and systematic reviews, and they are mentioned here partly for the sake of completeness, but the importance of patient preference, placebo effects, and the doctor-patient relationship outside trials should not be underestimated."[288]

Also observing the limits of RCTs, Sir Austin Bradford Hill* commented:

"At its best, a trial shows what can be accomplished with a medicine under careful observation and certain restricted conditions. The same results will not invariably or necessarily be observed when the medicine passes into general use."[290]

*"Sir Austin Bradford Hill (1897−1991), is the English epidemiologist and statistician, who pioneered the randomized clinical trial and, together with Richard Doll, demonstrated the connection between cigarette smoking and lung cancer." Quoted from Wikipedia.

1.13 Is there an ethical approach to surgical and invasive procedures within randomized controlled trials?

In 2009, Dr. Carol Ashton et al. from Methodist Hospital Research Institute and Department of Surgery, The Methodist Hospital, Houston, Texas, reflected on *the "double standard"* between novel medication approvals and evaluation of innovative surgical procedures. The Food and Drug Administration (FDA) monitors the development and approval of new drugs before public release by means of RCTs, while surgical and other invasive procedures have no official regulatory body, and often *hundreds of thousands* of procedures are performed *before* any RCTs are carried out with the claim that trial design and ethical concerns are prohibitive and limiting.[295] Furthermore, she and her colleagues aggressively argue for rigorous randomized trials for surgical and invasive procedures with specific design and reporting requirements recommended by her team. Reviewing the negative history of carotid artery surgery with the idea of "procedure first" and "evidence later" which for them is ethically repulsive. An important problem in surgical trials is when patients drop out or cross over during randomization, then the data lose its true authenticity. They propose that it is possible to reconcile medical ethics with rigorous research methods.[291]

Writing three years later, the same team from Methodist Hospital Research Institute and Department of Surgery *raised the alarm* about the quality and ethics of clinical research of surgical procedures. Their review covered January 1999−December 2008 and after an exhaustive literature search of *"… 37,944 unique articles across 33 medical subject headings. 2890 trials (7.6%) met our inclusion criteria (Table 2)."*[292] After that monumental review, Wenner et al. concluded that the quality of surgical trials and the reporting of those surgical trials,

"…is in need of significant improvement."[292] (Bold italics added)

The answer to the question is yes, there is an ethical approach to RCTs for surgical and invasive procedures; however, demands must be met. Wenner and associates cited five important papers discussing the unique barriers and difficulties related to surgical clinical trials, but they offered suggestions to vastly improve evidence from surgical trials including:

1. Application of **CONSORT,** which stands for, *CONsolidated Standards Of Reporting Trials,* requirements
2. Include a *research fellowship* into surgical training
3. Improve *research education* of independent review board members
4. Scientific rigor is possible as 90% of studies reviewed had successful randomization and only 16% of studies reviewed were blinded; however, to limit bias, blinding of the independent outcome assessors is possible
5. Regarding ethics: *"Clinical research ethics require that the risks of harm to participants be outweighed by the value of the knowledge to be generated."*

Finally, there are ethical imperatives because when surgical and invasive procedure trials are poorly constructed, absent bias reduction, and are inadequately conducted, then these trial results are of "questionable scientific value."[292]

We ask, when results from such trials that lack proof of efficacy or safety are applied to unsuspecting clinical patients, who is accountable?

1.14 What are the obligations and accountability to our patients regarding surgical *innovations*?

Yes, as physicians and surgeons, medicine, have the exquisite moral obligation to be accountable to the highest methodical standards, with essential ethical behavior especially as surgeons exploring surgical innovations. In a marvelous **three-part series** all published in *The Lancet,* in the September 26, 2009 issue, the entire topic of surgical innovation is intensely reviewed. Surgical innovation can result from evidence-based principles and not "trial and error" so as to avoid "innovations" that are ultimately deemed useless or harmful to patients.

The paradigm of critical appraisal arises before wide-spread adoption proceeds from innovation, development, exploration, assessment, long-term implementation, and monitoring. Essentially, ethical surgical innovation is **"staged development"** with unremitting ever continuous and endless evaluation.

Jeffrey Barkun and colleagues[293] discuss evaluation and the various stages of surgical innovations, Patrick Ergina et al.[294] cover the variety of challenges related to evaluating surgical innovation and RCTs, while Peter McCulloch and his associates[295] in their thoughtful discussion preferred the extensive use of *"prospective databases and registries."* Favoring, of course, RCTs with prospective design planning, pretrial statistical analysis with power calculations, and measures accounting for learning curves and other variables with rigorous results analysis including recording and reporting of late outcomes and complications. McCulloch et al. continued to emphasize ethics and safety over mercantile profits and cautioned that restrictive regulation must never negate imaginative creativity.[295]

1.15 What are the CONSORT requirements and what's their importance for researchers and journals?

McCulloch et al.[295] were certain that improvements in research reporting by investigators and acceptance by the journal editors would occur only after high standards are attained such as those of CONSORT. Having a uniform method of reporting RCTs would markedly improve trial methodological construction thereby avoiding publishing of flawed studies.[295] Thirteen years earlier, in 1996, Douglas Altman writing in *The British Medical Journal* recognized the critical importance of a well-executed RCT, which explicitly informs the readers as to precise methodology of the reported RCT.[296] That is, the purpose of the CONSORT statement which is a standard way for all interested parties, researchers, journal editors, and physicians of the general readership to know exactly how the RCT was performed, with a standardized check list for the authors of trials to adhere to and for journal editors to demand before the results of RCTs are published and disseminated.[296,297] In fact, *The Journal of the American Medical Association (JAMA), The British Medical Journal, The Lancet,* and *The Laryngoscope* all support the CONSORT check list with the hope that the research trialists will follow the checklist to improve RCTs reporting and now considered the correct conduct for future research.[296]

As recently as 2015, Peters et al.[213] used the CONSORT statement, which was developed to promote consistency, clarity, accuracy, and transparency of reporting of RCTs, reviewed and compared the five top general medical and ENT journals (by impact factor), assessing the number of CONSORT items adequately reported. They found that the reporting quality in the ENT journals was *"suboptimal,"* while the reporting of RCTs in the medical journals was of higher quality. (Bold italics added) They also suggested that the journal editors endorse using the CONSORT statement to improve reporting of the results from RCTs.[213]

As pointed out by Agha et al.,[269] the CONSORT statement which was first published in 1996 by Begg et al.[297] and revised in 2001 by Moher and colleagues[298] was intended to improve the overall value of RCTs by insisting on design and reporting standards through a specific checklist of 22 *essential* items and flow diagram that has the obligatory requirement of being included in the reporting of every RCT to each journal for consideration for publication.

More recently, in 2010, the checklist and flow diagram have been updated yet again and expanded to 25 *essential* items by the leading authorities Douglas Altman, David Moher, Kenneth Schulz, and others[299,300] with the details located at: www.consort-statement.org

CONSORT 2010 checklist of information to include when reporting a randomised trial*

Section/Topic	Item No	Checklist item	Reported on page No
Title and abstract			
	1a	Identification as a randomised trial in the title	_____
	1b	Structured summary of trial design, methods, results, and conclusions (for specific guidance see CONSORT for abstracts)	_____
Introduction			
Background and objectives	2a	Scientific background and explanation of rationale	_____
	2b	Specific objectives or hypotheses	_____
Methods			
Trial design	3a	Description of trial design (such as parallel, factorial) including allocation ratio	_____
	3b	Important changes to methods after trial commencement (such as eligibility criteria), with reasons	_____
Participants	4a	Eligibility criteria for participants	_____
	4b	Settings and locations where the data were collected	_____
Interventions	5	The interventions for each group with sufficient details to allow replication, including how and when they were actually administered	_____
Outcomes	6a	Completely defined pre-specified primary and secondary outcome measures, including how and when they were assessed	_____
	6b	Any changes to trial outcomes after the trial commenced, with reasons	_____
Sample size	7a	How sample size was determined	_____
	7b	When applicable, explanation of any interim analyses and stopping guidelines	_____
Randomisation:			
Sequence generation	8a	Method used to generate the random allocation sequence	_____
	8b	Type of randomisation; details of any restriction (such as blocking and block size)	_____
Allocation concealment mechanism	9	Mechanism used to implement the random allocation sequence (such as sequentially numbered containers), describing any steps taken to conceal the sequence until interventions were assigned	_____
Implementation	10	Who generated the random allocation sequence, who enrolled participants, and who assigned participants to interventions	_____
Blinding	11a	If done, who was blinded after assignment to interventions (for example, participants, care providers, those assessing outcomes) and how	_____
	11b	If relevant, description of the similarity of interventions	_____
Statistical methods	12a	Statistical methods used to compare groups for primary and secondary outcomes	_____
	12b	Methods for additional analyses, such as subgroup analyses and adjusted analyses	_____
Results			
Participant flow (a diagram is strongly recommended)	13a	For each group, the numbers of participants who were randomly assigned, received intended treatment, and were analysed for the primary outcome	_____
	13b	For each group, losses and exclusions after randomisation, together with reasons	_____
Recruitment	14a	Dates defining the periods of recruitment and follow-up	_____
	14b	Why the trial ended or was stopped	_____
Baseline data	15	A table showing baseline demographic and clinical characteristics for each group	_____
Numbers analysed	16	For each group, number of participants (denominator) included in each analysis and whether the analysis was by original assigned groups	_____
Outcomes and estimation	17a	For each primary and secondary outcome, results for each group, and the estimated effect size and its precision (such as 95% confidence interval)	_____
	17b	For binary outcomes, presentation of both absolute and relative effect sizes is recommended	_____
Ancillary analyses	18	Results of any other analyses performed, including subgroup analyses and adjusted analyses, distinguishing pre-specified from exploratory	_____
Harms	19	All important harms or unintended effects in each group (for specific guidance see CONSORT for harms)	_____
Discussion			
Limitations	20	Trial limitations, addressing sources of potential bias, imprecision, and, if relevant, multiplicity of analyses	_____
Generalisability	21	Generalisability (external validity, applicability) of the trial findings	_____
Interpretation	22	Interpretation consistent with results, balancing benefits and harms, and considering other relevant evidence	_____
Other information			
Registration	23	Registration number and name of trial registry	_____
Protocol	24	Where the full trial protocol can be accessed, if available	_____
Funding	25	Sources of funding and other support (such as supply of drugs), role of funders	_____

*We strongly recommend reading this statement in conjunction with the CONSORT 2010 Explanation and Elaboration for important clarifications on all the items. If relevant, we also recommend reading CONSORT extensions for cluster randomised trials, non-inferiority and equivalence trials, non-pharmacological treatments, herbal interventions, and pragmatic trials. Additional extensions are forthcoming: for those and for up to date references relevant to this checklist, see www.consort-statement.org.

Agha et al. commenting on the necessity for the CONSORT requirements in research, especially the reporting of RCTs in surgery was:

"There is a clear need to ensure that medical research, especially relating to clinical interventions, is carried out and reported to the highest possible standards."[296]

Douglas Altman (1948−2018) said it so succinctly and beautifully:

"To maximize the benefit to society, you need to not just do research, but do it well."

So, these CONSORT requirements are important for clinical investigators to have an accurate repeatable standard guideline to follow for performing valid RCTs of the highest quality, so ultimately practicing physicians and surgeons have proven principles to follow for effective clinical patient care.

Journal editors and peer reviewers should also demand that those investigators using RCTs follow the CONSORT requirements, so that the highest quality studies are transparently performed with the most accurate data published for their readership to consider when making clinical decisions. Even after a quarter of century of demand for following the CONSORT statement, many RCTs still do not adhere to those principles in their papers published in the ENT literature. Just a few years ago in 2018, the group from McGill University evaluating RCTs in otolaryngology and adherence to the CONSORT statement concluded that the reporting of RCTs in top nine ORL-HNS journals and in the top Canadian ORL-HNS journal is *"suboptimal."*[301] (Bold italics added)

1.16 What is propensity score matching all about?

Propensity score systems can be used in observational studies to decrease a confounding variable; an indication of bias. This technique is called propensity score matching (PSM). The PSM reputation has increased in the medical literature because improper methodology may lead to biased treatment effects or limited scientific reproducibility.

Prasad et al. aimed to study the quality of PSM methodology reported in the ENT literature.[302]

"Such analyses are able to measure and balance predetermined covariates between treated and untreated groups, leading to results that can approximate those generated by randomized prospective studies when such trials are not feasible."[302]

Since RCTs in the ENT literature is under 4%[205,207] because they are difficult, regularly expensive, and at times ethically challenging to perform, observational studies are utilized more frequently with a retrospective investigation to make connections concerning treatment effectiveness, which then can be followed by confirmatory studies. Regrettably, these observational studies are vulnerable to "treatment selection bias" owing to their lack of randomization; however, their results may become routine clinical practice without the same scientific scrupulousness as an RCT.

*"In an attempt to improve comparisons between cohorts in observational studies, statistical methodologies have been developed in order to reduce **confounding** when randomization is not possible. The most commonly employed statistical technique to reduce bias is multivariable regression."*[302] *(Bold italics added)*

A confounding variable is an "extra" variable not accounted for that can ruin an experiment giving flawed results. For example, suggesting a correlation when in fact there isn't one or even unwittingly introducing bias is a confounding variable. That's why it's important to know confounding factors and how to avoid getting those factors into a research experimental design in the first place.

Prasad el al. provided pivotal recommendations to future authors regarding reporting of PSM at the same time they critically concluded that although PSM has increased in frequency in the ENT literature, the ***quality of those reports*** can be ***"improved."***[302] *(Bold italics added)*

In a competent comparison study writing from Paris, France, in the *Annals of Surgery*, Lonjon et al., in a metaepidemiological study, compared the treatment effect from prospective nonrandomized studies (NRSs) with PSM analysis and RCTs of surgical procedures and found that:

"There was no statistically significant difference in treatment effect between NRSs with PS(M) analysis and RCTs. Prospective NRSs with suitable and careful PS(M) analysis can be relied upon as evidence when RCTs are not possible."[303]

In other words, if performed accurately, analysis of outcome differences between treated and untreated participants following PSM can imitate an RCT.[303,304] Note: the (M) is added to the quotation and for clarity, stands for the word "matching."

1.17 What about using clinical practice guidelines and associated conflicts of interest?

It is well recognized that comprehensive clinical practice guidelines (CPGs) can provide significant information to busy "overworked" physicians and surgeons seeking advice regarding diagnosis and treatment of an assorted mix of medical and surgical disorders. The primary motivation for these recommendations offered by CPGs is for the enhanced improvement of patient care based on the "best available solid evidence" usually from RCTs. Developing even one CPG requires authoritative judgments from various individuals, thereby potentially introducing bias. At times, members of a guideline development team lack solid evidence requiring dependence on individual "expert" interpretations positioning some members into a COI. The legions of healthcare providers including physicians and surgeons as well as the public all depend upon the integrity, honesty, and transparency of all those individual members involved in creating CPGs. It's all about the belief in the expectation and conviction, in the confident certainty of trust.

According to Sniderman et al.[180] when and if the data from RCTs are limited, incomplete, inconclusive, conflicting, or starkly nonexistent, then contemporary

CPGs or advisories are often still relied upon for a reliable and trusted expert opinion.[180]

Loss and Nagel writing from Germany favored evidence-based guidelines which were supportive of free decision-making, yet were cautious about the confining influence of *evidence-based clinical guidelines* in surgery fearing the restrictive influence on independent thinking which "*…may lead to an oversimplified and **rigid** standardization in medical care ('cook book medicine'). In addition, scientific progress might be prevented by **inflexible** guidelines.*"[305] (Bold italics added)

Dr. Bruce Barrett at the University of Wisconsin, Madison writing in *The Journal of General Internal Medicine* in 2012, continues the discussion by supporting the notion that medical decision-making is really an individualized process between physician and patient, and because decisions are between doctor and patient that *patient guidelines* are beyond the rigidity and inflexibility that Loss and Nagel spoke of, but that guidelines are irrational.

> "*…and because the ethical principle of autonomy mandates informed choice by patient, medical decision-making is inherently an individualized process. It follows that the practice of aiming for universal implementation of standardized guidelines is irrational and unethical. Irrational because the possibility of benefits is implicitly valued more than the possibility of comparable harms, and unethical because guidelines remove decision making from the patient and give it instead to a physician, committee or health care system. This essay considers the cases of cancer screening and diabetes management, where guidelines often advocate universal implementation, without regard to informed choice and individual decision-making.*"[306]

Woolf and colleagues from the Department of Family Practice, Virginia Commonwealth University, Fairfax, Virginia noted the assured benefits of clinical guidelines as improving outcomes, reducing morbidity and mortality while enhancing the quality of life and consistency of medical care for patients regardless where they are treated or by whom.[307] All positive. Guidelines that are based on scientific evidence (evidence-based guidelines) simplify which interventions are proven to be of benefit with substantiating supporting data. All good. Now Woolf et al. also discussed the limitations with the most important limitation of the guideline recommendation is that it might be wrong. Wrong because the scientific evidence maybe flawed, ineffective, or even harmful, and with the promotion of flawed guidelines, the greatest danger is to the patients. What is helpful and best for patients "globally" as recommended by the guidelines may be inflexible and inappropriate for a specific individual patient. Flawed guidelines harm not only the patient but also the physicians and surgeons practicing from fallacious science.

Clinical guidelines are not the ultimate panacea but only an option to consider, especially when a clinical care dilemma needs clarity, then a set of guidelines based on accurate unbiased solid scientific evidence (evidence-based guidelines), then those guidelines make sense to consider for our patients.[307]

David Jevsevar and Kevin Bozic in the Department of Orthopedics at Dartmouth-Hitchcock Medical Center, Lebanon, New Hampshire, in the context of decision-making, defined CPGs as:

> "…a systematic approach to exploring, evaluating, appraising, and synthesizing the literature so that the individual reader need not perform each of these time-consuming activities."[308]

The Institute of Medicine (IOM) defines a CPG as a *"systematically developed statement to assist practitioner and patient decisions about appropriate healthcare for specific clinical circumstances."*[308] Wisely, because of the well-known quality variability of any specific CPG, the Orthopedic Academy suggests grading the authority and strength of any CPGs as: strong, moderate, limited, and consensus. That a CPG should be considered no more than a well-thought-out reference tool, ultimately serving for proficient patient care, integrating physician expertise with a unique patient's situation and preferences.[308]

In a very interesting facet of CPG Stefan Timmermans from the Department of Sociology, University of California-Los Angeles traces the evolution and impact of CPGs, on clinicians by addressing ambiguities of patient care with a set of standardized CPGs and yet recognizing the commanding power transfer from physician autonomy to physician accountability.[309] Timmermans like Loss and Nagel[305] was concerned about rigidly constructed CPGs that may inflexibly stipulate how medical care should be accomplished, threatening professional freedom, our sovereignty.[309] In reality, studies have shown that there is only "modest" physician behavior change regarding rigidly following CPG directives, but this "nonobedience" to CPGs may mark the physician susceptible to third-party "oversight" and eyes from legal circles with all that entails.[309]

As has been noted, CPGs are costly to create, and most recently, CPGs have been seriously discussed by various participants and stakeholders including physicians, surgeons, third-party payers, legal experts as a means of measuring performance, ranging from reimbursement to malpractice litigation. With the trustworthiness of the CPGs creators, the authors of any given group of CPGs need to have impeccable credentials for integrity, free from any fragrance of fiscal COIs. The University of Michigan otolaryngologist, Gordon Sun, MD, a Robert Wood Johnson Foundation Clinical Scholar, extolling the American Academy of Otolaryngology—Head and Neck Surgery Foundation wrote in 2013 that:[310]

> *"Since 2004, the 9 CPGs sponsored by the American Academy of Otolaryngology-Head and Neck Surgery Foundation have been developed with **full disclosure** and appropriate management of potential pecuniary conflicts of interest. This commentary discusses the potential for conflict of interest in otolaryngology CPGs and how the otolaryngology guideline development process **can serve as a model** for other professional medical organizations."[310] (Bold italics added)*

Firestorm! Flash! Five years later, in 2018, three medical students and a PhD clinician from the Department of Psychiatry Oklahoma State University Center for Health Sciences, Tulsa, Oklahoma, using both the ***Open Payments database and the Dollars for Docs website***, which identifies industry payments to physicians, investigated the relationship between physicians developing CPGs and industry. This faction of four exploded the myth of candid and reliable integrity in their COI statements in the development of CPGs by guideline development groups (GDGs) of the American Academy of Otolaryngology—Head and Neck Surgery (AAO-HNS).[311] (Bold italics added)

The findings of Horn et al.[311] are so striking and arresting; to avoid any suggestion of misrepresentation, we quote entirely from both their Key Points and Abstract:

1.17.1 "Key Points
1.17.1.1 Question
What is the extent of potential financial conflicts of interest among physicians who author otolaryngology clinical practice guidelines?

1.17.1.2 Findings
*In this cross-sectional analysis of 49 authors of otolaryngology clinical practice guidelines, 39 received industry payments and **three did not accurately disclose financial relationships.** Of the three Institute of Medicine standards assessed, only one was being enforced.* (Bold Italics added for emphasis)

1.17.1.3 Meaning
Guideline authors received significant industry payments, and most panel members received payments from industry, which raises concern about potential financial conflicts of interest in the otolaryngology guideline development process"

1.17.2 Abstract
Importance: *Financial relationships between physicians and industry have influence on patient care. Therefore, organizations producing clinical practice guidelines (CPGs) must have policies limiting financial conflicts during guideline development.*

Objectives: To evaluate payments received by physician authors of otolaryngology CPGs, compare disclosure statements for accuracy and investigate the extent to which the American Academy of Otolaryngology—Head and Neck Surgery complied with standards for guideline development from the **IOM.**

Design, setting, and participants: *This cross-sectional analysis retrieved CPGs from the American Academy of Otolaryngology—Head and Neck Surgery Foundation that were published or revised from January 1, 2013, through December 31, 2015, by 49 authors. Data were retrieved from December 1, 2016 through December 31, 2016. Industry payments received by authors were extracted using the Centers for Medicare & Medicaid Services Open Payments database. The values and types of these payments were then evaluated and used to determine whether self-reported disclosure statements were accurate and whether guidelines adhered to applicable IOM standards.*

Main outcomes and measures: The monetary amounts and types of payments received by physicians who author otolaryngology guidelines and the accuracy of disclosure statements.

*Results: Of the 49 physicians in this sample, 39 (80%) received an industry payment. Twenty-one authors (43%) accepted more than $1000; 12 (24%) more than $10 000; **7 (14%) more than $50 000; and 2 (4%) more than $100 000.** Mean (SD) financial payments amounted to $18 431 ($53 459) per physician. Total reimbursement for all authors was $995 282. **Disclosure statements disagreed** with the Open Payments database for **three authors,** amounting to approximately $20 000 among them. **Of the three IOM standards assessed, only one was consistently enforced.***

*Conclusions and relevance: **Some CPG authors failed to fully disclose all financial conflicts of interest,** and **most** guideline development panels and chairpersons had conflicts. In addition, adherence to IOM standards for guideline development was lacking. This study is relevant to CPG panels authoring recommendations, physicians implementing CPGs to guide patient care, and the organizations establishing policies for guideline development."*[311] (Bold italics added)

David Tunkel in the Department of Otolaryngology—Head and Neck Surgery, Johns Hopkins University School of Medicine, Baltimore, Maryland writing in *JAMA Otolaryngology Head Neck Surgery* commented on trustworthiness of CPGs and COI of those involved in creating those recommendations after reading Horn et al.[311] He said:

> *"Clinical practice guidelines must be trustworthy, and the Institute of Medicine (IOM) and the Guideline International Network have provided standards for CPGs.[1] A major threat to the creation of trustworthy guidelines is conflict of interest (COI) among the organizations and the committee members who create CPGs."[312]*

Dr. Tunkel adroitly observed that COIs may be threefold: (1) Financial, (2) Intellectual, i.e., by holding exclusive and specific views precluding dispassionate objective judgment, and (3) Professional COI where the guideline developer has a clinical practice affected directly by guideline proposals. Tunkel was similarly troubled by the fact that:

> *"…several AAO-HNS guideline authors received large payments from companies related to their guideline topic and even more troubling that disclosure of conflicts for a few was not accurate."[312]*

David E. Tunkel's comment that several guideline authors' disclosure of COIs "were not accurate" is undeniably troubling.[312] The honor system runs amuck; obsessed with mammon and with cynical ruefulness, the letters "**CPG**" might now stand for ***clinician payment guidelines (CPGs),*** especially for those colleagues who accepted funding and otherwise without the integrity of direct disclosure of their conflict(s) of interest.

Some "good" news arrived from the Yale University group with the work of Pathak et al.[313] who found that: *"Otolaryngologists continue to demonstrate limited industry ties when compared with other surgical specialists."* Once again, a year later the Yale group from the Division of Otolaryngology, Yale University School of Medicine, New Haven, Connecticut, comparing drug and device industry year to year payments "opened our eyes" about those disbursements to otolaryngologists with a final flourish from their 2019 paper:

> *"Conclusion: Industry payments to otolaryngologists decreased to $11.2 million in 2017 from $14.5 million in 2016. Much of the decrease can be attributed to decreases in consulting fees and ownership payments. It is important that otolaryngologists remain aware of changes in industry funding with each release of the Open Payments Database."[314]*

Very recently, in April 2021, a powerful paper from the Department of Medicine, Center for Biomedical Ethics, and the Law School, at Vanderbilt University, Nashville, Tennessee, J. Henry Brems and colleagues skillfully and punctiliously studied the COI public policies statements among 46 organizations producing five or more CPGs since the IOM, now the National Academy of Medicine, publicized their COI policies 10 years ago in 2011.[315]

These 46 organizations were identified by CPG databases, and their COI policies were acquired after a public internet search. Among the 46 organizations that trumpeted five or more CPGs, 36 (78%) had a COI policy but **only** two of the 36 (6%) met the divestment requirement for a financial COI. Cheerfully, the disclosure requirement of a COI had the highest frequency of compliance with 33 of 36 (92%) organizations with a COI policy disclosed a COI. Nevertheless, the Vanderbilt team concluded that:

> *"Among organizations producing CPGs, COI policies frequently do not meet IOM standards, and organizations often violate their own policies. These shortcomings may undermine the public trust in and thus the utility of CPGs. CPG-producing organizations should improve their COI policies and their strategies to manage COI to increase the trustworthiness of CPGs."[315]*

Dr. J.C. Denneny 3rd from the American Academy of Otolaryngology—Head and Neck Surgery Foundation, Alexandria, Virginia, writing from his pivotal post as Executive Vice President/CEO of the American Academy of Otolaryngology— Head and Neck Surgery and its Foundation representing about 12,000 otorhinolaryngologists—head and neck surgeons in the United States, explaining the CPG development process at the academy while tackling the COI situation by Horn et al.[311] who were critical of the practices at the academy by some who failed to honor their commitments to their integrity regarding COI. Denneny et al. referring to the academy's CPG development process postulated that:

> *"By focusing only on conflict of interest and related potential bias, the authors (Horn et al.[311]) do a disservice to the process as a whole."[316]*

Dr. Denneny and coauthors[316] submitted that COIs cannot be totally circumvented or entirely prevented, so their answer is "proper management," which includes total transparency and the responsibility of the chair and the members of the GDG to recuse themselves from discussions, voting or even removal from the entire group process should conflicts arise. The authors also pointed out that:

> *"Questions regarding the accuracy of the Open Payments Database (OPD)* have been reported, with a 2014 estimate **suggesting** that about 30% of data collected **may** be inaccurate. 10,11. References 10 and 11 listed by Denneny et al. are: (Bold Italics added)*

10. Maddux D. Open payments: CMS data makes headlines. Acumen Physician Solutions website.https://acumenmd.com/blog/open-payments-cms-data-makes-headlines/. Published October 6, 2014. Accessed January 16, 2018.
11. Babu MA, Heary RF, Nahed BV. Does the open payments database provide sunshine on neurosurgery? *Neurosurgery.* 2016;79:933–938.

*Note: Reference 10. Above: The article by Dugan Maddux, MD Vice President, Kidney Disease Initiatives written October 6, 2014 thought that the data did not specify enough information to make intelligent comments about industry and physician relationships plus data could be misleading and there were "**significant concerns about inaccurate data."** Reference 11. Above: *"The Open Payments Database (OPD) was launched by the Centers for Medicare & Medicaid Services in 2014. Through this online searchable database, the public can explore physician-industry interactions."* Babu et al. concluded: *The OPD details physician interactions with industry and has **multiple inaccuracies**.*

The simplest way to answer the matter is for the officials at the American Academy of Otolaryngology—Head and Neck Surgery to unequivocally ask the involved individuals about the accuracy of the allegations, emphasizing that COI can be threefold: (1) Financial, (2) Intellectual, and (3) Professional, as pointed out by David Tunkel.[312]

Digesting these revelations amid allegations of *inaccurate data* and *multiple inaccuracies*, from the *Open Payments database and the Dollars for Docs website* we think as a profession, there is much to contemplate, ruminate, and ponder, prior to ultimate action, since the underpinning of medical care is all about, as previously stated, the expectation and conviction, in the confident certainty by colleagues and the general public of trust in our unmitigated total integrity; integrity matters.

Lastly, this section is closed with a fascinating and intriguing corollary paper regarding the use of CPGs written by Dr. Chris Taylor, in 2014, a neurosurgeon and Vice Chairman of the Department of Neurosurgery at the University of New Mexico School of Medicine contributing to the *Journal of Legal Medicine* about using CPGs in determining the standard of care in the medicolegal sense.[317] He reviewed a number of legal cases determining that since CPGs are numerous and variable in quality, with some CPGs established on evidence-based RCTs and meta-analyses and others based purely on the "consensus opinions" of "experts" who have, none the less, reviewed the scientific basis of their opinions, regarding a specific clinical situation but without the rock-solid evidence of RCTs. The entire concept of "evidence-based-medicine" is the distinction between decisions based on hard scientific evidence, RCTs as opposed to decisions based on expert opinion. Certainly, our legal system allows for CPGs to be presented to judge and jury by expert medical witnesses representing both sides of a litigation for bolstering their position. While there are some CPGs that *approximate* the "standard of care" in the medicolegal definition but considered alone, CPGs do not equate or legally represent the "standard of care" in a court of law.[317]

1.18 What about practice replacement, reversal, and the nature of medical progress?

Ever since Hippocrates, the gravitational principled core of medicine which maintains moral authority is: *the interest of the patient is the only interest of concern*. With the enormity of that gravitational moral and ethical pull, physicians and surgeons are obligated to continuously scrutinize, evaluate, and reevaluate their current practices ever searching for improvements, for optimal patient care procedures and techniques. As a profession, we are ever wary of practices that are useless or harmful searching for validated therapies to safeguard and protect the best interests of our trusting patients. Unvalidated therapies need scrutiny with attempts at verification to be embraced and approved as sensible and successful or discarded as useless or harmful.

Viny Prasad and Adam Cifu writing in the *Yale Journal of Biology and Medicine* cited the twofold reasons that medical therapies decline in esteem and are no longer used: (1). *Replacement* or (2). *Reversal*

1. *Replacement* occurs when a practice is displaced by one that is better.
2. *Reversal (discontinued)* occurs when a practice is discontinued not by being exceeded and replaced by something better, but when it is realized that the practice was never really successful or it was discovered to be harmful, it is then reversed.[318]

Reversal produces a loss of trust for the entire medical system by both patients and physicians. The solution to a reversal is finding the answer by randomized controlled trials (RCTs) for newer effective practices or RCTs can be used to reevaluate practices currently in existence.[318] RCTs avoid bias and are absolutely indispensable for intelligently comparing competing medical practices.[214] By comparison, *replacement* represents a coherent and logical progression in medical care, while *reversal* exposes errors which by its very nature damages trust.

Prasad and Cifu cite examples including Atenolol that "...*is no better than placebo in increasing survival*."[318] Some other examples offered included Class 1C antiarrhythmics, vertebroplasty, mammographic screening does not benefit women in their 40s, hormone replacement therapy for treating menopausal symptoms, and others.[318] A common sense understanding of science or that a treatment objective "makes sense" does not assure investigational experimental confirmation, proof.

Proof is obtained though good evidence, and good evidence is obtained through well-conceived and well-done RCTs.

"Well-done means a strong methodology, adequate power, and blinding, such trials are appropriately controlled (in certain cases, sham-controlled) and address proper endpoints."[318] This applies not only to medical and surgical procedures but to new technologies too "...since we continue to adopt new technologies not because they are supported by the strongest evidence base, but based on a common sense appeal that they should work."[318]

These authors cited a recent article announcing that only 27% of new and novel cardiac devices had randomized testing prior to the United States FDA approval. Straightforward testing would be a blessing to both patients and physicians alike. Reversal reminds us all that failure to do the straightforward testing, exposes patients to possible profound and permanent damage.[318] Preferably, questionable medical practices are replaced by better ones, based on strong and substantial comparative trials RCTs where new practices overtake older ones inaugurating novel canons and new standards of care.[319] As previously presented, Vinay Prasad and associates reviewed over 2000 new articles with over 1000 covering medical practice. Over 900 articles tested new practices, while 363 articles tested established standard of care practices, ***146 (40.2%) of 363 reversed (discontinued)*** the established standard of care practice, whereas 138 (38.0%) of 363 ***reaffirmed*** and 79 were inconclusive regarding the established standard of care practice.

*"The **reversal** of established medical practice is common and occurs across all classes of medical practice." "Reversals included medications, procedures, diagnostic tests, screening tests, and even monitoring and treatment guiding devices. We were unable to identify any class of medical practice that did not have some reversal of standard of."[271](Bold Italics added)*

A comment, of the 981 articles testing new practices, 77% were ***replacements*** (improvements-betterment) and 17% no better or worse, so back to the "drawing board" and 6% were inconclusive.[271]

Following Prasad et al. with the demands that all, or almost all, practices, techniques, and devices be studied in well-designed trials (RCTs) to solve clinical problems with dictum, "evidence first."[271] In that way, medicine advances, progressing toward a loftier perch with safer and more predicable positive outcomes for patients. Surgeons began noticing that data from many scientific studies including RCTs were not widely or easily assignable to a given unique individual surgical patient leading to the receding enthusiasm among surgical constituents for RCTs and its generalizability.

In a dazzlingly provocative paper published in 2016, John Ioannidis from the Departments of Medicine, Health Research and Policy, and Statistics, and Meta-Research Innovation Center at Stanford (METRICS), Stanford University, Palo Alto, California, defended his assertion that ***most clinical research is not useful*** by arguing that for clinical research to be useful, it must have unbiased transparent pragmatic utility for a patient's well-being. After listing a number of "utility features" (Table 8.1 below) that must be met for clinical research to be useful, he concluded by announcing that:

> *"Overall, not only are most research findings false, but, furthermore, most of the true findings are not useful. Medical interventions should and can result in huge human benefit. It makes no sense to perform clinical research without ensuring clinical utility. Reform and improvement are overdue."[320]*

In closing this section, we read from the perspicacious philosophical pen of Sergio Cocchei, University of Bologna School of Medicine, Bologna, Italy, writing in 2017 about error and contradictions in medicine proposing that the occurrence of adverse events is not totally damaging since, quoting the 17th century words of Sir Francis Bacon, *"truth emerges more readily from error than from confusion."*

Cocchei paraphrasing the work of the late Professor Sir Karl R. Popper, the 20th century Austrian philosopher of science, from his 1959 book *"The Logic of Scientific Discovery,"* who:

> *"introduced the concept of an '**approximate temporary truth**' that constitutes the engine of scientific progress."[321] (Bold italics added)*

Cocchei further invites us to consider the temporal quality of "truth" since biomedical research and clinical practice have witnessed many, as Prasad et al.[271] has revealed, reversals and rejections of once dearly held beliefs. Medicine utilizes the "best information available" at the time, allowing for "educated guesses," which, of course, is subject to change. That we physicians and surgeons should tolerate "uncertainty" acknowledging the reality that medical theories and practices are subject to dislocation, disruption, continuous change, and improvements since that's the nature of medical progress.[321]

Table 8.1 Features to consider in appraising whether clinical research is useful.

Feature	Questions to ask
Problem base	Is there a health problem that is big/important enough to fix?
Context placement	Has prior evidence been systematically assessed to inform (the need for) new studies?
Information gain	Is the proposed study large and long enough to be sufficiently informative?
Pragmatism	Does the research reflect real life? If it deviates, does this matter?
Patient centeredness	Does the research reflect top patient priorities?
Value for money	Is the research worth the money?
Feasibility	Can this research be done?
Transparency	Are methods, data, and analyses verifiable and unbiased?

Table 8.1 from: Ioannidis JP. Why most clinical research is not useful. PLoS Med. 2016;13(6): e1002049. https://doi.org/10.1371/journal.pmed.1002049. PMID: 27328301; PMCID: PMC4915619.[320]

Children and inferior turbinate reduction

Principally, this book is about the **Empty Nose Syndrome** and **Inferior Turbinate Management in Adults** and not about the pediatric population with enlarged inferior turbinates. However, because of the enormity of a possible lifespan of the surgical consequences in children, we think some cosmic frame of reference is vital to the childhood turbinate debate; therefore, a very succinct overview concerning children and inferior turbinate reduction is warranted; we are speaking about our children and a possible lifetime handicap!

When compared to adults, turbinate reduction surgery in children is beyond *debatable, it's contentious*. Anxiety centers around complications such as excessive bleeding, mucosal damage with synechia, possible alterations of future facial developmental growth plus long-term disruption of nasal physiologic function.

Numerous papers have been published in the medical literature touting one method or another for turbinate reduction in children from the "maximist" hair-raising terrifying total turbinectomy to a "minimalist" out-fracture (lateralization) of the inferior turbinate with submucous inferior turbinoplasty with or without tonsillectomy and adenoidectomy.

Often these procedures are associated with a totally truncated follow-up of less than five years, sometimes merely months. In 2010, Leong and colleagues contributed to the *International Journal of Pediatric Otorhinolaryngology* knowing full well that the subject of surgical management of turbinates in children was still patently prickly and considerably controversial. Their stated goal was: *"To evaluate the 'evidence' for inferior turbinate surgery in children suffering with chronic nasal congestion."* After their extensive literature search, only 11 selected studies fulfilled their inclusion criteria with ages ranging from one-year-old to 17 years of age and follow-up from a paltry 3 months to a substantial 14 years after surgery. With ($n = 730$) patients, 79.1% had turbinate surgery exclusively, as a "standalone procedure," while the other 21.9% had other procedures with an additional adenotonsillectomy, performed most frequently. Unfortunately, the outcome measures varied so significantly between studies that cross-study comparisons were impossible. However, after serious study and rightful reflection regarding turbinate surgery in children, Leong, Kubba, and White concluded:

> *"There is currently little evidence to support turbinate reduction surgery in children. The role of surgery, if any, has not been properly examined. Furthermore, the long-term effects on nasal airflow dynamics, nasal physiology, and long-term complications remain to be studied."*[322] *(Bold italics added)*

Empty Nose Syndrome. https://doi.org/10.1016/B978-0-443-10715-3.00009-3

Just a few years ago, in 2019, nine years after Leong et al.[322], a group from the Department of Otolaryngology-Head and Neck Surgery, Boston University, School of Medicine, and the Department of Surgery, Veterans Administration Medical Center, Boston, Massachusetts, stated their desire to compare the *"efficacy, duration, and complications"* while charting the evolution of different pediatric surgical methods (turbinectomy, electrocautery, lasers, submucous microdebridement, and radiofrequency) for managing pediatric inferior turbinate hypertrophy. We chose to report this paper because of the number ($n = 1,012$) of children involved. After a comprehensive literature review, they noted that pediatric surgeons are now thinking past "conservative" *medical* options in pursuit of surgical management. These authors acknowledge that surgery in children is an *"escalation"* in the management of inferior turbinate *"hypertrophy."* On the other hand, being ethically honest, these authors also acknowledged that in 2019:

> *"Still, no guidelines currently exist to help guide the escalation of management in children."*[323] (Bold italics added)

Yet, they pushed forward, justified by the gathering assembly of "medical failures" when 16 reviews (1989–2019) fulfilled their inclusion criteria ($n = 1,012$) children ranging from 1 to 17 years of age. Their study's *procedural characteristics* and *outcomes* are summarized in Tables 9.1 and 9.2 below.

It is clearly seen, Table 9.2, that the radiofrequency volumetric tissue reduction (RVTR) method has a short-lived follow-up from 6 weeks to 12 months. Komshian et al. drew support from their reference number 36. Bhattacharyya and Kepnes touting the advantages of coblation in adults with long-lasting reduction in nasal volume, subjective nasal airway improvement, and low complication rates all credited to mucosal preservation. RVTR steadily gained acceptance as a low-risk method in children as well, supported by reference number 36. Bhattacharyya N, Kepnes LJ. Clinical effectiveness of coblation inferior turbinate reduction. *Otolaryngol Head Neck Surg.* 2003;129(4):365–71. https://doi.org/10.1016/s0194-5998(0300634-x). PMID: 14574290.

Bhattacharyya and Kepnes simply had a modest ($n = 24$) patients with follow-up evaluations at 3 and 6 months. Nonetheless, they boldly and confidently concluded that:

> *"Coblation inferior turbinate reduction is an effective procedure for inferior turbinate hypertrophy. The clinical benefit persists at 6 months after the procedure."*

Of the papers contributed to the literature subsequent to the cautionary and analytical paper of Leong, Kubba, and White, in 2010, cited above,[322] many are cheering a *"conservative inferior turbinoplasty approach."*[323–328] Their canons were often, unfortunately and regrettably, rife with limitations, for example, retrospective results, limited patient numbers, limited follow-up, often less than one

Table 9.1 Overview of study characteristics.

Method	Number of studies	First author	Year	Study Types[a]	Number of patients	Patient age range
Turbinectomy	5	Thompson	1989	1	22	9–15
		Percodani	1996	1	38	9–16
		Weider	1998	1	64	3–15
		Segal	2003	1	227	3–10
		Arganbright	2015	2	21	1–17
Submucosal diathermy	2	Rejali	2004	2	11	6–16
		Montgomery	2011	1	47	3–14
Laser cautery	3	Pang	1995	1	20	6–15
		Araki	2001	3	22	9–15
		Rejali	2004	2	8	6–16
Submucous microdebridement	4	Chen	2007	3	120	9–14
		Cheng	2008	4	51	3–12
		Arganbright	2015	2	19	1–17
		Manzi	2017	1	43	5–17
Radiofrequency volumetric tissue reduction	5	O'Conner-Reina	2007	3	93	2–9
		Sullivan	2008	4	86	1–17
		Simeon	2010	3	9	6–16
		Bitar	2014	4	32	6–17
		Arganbright	2015	2	79	1–17

[a] (1) Retrospective case series, (2) retrospective comparative case series, (3) prospective case series, and (4) prospective cohort study.
Table 9.1 from Komshian SR, Cohen MB, Brook C, Levi JR. Inferior turbinate hypertrophy: a review of the evolution of management in children.[323]

Table 9.2 Pooled outcomes for each surgical technique.

Method	Subjective Improvement[a]	Follow-up	Complications
Turbinectomy	68%–93.4%	12–26 months	Bleed (0%–2.6%) Crusting (0%–3.1%) Synechia (0%–6.6%) Facial bone malformation (0% –0.44%)
Submucosal diathermy	36%–51%	23–72 months	Bleed (13%–18%) Pain (4%) Anosmia (7%)
Laser cautery	50%–90%	18–32 months	–
Submucous microdebridement	93%	3–12 months	–
Radiofrequency volumetric tissue reduction	93.6%–100%	6 weeks–12 months	Bleed (0%) Crusting (0%–8.6%) Synechia (0%)

[a] Outcomes are from reports from parental questionnaires and interviews.
Table 9.2 from Komshian SR, Cohen MB, Brook C, Levi JR. Inferior turbinate hypertrophy: a review of the evolution of management in children.[323]

year, merely months, some devoid of objective and or subjective outcome measures of "success," and others using simply subjective "symptom grading tools." Sadly, in the present era, that's just what's available; however, some papers require mention for their "conservative" mucosal preservation preference, necessarily functioning in lieu of randomized controlled trials (RCTs), which similarly are currently nonexistent for children.

The 2015 paper of Jill Arganbright and colleagues from Children's Hospital Colorado, Denver, University of Colorado (affiliated), presented a *"conservative inferior turbinoplasty approach"* from a pediatric population chart review from August 1, 2003, through August 1, 2013.[328] The mean age of the 107 children studied was 10.5 years (range, 1.2–17.9 years). They appraised three different isolated inferior turbinoplasty procedures which included:

(1) radiofrequency ablation in 72 children (67.3%)
(2) partial turbinate resection in 21 children (19.6%)
(3) microdebridement in 19 children (17.8%)

They observed no major complications and of the 107 patients, 63 parents (58.8%) accomplished a postoperative telephone interview with a mean follow-up of 4.55 years (range, 0.63–10.68 years). They documented that 34 patients

(54.0%) required persistent postsurgical symptomatic medical management. At the close, they concluded that:

> *"Inferior turbinoplasty showed overall utility and was safe and effective in the treatment of nasal obstruction in children for whom medical management had failed."[328]*

As previously presented, the honored work of Haight and Cole published in *The Laryngoscope* in 1983,[5] titled, "The site and function of the nasal valve" substantiated that the *head of the inferior turbinate* is the posterior portion of the internal nasal valve which acts as a flow limiting segment, an upstream resistor, which is much more significant in altering air flow, capable of producing nasal obstruction than an "obstructing adenoid" which is a downstream resistor. Unless an adenoid *"totally"* obstructs the nasopharynx, an anterior inferior turbinate enlargement is more significant than the adenoid in producing nasal airway obstruction and difficulty breathing.

Regarding aggressive pediatric inferior turbinate reduction procedures, we note the strikingly stunning 2003 paper of Samuel Segal and colleagues[113] writing in *American Journal of Rhinology,* March–April edition, page 72, the last sentence of their paper reads:

> **"Complete inferior turbinectomy should be considered in children** *who suffer from extremely enlarged inferior turbinates and who have failed to benefit from medical treatment or a more conservative surgical approach." (Bold italics added)*

We *vociferously and stridently* support the adroit comments of David Kennedy, then Editor-in-Chief of the *American Journal of Rhinology,* who in that same March–April edition, remarked, on page 69, regarding the work of Segal et al.[113]

> **"This study by Segal et al. reports no significant adverse effects from total inferior turbinectomy in 227 children with nasal obstruction."** *(Bold italics added)*

Kennedy carefully yet purposefully continues cautioning the reader as follows:

> *"Although it is appropriate for the Journal to present alternative opinions and ideas, it would seem appropriate for the reader to be **cautious in considering total inferior turbinectomy in children** until this cohort has been followed for a significantly longer period of time." (Bold italics added)*

The follow-up period that Segal et al. reported was:

> *"… of whom 179 children had significant relief of nasal obstruction at the 1-year follow-up."*

We add to Kennedy's sagaciously reproving position by arguing that ***all authors*** who operate on children have an ***explicit moral and ethical obligation*** *to the follow, report, and publish on the trajector*y of these *children* as they passage into adulthood. This "rational" demand is obvious, as firm long-term follow-up data can be the sure-footed guide for all future surgeons when weighing the therapeutic options for any and all future pediatric patients with symptomatically enlarged inferior turbinates.

Until proof by *solid evidence,* with well-executed RCTs, we along with Leong, Kubba, and White brashly and boisterously broadcast:

> *"Do not remove turbinates in children, since there is little evidence to support turbinate reduction surgery in childhood!"*[322] *(Bold italics with exclamation mark added)*

Unless there are a series of serious contradictory papers with powerful solid evidence challenging the cautions announced by Leong et al., we hold that their strongly held truths are self-evident and must be maintained until reversed and thrown asunder, replaced by a newly minted *"approximate temporary truth."*[322] (Bold italics added)

Ultimately the question is, what's the surgeon to do, when pressed to act, before solid evidence from a well executed RCT arrives to successfully manage the enlarged inferior turbinates of a child?

Remarkably, the mucosal-sparing approach has been "assumed" and "shown" to be safe and efficacious for the time being and can, apparently, as some suggested, be performed safely concurrently with other procedures such as tonsillectomy and adenoidectomy or with adenoidectomy alone. Due to the very limited and likely currently biased data and with marked uncertainty, regarding the "likelihood" of possible long-term adverse effects, the decision to perform surgical turbinate reduction in children depends on individual circumstances and surgical "clinical judgment," because we lack the evidence from well-conceived and well-performed RCTs.

For now, our preference is to respectfully follow the patients' parents (or responsible adult) holding authoritative dominance, along with courteously accepting the "clinical judgment," of a wise and honorable pediatric rhinologic surgeon.

Today, some type of *"conservative"* mucosal preserving turbinoplasty procedure is the plausible treatment of choice, for children who fail the obligatory three-month trial of intense medical management, as suggested by Argenbright et al. in their 2015 paper.[328] Microdebrider submucosal inferior turbinoplasty (**without** bony resection) with additional out-fracture (lateralization) of an inferior turbinate makes the most sense at this juncture without guidance from any RCTs.

Medical journals: judging the quality of the editors, the peer reviewers, plus the issue of plagiarism

10

Journals can be and often are extremely influential voices in setting standards of accepting and adjudicating submitted research to accurately and unbiasedly update and inform the profession. We depend upon the editors and the legions of peer reviewers for supreme sagacity with soaring standards of integrity when reviewing the submitted texts of thinking and data-rich experimental findings. Our unwritten covenant with the peer reviewers and their editors is they all act in the best interest of the profession, ultimately that is translated into, for the best interest of the patient. In a 2016 paper, "Why Most Clinical Research Is Not Useful," by John Ioannidis,[320] physician and professor at Stanford School of Medicine and codirector of Meta-Research Innovation Center at Stanford, claims that practicing physicians among others in the profession find very little useful information in medical journals.[320] He states that these medical journals can affect the standards of acceptable research by having an external group of reviewers assessing the clinical usefulness of papers to be published by some objective "Journal Clinical Usefulness Factor" by saying:

> "Overall, not only are most research findings false, but, furthermore, most of the true findings are not useful. Medical interventions should and can result in huge human benefit. It makes no sense to perform clinical research without ensuring clinical utility. Reform and improvement are overdue."[320]

> With that said, he does not blame the medical journal editors for useless research but sees that as an "opportunity" for improvements involving not only investigators "… but also institutions, funding mechanisms, the industry, **journals**, and many other stakeholders, including patients and the public."[320] (Bold italics added)

Previously, in a 2005 essay, *"Why Most Published Research Findings are False"* Ioannidis asserted,

"Simulations show that for most study designs and settings, it is more likely for a research claim to be false than true. Moreover, for many current scientific fields, claimed research findings may often be simply accurate measures of the prevailing bias."[329]

According to Wikipedia, as of 2020, "Why Most Published Research Findings are False" is the most widely accessed article from the Public Library of Science with over three million views.

Additionally, Ioannidis in his 2014 article "How to Make More Published Research True" he offers a thoughtful solicitous summary:

"To make more published research true—possibilities include the adoption of large-scale collaborative research; replication culture; registration; sharing; reproducibility practices; better statistical methods; standardization of definitions and analyses; more appropriate (usually more stringent) statistical thresholds; and improvement in study design standards, peer review, reporting and dissemination of research, and training of the scientific workforce."[330]

While the opinion of John Ioannidis regarding the responsibilities of medical journals was an oblique charge, a glancing tangential knock at medical journals in general, a coalition of diverse investigators from Croatia, France, and Spain, endeavored a straightforward direct inquiry of the medical journal collective with the candid inquiry: *"Is judging the quality of the editors and reviewers an legitimate area of inquiry?"*[331] This March 2019 paper by Cecilia Superchi and associates[331] "was the first comprehensive review" searching for tools for determining the quality of peer review reports. They cited references reaching from the original peer review referees of 18th century scientific journalism to the present day, offering dispassionate judgements for evaluating and improving scientific submissions. Numerous critics of the review process asked piercing perspicacious questions such as:

1. Is peer review: a flawed process at the heart of science and journals?
2. Who reviews the reviewers?
3. Editorial peer reviewers' recommendations at a general medical journal: are they reliable and do editors care?
4. Rereviewing peer review.
5. Peer review for biomedical publications: we can improve the system.
6. Make peer review scientific.
7. Custodians of high-quality science: are editors and peer reviewers good enough?

Realizing the need for validated tools that define the quality of peer-reviewed research reports, Superchi et al.[331] scoured PubMed, EMBASE (via Ovid), and The Cochrane Methodology Register (via The Cochrane Library) as well as Google finding 24 tools: 23 scales and one checklist, which could define the quality of peer review reports although, not one tool defined the word "quality." They concluded that while:

"Several tools are available to assess the quality of peer review reports; however, the development and validation process is questionable and the concepts evaluated by these tools vary widely."[331]

One out of four tools (25%) presented only one item asking the reviewer for the "overall quality" of the work. Those tools with more items gave a "summary score" without weighting of each individual scale. After all, how do you weight a scale? And what do the tools measure? To complicate matters, scales are considered controversial tools at best by some critical biostatisticians. The Risk of Bias tool clearly measures the trial conduct by providing clear support for adjudication. Of course, Superchi et al. pointed out that bias and uncertainty may occur using poorly designed tools:

"... that ("those tools") are not evidence-based, rigorously developed, validated, and reliable, and this is particularly true for tools that are used for evaluating interventions aimed at improving the peer review process in RCTs, thus affecting how trial results are interpreted."[331] ***Note ("those tools")*** *are added for clarity.*

The serious effort for this critical work comes down to the importance of the peer reviewer's comprehension and understanding of the scientific work offered in the paper under review. The consequences of the reviewer's findings are obviously critical, requiring astute interpretative rigor, so the editorial decision is scientifically justified. Admirably, the authors plan to continue the quest for new *validated quality assessment tools for peer review reports* in biomedical research. Their plans involve surveying journal editors and authors alike by initiating and managing an international online survey regarding the quality of peer reviewer's reports for developing new evaluation tools that can be used for appraising interventions aimed at improving the peer review process especially in the analysis of randomized controlled trials (RCTs).[331]

Since the first international Peer Review Congress, about 30 years ago, Drummond Rennie former member of the Commission on Research Integrity for the US Public Health Service, and former president of the World Association of Medical Editors writing in *Nature* in 2016 made his plea in the paper's title: "Let's Make Peer Review Scientific."[332]

There are problems in medical journal paradise. There are accusations that almost any hypothesis of trivia or a tattered fragmented thread of an idea can be published because evidence abounds revealing that peer reviewers rarely receive formal preparation for their responsibility. Therefore, it's not surprising that their competence, especially in biostatistics, and overall capability to uncover errors and detect reporting deficiencies is unacceptably wanting. Other studies showed that:

"... there is still a lack of evidence supporting the use of interventions to improve the quality of the peer review process."[332]

Therefore, the need is urgent for improving the quality of peer review reporting and for finding instruments (tools) for evaluating and improving the quality of those reports.[332]

Merely a few years ago in 2017, in Chicago, Illinois, David Moher presented a plenary talk at the eighth International Congress on Peer Review and Scientific Publication (below) entitled:

Custodians of High-Quality Science: Are Editors and Peer Reviewers Good Enough? which is available at: https://www.youtube.com/watch?v=RV2tknDtyDs&t=454s.

Eighth International Congress on Peer Review and Scientific Publication

Enhancing the quality and credibility of science

September 10-12, 2017 | Swissôtel, Chicago, IL, USA

Finally, a closer look at the dark side of medical journal's lunar landscape, scrutinized for sure, as there are malevolent forces in our medical solar system even among us in their guise as nobles in our glorious profession. Enter the sanguine orthopedic honorable triad of Joseph Buckwalter, Vernon Tolo, and Regis O'Keefe orthopedists all, asking *"How do you know it is true? Integrity in research and publications: AOA critical issues."* These three musketeers, armed with truth, blasted some of the notorious evil perpetrators and perverts of the sacred scientific trust. Note: *The Three Musketeers* was written[333] by the French novelist Alexandre Dumas in 1844 about heroic, honorable, moral men fighting for justice. As surgeons, Buckwalter, Tolo, and O'Keefe focused on orthopedic practice, but their cautions and admonitions apply to all in medicine. Explicitly, and without question, we all acknowledge that scientific research findings have led to momentous changes in medical and surgical practice to the betterment of our human kind. Research can certainly be deliberately biased owing to lucrative patents owned by investigators with commercial consulting arrangements within the high drama of a competitive research environment.

Disgustingly, some current research has been characterized:

"… by an increase in plagiarism, falsification or manipulation of data, selected presentation of results, research bias, and inappropriate statistical analyses." [333] *(Bold italics added)*

In homage to the exquisitely laudable efforts of Buckwalter, Tolo, and O'Keefe, we have chosen to reproduce a portion of their applicable text, citing the maleficence we must all be alerted to, *never naïve please*, always aware to the possibility of crimes and misdemeanors in the revered name of medical research.[333]

*"The misrepresentation of natural observation has existed for as long as scientific research has been recorded. Ptolemy, the renowned second-century Egyptian astronomer, recorded astronomical measurements that he could not have made. **Ptolemy's work,** purporting to prove that Earth was the center of the universe, influenced science and philosophy for centuries. **Copernicus,** who revolutionized our understanding of both Earth and man's place in the universe, was accused of heresy when he reported a conflicting celestial configuration based on appropriate scientific methods and accurate measurements. The legendary physicist and **Nobel laureate Robert Millikan (1868−1953),** who discovered the negative charge of the electron, selected only 58 of 140 observations for inclusion in his scientific presentations. While this selective use of data likely improved precision and the credibility of his claims, it did not truly represent his actual scientific findings. **Sir Cyril Burt (1883−1971),** a noted British psychologist, fabricated (extrapolated) data to show that human intelligence is 75% inherited. His work influenced educational programs and policies for generations."[333](Bold italics added)*

*"From 1996 to 2008, **Dr. Scott Reuben** published a series of articles that examined the potential role of cyclooxygenase-2 (COX-2) specific inhibitors in controlling postoperative pain following orthopedic surgery. In a series of carefully designed and double-blind placebo-controlled studies, Dr. Reuben established that Celebrex (celecoxib; Pfizer), Bextra (valdecoxib; Pfizer), and Vioxx (rofecoxib; Merck) dramatically improved pain management for patients undergoing joint replacement, spine fusion, and anterior cruciate ligament reconstruction and decreased the complications associated with the standard use of opiates.[3] Dr. Reuben, a Professor of Anesthesiology and Pain Medicine at Tufts and the Chief of Acute Pain at Baystate Medical Center, was widely recognized for revolutionizing pain management for orthopedic patients. A 2007 editorial in Anesthesia and Analgesia stated that Reuben had been at the "forefront of redesigning pain management protocols" through his "carefully planned" and "meticulously documented studies.[(333)"4](Bold italics added)*

*"In 2008, it was discovered that two abstracts submitted by **Dr. Reuben** for Baystate Medical Center's Annual Research Week lacked institutional review board approval. Investigation showed that **Dr. Reuben** had never enrolled patients or performed the studies described in the manuscripts. Further review resulted in Baystate requesting medical journals to retract a combined total of 21 of **Dr. Reuben's** papers. **Dr. Reuben's** advocacy for COX-2 inhibitors to treat postoperative pain appeared in reviews, textbooks, and practice guidelines. Beginning in 2000,*

*Reuben advocated that physicians should shift from the use of first-generation nonsteroidal antiinflammatory drugs to the use of Vioxx, Celebrex, and Bextra to treat musculoskeletal pain.[3] **Reuben** urged the United States Food and Drug Administration (FDA) not to restrict use of the drugs he studied, citing their efficacy and safety. Drug companies organized educational programs and symposia on the basis of Reuben's reports. Various editorials noted that "millions of orthopedic patients' pain management has been affected by Dr. ha ha Ha ha-ha did you have dinner ready Reuben's research" and "Reuben's studies led to the sale of billions of dollars of Celebrex and Vioxx."[5,333](Bold italics added)*

Authors' (EBK, OF) note from Wikipedia: **"Scott Reuben plead guilty to "health-care fraud" and was convicted on February 24, 2010 and served six months in federal prison. His Massachusetts medical license was permanently revoked."**

"Reuben's *work had actually come under scrutiny as early as 2007, when several anesthesiologists noticed his studies never showed negative results [4]. Greg Koski, former director of the Office for Human Research Protections, said the* fraud *was unusual because* **Reuben was able to carry it on for almost 13 years without being caught by the peer review process."**(Bold italics added)

"In 1998, **Dr. Andrew Jeremy Wakefield and coauthors published a study in** *The* Lancet **of 12 children, suggesting a link between the measles, mumps, and rubella (MMR) vaccine and autism.**[6] *The results were widely reported by the media, were popularized on a variety of web sites, resulted in the refusal of vaccination by many parents, and led to lawsuits by parents of autistic children against vaccine manufacturers. The Lancet and the press later learned that* **Wakefield had received a $110,000 payment from the Legal Aid Board prior to publishing the paper. The Legal Aid Board was seeking evidence** *that could be used in lawsuits against vaccine manufacturers and, following publication of the article, provided an additional* **$674,000 payment to Wakefield. A retrospective review of the data used by Wakefield revealed that the diagnosis and/or dates of records were changed for all 12 children in the publication report so as to support the author's conclusions.**[7,8] *The Lancet partially retracted* **Wakefield's** *paper in 2004 and later issued a full retraction. The General Medical Council of the United Kingdom found* **Wakefield guilty of professional misconduct** *(autism fraud) and* **revoked his medical license.** *However, public suspicion that vaccinations can cause autism persists. Vaccination rates have dropped sharply in many countries, including the United States, and this drop in vaccinations is a major contributor to the increased incidence of measles and mumps, resulting in outbreaks of the diseases and deaths in multiple countries.*[9] *Subsequent studies have demonstrated* **no link between the MMR vaccine and autism.** *Position statements supporting* **vaccination and the absence of a link with autism have been released by the Centers for Disease Control and Prevention, the American Academy of Pediatrics, the Institute of Medicine, the National Academy of Sciences, and the UK National Health Service"**.[333] **(Bold italics added)**

Review, finishing touches, and closure

11

Following our literature review, apparently other observers also agree with us that the empty nose syndrome (ENS) is a strikingly important yet uncommon clinical entity because of the profound physical suffering especially with breathing difficulties and a surprisingly high incidence of disabling emotional anguish experienced by so many of these patients.[2–4,18–28,33,73,76,214,335,345,353,355]

The difficulty of breathing is frequently associated with dyspnea (breathlessness), the so-called paradoxical nasal obstruction with a sense of suffocation despite a "wide open" nasal airway.[18–21,55,347] The emotional torment encountered by ENS patients is astonishingly high, over 50% in the Mayo study[18], and in most other accounts also, with anxiety, depression, and suicidal ideation (near 43% in one study[340]) are the usual; mental misery an unexpected comorbidity.[20,33,62,73,74,76,334–350]

ENS, a secondary atrophic rhinitis (AR), is almost always iatrogenic in origin excluding those resulting from the inexorable and inevitable aging process which we have documented or from an infectious process produced by *Klebsiella pneumoniae ozaenae*, which we consider as primary AR.

Yes, ENS, most often, occurs secondary to an iatrogenic reduction of turbinate tissue, secondary to therapeutic turbinate trauma (TTT), with symptoms that are of unpredictable intensity. Fundamentally, this occurs secondary to a procedure on the turbinate(s) which injures immeasurable amounts of functioning turbinates mucosal and submucosal (lamina propria-stroma) tissue. The intervention is usually and predominately designed to reduce an enlarged inferior turbinate to improve a patient's breathing function; however, in some individuals the turbinate procedure of puzzling and inexplicably produces ENS. In the section below, we will explore some theories regarding the etiology and pathophysiology of ENS.

We have personally cared for more than 300 ENS patients. Based on our reading of the literature, to avoid ENS, we have emphasized the need for conservative surgical intervention when treating patients with inferior turbinate enlargement ("hypertrophy") who failed intense medical management. When treating those souls suffering from ENS, our required responsibility is for sensitive compassionate comprehensive care which we will proffer for you in detail below.

Unfortunately, currently (2022) there are no curative or even subtotally restorative therapies for ENS though we will present recent results, promising pronouncements from the literature, regarding surgical options assuring favorable "long-lasting" or "long-term" benefits for our ENS patients, although there is no long-term follow up, usually in months not years.

Empty Nose Syndrome. **https://doi.org/10.1016/B978-0-443-10715-3.00011-1**

We condensed and concentrated much, certainly not all, of the currently known knowledge regarding ENS (up to the first of November 2022), with an exhaustive extensive bibliography, into a single "comprehensive" resource so each practitioner may reach their own conclusion(s) about this underappreciated syndrome along with the inestimable risks associated with any turbinate reduction procedure for improving nasal breathing, especially when nasal function (physiology) is often seemingly unseemly slighted or ignominiously grossly and deliberately ignored. Oddly, even presumably "minor" turbinate trauma may subsequently result in ENS, weeks, months to years later, superimposed, as it were, on the aging process with its inexorable dwindling capacity for fulfilling fundamental functional processes.

After initial recognition, preliminary treatment for ENS usually involves topical medications for crust and odor control along with pain management (post-traumatic neurogenic pain) and psychiatric evaluation with treatment, when required, since the psychologic burden and emotional suffering are significant, as over 50% of ENS patients experience emotional distress, anxiety, and depression, many with suicide ideation, which, in some cases, was not evident prior to the onset of ENS.

Possible surgical intervention is considered as a last resort since, currently, the postsurgical data lack long-term (years) proof of "permanent" success (relief of symptoms), although most recently (2020−22) a number of reports have assured, with data, a reduction in symptoms after specific surgical intervention(s), which we will analyze and discuss in Section 8, Surgical treatment of ENS, below.

We offer deliberations and reflections regarding safe management of nasal airway obstruction secondary to pathology of the inferior turbinate. We present four different classification systems for inferior turbinate enlargement ("hypertrophy") and summarize the "latest thinking" with a few evidence based proposals for inferior turbinate management from the literature; intending and expecting to avoid ENS.

Presently, ENS is best prevented by minimizing inferior and middle turbinate tissue trauma during turbinate reduction (modification) procedures, period. Future randomized controlled trials (RCTs) are indispensable to definitively answer the inferior and middle surgical treatment questions.

With the opening sentence to Chapter 4 "Treatment options for ENS," we are confronted with the reality as to why the "empty nose syndrome" is so challenging; not only the challenge of accurate diagnosis and the fact that the mean time from therapeutic turbinate trauma to diagnosis is often measured in months to years, and as a consequence, we emphasize the need for prevention by intelligent management of symptomatic inferior turbinate hypertrophy. These facts require you, dear readers, to enter into the world of the turbinate anatomy, physiology, surgical debates, evidence-based medicine (EBM), and the moral and ethical search for data-driven turbinate studies that will guide we surgeons to provide successful patient care.

With our wide-ranging bibliography of almost 400 references and our historical journey over the past 100 years of turbinate surgery, in Chapter 5, plus the variety of

contemporary management options for treating enlarged symptomatic inferior turbinates are presented in Chapter 7 as we endeavored to give the text the extensive
comprehensive sense of accurate authoritativeness.

The literature review was the consequential harbinger for necessarily enter-
taining EBM. EBM advised, rather demanded, a most sensible and logical approach
to inferior turbinate reduction which to date (2022) is based on the landmark work of
Professor Desiderio Passali, MD, and his co-workers who performed a randomized
turbinate study, following their 382 patients, carefully collecting objective breathing
and physiologic data, at four years and six years after surgery. Passali et al.[211,216]
concluded:

> *"After 6 years, only submucosal resection resulted in optimal long-term normal-
> ization of nasal patency and in restoration of mucociliary clearance and local
> secretory IgA production to a physiological level with few postoperative compli-
> cations. We recommend, in spite of the greater surgical skill required, submucosal
> resection combined with lateral displacement as the first-choice technique for the
> treatment of nasal obstruction due to hypertrophy of the inferior turbinates."[211]*

Chapter 8 is a uniquely interesting chapter as we grappled with ethical issues
related to advances in medicine especially concerning introducing new and novel
surgical procedures including the potential role of sham surgery and its application
to RCTs when an operation is indicated.

We present an up-to-date discussion of the Consolidated Standards of Reporting
Trials (CONSORT) requirements, propensity score matching (PSM), clinical practice guidelines (CPGs), and the entire issue of conflicts of interest (COI) as these
topics are all considered, deliberated, and explored in depth since rhinology is still
coping with these issues in a very practical every-day sense.

We endeavored to broaden the discussion beyond the diagnosis and treatment options of the "empty nose syndrome" as we explored EBM its origins, its applications,
and limitations especially as related to the direction of future rhinologic research investigations resulting in an enlightened approach to practical clinical practice.

The dilemmas of the rhinologist are examined when data from RCTs are unavailable since "the crucial study" was never performed. The argument of empiricism
(evidence first) versus rationalism (clinical judgment) takes center stage specifically
when data from a "definitive" RCT are "limited, incomplete, inconclusive, conflicting, or starkly nonexistent." We, authors, argue and maintain that when empirical
data are unavailable, then experience and clinical judgment governs as the indispensable key rational alternative. The ethics of using placebos are also considered
along with the distinction and differentiation between "research" and "care" as in
surgical research trials and **surgical clinical care**. The nature of medical progress
is a subject that is also examined especially since the cited work of Prasad et al. from
the National Institute of Health (NIH) revealed that *"the reversal of established medical practice is common and occurs across all classes of medical practice."*[271] In
fact, Prasad et al. found that 40.2%, of established practices they reviewed (2044

original articles), was reversed (discontinued) because that practice was *either useless or harmful*.[271]

The work of Prasad et al. clarified the fact that medicine aspires to apply the finest, most accurate, information obtainable at the time, which allows for "knowledgeable guesses," which of course, is subject to change.

We, as physicians and surgeons are obliged to endure "uncertainty" acknowledging the reality that medical theories and practices are subject to dislocation, disruption, continuous change, and improvements since that is the nature of medical progress. Realize that there is a temporal quality to truth as the work of Sir Karl R. Popper, the 20th century philosopher of science, instructed us, by introducing the concept of an "approximate temporary truth".

Regarding children, Chapter 9, again there is a shockingly scandalous lack of RCTs for guiding the surgeon toward intelligent inferior turbinate surgical decisions for the pediatric populations. Leong and colleagues (2010) thought that:

> *"There is currently little evidence to support turbinate reduction surgery in children. The role of surgery, if any, has not been properly examined. Furthermore, the long-term effects on nasal airflow dynamics, nasal physiology and long-term complications remain to be studied."*[322]

Despite that fact of "little evidence" and "no guidelines," we suggest a "rational" surgical approach, for now, which, after our literature study, we, your authors (EBK, OF), advocate for children that:

> *"Some type of "conservative" mucosal preserving turbinoplasty procedure with an additional out-fracture (lateralization) for children who fail the obligatory three month trial of intense medical management without guidance from any RCT."*

At a minimum, until the arrival of convincing rational guidelines from a well-conducted RCT, we make the "moral and ethical" demand that surgeons who operate on these youngsters, must follow, reported and published on the trajectory of these children as they passage into adulthood. It's critical that we establish and set a "high bar" before approving and accepting any new surgical procedures or technologies.

An academically yet ultimately pragmatic and consequential Chapter 10 deals with medical journals and issues regarding judging the quality of peer reviewers which of course has consequence as to which articles are published which in turn can profoundly influence our medical and surgical practices. The all-inclusive challenging question of evaluating journal editors and peer reviewers is addressed, and the need for validated tools for assessing the quality of peer review reports is presented and considered.

We cite, demanding reflection, the 2016 provocative paper by John Ioannidis, MD, professor at Stanford School of Medicine, in which Ioannidis argues that most clinical research is "Not Useful."[320]

In this, our last chapter, Chapter 11 Review, Finishing Touches, and Closure, we journey through and beyond the "empty nose syndrome," appropriately so, as we contemporaneously, almost up to the very minute, offer the overview as to where we are and where we, as a profession, need to go first protecting patients by preventing ENS when we operate on turbinates and when needed, treating those patients plagued with "empty nose syndrome."

We demand lofty goals for medical science to seek and achieve that any noble future direction in medicine must be based on high-quality validated evidence-based published studies that provide actionable steps to protect the interest of all of our past, present, and future patients, short of that lofty moral aspiration, we rely on experienced clinical judgment, realizing that it may eventually prove to be biased and flawed requiring revision, "safety" first followed by "useful" in all her glory.

1. Managing the empty nose syndrome patient—summary

1.1 Empty nose syndrome exists

In 2020, the American Rhinologic Society (ARS) website stated:

> *"The exact incidence of ENS is currently unknown. There are still thousands of patients experiencing ENS."*

Apparently, ENS is more common than originally thought, with over 80 literature citations listed in our Table 1.1 from 2001 to November 1, 2022 acquired from the PubMed database. ENS appears on numerous worldwide websites and in multiple languages including: Arabic, Chinese, Dutch, French, German, Hebrew, Italian, Korean, Portuguese, Russian, Spanish, and Turkish among others. The evidence is mounting that ENS is now recognized as a valid (authentic) physiologic disorder with a rising flood of research and clinical interest with over 40 papers listed on the PubMed database with Empty Nose Syndrome in the title over the past four years alone, 2019–22, Table 1.1.

1.2 Pertinent nasal physiology

The mucosa is the organ of the nose. Nasal anatomy is created to serve our physiological needs. Olfaction, breathing (respiration), and defense are optimized when air flows through the nose. Regarding nasal breathing, the nose offers a critical upper airway resistance, provided by the internal nasal valve area, which includes the head of the inferior turbinate. The nose creates the proper resistance ("**resistor function**"—the internal nasal valve area) for breathing; lung expansion, enhancing venous return. Charging the inspired air ("**diffusor function**"—turbulent air flow) for the sense of breathing, providing warmth (temperature) and moisture (humidity) to the inspired air enabling ideal CO_2 and O_2 exchange to occur optimally at the alveolar level, which is after all, respiration.

The trigeminal nerve mediates the perception of normal nasal airflow by action potentials from the transient receptor potentials melastatin 8 (TRPM8) receptors that are located in the mucosa, goblet cells, and vessels, not in the connective tissues. These TRPM8 receptors, the trigeminal "cool" thermoreceptors, are triggered by the wall shearing stress effects of the inspired air currents cooling of the nasal mucosa providing the sense of normal breathing.[33,74,353−355]

The surface area of the nasal mucosa and submucosa (lamina propria, stroma) is increased with intact turbinate tissue, allowing the defensive mechanisms of the nose to protect (defend) us in the following four ways: mechanical, humoral, cellular, and various nasal reflex defenses, which we have summarized and presented for the reader earlier in the text in Chapter 1. Especially interesting are the humoral defenses that include immunoglobulins IgA and IgG and the cytokines that are released by white blood cells and fibroblasts including the important interleukins (Il) include: Il-4, Il-5, Il-8, and Il-13. Antimicrobial secretory proteins include: lactoferrin (Lf), lysozyme (Ly), and human beta-defensin 1 (hBD-1) are also components of the nasal humoral defense system.

The other interesting defense system is the cellular defense living and breathing within the submucosa (lamina propria, stroma) including the dendritic cells that present foreign proteins to T and B lymphocytes designed for initiating immune responses. Remarkably dazzling.

1.3 Symptoms of ENS

The hallmark symptoms of ENS are fluctuating, variable, and protean including many of the following symptomatic indicators of ENS listed below:

1. Paradoxical nasal airway obstruction (nasal "congestion," difficulty breathing, "breathlessness," *often with a sense of suffocation*)
2. Nasal crusting, nasal dryness ("rhinitis sicca"), bleeding (varying degrees of epistaxis)
3. Inability to feel nasal airflow
4. Foul (fetid) odor (often noted by others) with thick nasal discharge and post-nasal "drip"
5. Anosmia or hyposmia
6. Headache
7. Pain, localized nasal facial pain (post-traumatic neuropathic pain)
8. Disturbed sleep (with secondary symptoms of fatigue and lethargy)
9. Aprosexia nasalis (inability to concentrate)
10. Disturbance in the sense of "well-being"
11. Impaired quality-of-life
12. Emotional comorbidity (anxiety, clinical depression, suicidal ideation)

Remarkably, not astonishingly, the mental health burden (emotional comorbidity) experienced by ENS patients is generally over 50%, including anxiety, depression, and suicide ideation approaching 43% in one study.[18,20,33,62,73,74,76,334−350]

ENS patients with suicidal ideation (thoughts) consistently experienced and interpreted their symptoms as severe, and as such these patients must be identified to avert a catastrophic tragic ending. As a consequence of this reality, systematic "routine" psychological evaluation is mandatory as part of the medical assessment and management of all diagnosed ENS patients; unquestionably needed before any contemplated surgical intervention as the effect of "surgical failure" could profoundly and adversely impact a peak psychologically vulnerable person. The self-rated questionnaires such as Beck Anxiety Inventory (BAI) or Generalized Anxiety Disorder (GAD-7) for anxiety or the Beck Depression Inventory, updated version, (BDI-II) or Patient Health Questionnaire (PHQ-9) for depression are reliable diagnostic tools and aids for determining anxiety and depression.

Summary of applicable diagnostic investigations for ENS:

1. History of previous turbinate surgery and symptoms—can be strongly suggestive for ENS
2. Endoscopy-nonspecific, but can document turbinate surgical resection
3. Imaging-nonspecific, but can document turbinate surgical resection
4. Testing/questionnaire for ENS
   a. Breathing tests-nonspecific
   b. Computational fluid dynamics (CFD)—can be strongly suggestive for ENS
   c. *Cotton test-specific for ENS
   d. Menthol test-impaired in ENS
   e. Nasal nitric oxide (nNO) test levels—reduced in ENS
   f. Olfactory testing-nonspecific
   g. Tissue biopsy—can be strongly suggestive of ENS
   h. *Questionnaire-empty nose syndrome 6 item questionnaire (ENS6Q)—can be strongly suggestive of ENS
   i. *Questionnaire-the 22-item Sinonasal Outcome Test (SNOT-22)
   j. *Questionnaire-the Nasal Obstruction Symptom Evaluation (NOSE) Instrument—grading the degree of nasal obstruction
   k. Psychological testing—with self-rated questionnaires are nonspecific but supportive
      1. * Generalized Anxiety Disorder (GAD-7) for anxiety
      2. * Patient Health Questionnaire-9 (PHQ-9) for depression

* See Appendix for details: The appendix contains seven items: (1) a brief history of Professor Maurice H. Cottle, MD; (2) the Empty Nose Syndrome 6 questionnaire (ENS6Q); (3) the Sino-Nasal Outcome test 20-25 (SNOT20-25) for ENS; (4) Nasal Obstruction Symptom Evaluation (NOSE) Instrument; (5) the cotton test, and how to perform it; (6) the questionnaire Generalized Anxiety Disorder (GAD-7); (7) the Patient Health Questionnaire-9 (PHQ-9) for depression.

Consider the "spectrum of disease" concept. The diagnosis of any illness or disease process is made when that particular process becomes manifest, obviously symptomatically observable, first to the patient, then to the physician. Most often termed, the onset, as the initial stage of the clinical presentation of any illness. In some, disease development evolves, becoming a clear clinical illness. In others, the disease process may remain subclinical, somewhat asymptomatic, or range from mildly manifest and manageable to severe and intractable or even fatal (suicide); as was the case with four of our patients (neither of us operated on any of these unfortunate despondent suicidal ENS patients). This range and scope of illness is titled the "spectrum of disease."

When considering and processing the range of symptoms and treatment options for ENS patients, it is valuable to adopt this longitudinal "spectrum of disease" view about this protean, fluctuating, oscillating disease process; trying to identify the "precise" stage within the "continuum of disease" that you are meeting in a particular ENS patient can be of tremendous utility. If early in the course of illness you may initially choose medical management including psychologic support and referral after positive psychological screening tests, as this emotional component may require the most aggressive management at this juncture or at any time you meet the ENS patient during the continuum of their disease development, especially before contemplating any invasive treatment plan, especially surgery, but including injections.

Thinking broadly, we classify ENS as an overlapping physical, emotional, primarily noninfectious, secondary AR, iatrogenic disorder.

Currently there are *no absolute* diagnostic standards for ENS; however, the diagnosis is practically and predictably established by the patient's exclusive history of previous nasal turbinate reductive treatment, symptoms of paradoxical nasal airway obstruction (difficulty breathing despite a nonobstructing "open airway"), crusting, dryness, feeling of an open airway, and suffocation with frequent emotional symptoms of anxiety and depression. The intranasal examination with nasal endoscopic inspection is supplemented by computed tomography (CT) of the nose and paranasal sinuses, which is suggestive but not diagnostic, unless the turbinates have been surgically removed (resected) clearly leaving the telltale remaining surgical stumps as evidentiary proof.

1.4 History and symptoms

The history of previous nasal surgery explicitly turbinate surgery more specifically an inferior turbinate procedure although middle turbinate modification may also herald the arrival of ENS although less frequently than inferior therapeutic turbinate trauma. The 22-item Sinonasal Outcome Test (SNOT-22) is extremely helpful in diagnosing ENS as it is a validated patient symptom questionnaire.[350] The empty nose 6 item questionnaire (ENS6Q) is valuable, very strongly suggestive for ENS when the symptom score exceeds 10.5 (>11) of their subjective symptoms on the ENS6Q.[31] For the empty nose 6 item questionnaire (ENS6Q), the scoring ranges from 0 to 5 with 0 meaning no symptoms to 5 with extremely severe symptoms and with a total score over 10.5 (>11) is suggestive of ENS.[31]

1.5 Nasal endoscopy

Nasal endoscopy with the frequent finding of surgically truncated turbinates found on intranasal examination correctly correlates with the patient's history in many cases, although not all.

1.6 Imaging

Imaging, especially CT is exceptionally effective in visually documenting resected turbinate tissue(s). The CT scan often displays a cavernous expansion of the intranasal airway with the absence or reduction of various amount of one or both inferior turbinates and reduction or absence of one or both middle turbinates which have been previously surgically reduced or resected. On the other hand, at times, the CT appears "normal," yet the patient has had a previous turbinate procedure or procedures and the functional integrity of the turbinate(s) has been functionally compromised; a blatant case of ENS may exhibit normal appearing intranasal structures, especially when a submucosal turbinoplasty or **n**on-surgical **T**urbinate **R**eductive **A**djunctive **P**rocedure (n-s TRAP) has been performed.

1.7 Testing in ENS

1.7.1 Cotton test—specific for ENS

There are specific and nonspecific tests for ENS, and the cotton test is considered specific, which involves placing a dry cotton (plug) pledget (in an unmedicated nose) in the region of the previously resected structure(s), usually in the region of previously resected head(s) of the inferior turbinate(s). The test is "positive" if the patient reports a reduction (lessening) of their nasal symptom severity score on repeat ENS6Q (compared to pretest ENS6Q score), while the cotton (plug) pledget is in place.[32]

1.7.2 Olfactory test—nonspecific for ENS

Olfaction tests are nonspecific, suggestive but not diagnostic. We use the modified Sumner olfactory test for all our rhinology patients.[147]

1.7.3 Menthol test—impaired in ENS

In a number of separate studies, the menthol detection test was established to be lower in patients with ENS.[43,335,355,358–359]

1.7.4 Breathing tests—nonspecific for ENS

The breathing tests, including rhinomanometry and acoustic rhinometry, are nonspecific and not diagnostic of ENS.[333,345]

1.7.5 Nasal nitric oxide test levels—reduced in ENS

Low nNO levels are usually seen in ENS.[344]

1.7.6 Computational fluid dynamics—strongly suggestive for ENS

Currently there are a number of CFD studies for ENS patients.[335,354,361−364] The results are specific for ENS in that patients with ENS demonstrated reduced nasal air flow rates at the inferior regions of the nasal cavity, where they should normally be higher, as the airflow distribution shifts upward toward the region of the middle meatus. The intimate interaction between the air flow column and the nasal mucosa, measured as wall sheer stress, was decreased. These findings of lower flow rates with lower resistance values strongly suggest ENS; although they are not absolutely diagnostic, these findings are consistent in ENS patients.[335,354,361−364]

1.7.7 Psychological testing—nonspecific but supportive

*"*Self-rated questionnaires such as Beck Anxiety Inventory, (BAI) or Generalized Anxiety Disorder (GAD-7) for anxiety or the Beck Depression Inventory, updated version, (BDI-II) or Patient Health Questionnaire (PHQ-9) for depression are reliable diagnostic tools and aids for determining anxiety and depression. The Minnesota Multiphasic Personality Inventory (MMPI) assesses personality style rather than explicitly designed for depression/anxiety. If patients are outpatients and not severely compromised, the self-rated scales are adequate and acceptable. However, if a person is psychiatrically or neurologically ill requiring intensive services such as hospitalization, then the patient should be assessed with an observer-rated scale such as the Hamilton Anxiety Scale or the Hamilton Depression Scale."*

*Personal communication: Teresa A. Rummans, MD.
Donald and Lucy Dayton Professor of Psychiatry, Mayo Clinic.

The following self-rated questionnaires are very valuable in managing ENS patients as they help identify anxiety and depression which may require professional emotional support:

1. Generalized anxiety disorder (GAD-7)
2. Patient health questionnaire (PHQ-9)
3. Beck anxiety inventory (BAI)
4. Beck depression inventory, updated version (BDI-II)

Note: The BAI is not in the public domain, but it is a copyrighted measure by the developer, Dr. Aaron T. Beck. The measure can be purchased from Pearson Assessment at www.pearsonassessments.com.

1.7.8 Tissue biopsy—strongly suggestive

Wu et al. (2021) presented the histological review of some 17 ENS patients and a control group of six people.[365] Tissue biopsies were performed at the midpoint of the inferior turbinate revealing squamous metaplasia (76%), submucosal fibrosis (94%), and a lower submucosal gland population when compared to controls. In their ENS patients' samples, the nasal respiratory epithelium was characteristically intact. Additionally, a unique histological change called goblet cell metaplasia was found in the ENS group, and this ENS group had a significantly lower expression level of transient receptor potential melastatin subtype 8 (TRPM8).* Immunohistochemical staining was performed for TRPM8 and is found in the epithelium, goblet cells, and in the submucosal vessels.

*The transient receptor potential melastatin subtype 8 (TRPM8) is a nonselective, multimodal ion channel, activated by low temperatures (<28°C), pressure, and cooling compounds (menthol, icilin). Experimental evidences indicated a role of TRPM8 in cold thermal transduction … From González-Muñiz R, Bonache MA, Martín-Escura C, Gómez-Monterrey. Recent Progress in TRPM8 Modulation: An Update. Int J Mol Sci. 2019 May 28; 20(11): 2618. https://doi.org/10.3390/ijms20112618. PMID: 31141957; PMCID: PMC6600640.

Gill et al.[33] believing ENS as a true physiologic disorder involving altered nasal airflow, not primarily an "uncloaked psychiatric problem," held that the major advances for assessing and diagnosing ENS patients included the following:

> *"ENS is increasingly becoming recognized as a legitimate, physiologic disease entity. As such, it is important for clinicians to understand the most up-to-date diagnostic tools to assess ENS, confirm the diagnosis, and create a more standardized means to counsel these complex patients. For the purposes of this review article, we assume that ENS is a true sinonasal disease with a physiologic foundation consistent with altered nasal airflow. We review these diagnostic techniques as well as mental health comorbidities associated with ENS".[33]*

Emphasized above, the empty nose 6 item questionnaire (ENS6Q) is valuable as it's very strongly suggestive for ENS when the symptom score exceeds 10.5 (>11) of their subjective symptoms on the ENS6Q.[31] The cotton test reported by Thamboo et al. used the ENS6Q to validate an office-based physical examination maneuver as another provocative supportive adjunct in confirming the diagnosis of ENS. The test itself was accomplished in the absence of any topical intranasal sprays, where a fashioned plug (pledget) of cotton was placed in the patient's inferior meatal space that was partially or completely devoid of inferior turbinate tissue. The cotton remains in place for approximately 20—30 min, and the ENS6Q is performed prior to testing; after 20—30 min while the cotton is in place (situ), the ENS6Q is repeated and for one final time after cotton removal, a third time.[32]

To review, the ENS6Q is obtained prior, during, and after the insertion of the cotton for the cotton test ENS6Q which occurs during three conditions:

a. Precotton placement, ENS6Q testing
b. Cotton in place (situ), after 20—30 min, ENS6Q testing
c. Postcotton (after removal), ENS6Q testing
  1. The ENS6Q, which is a patient reported outcome measure that was validated using the SNOT-22.[31]
  2. The cotton test helps confirm the diagnosis of ENS using the ENS6Q specifically and especially if the patient has an improvement (reduction) in

symptoms with the cotton in place. A patient with a positive cotton test *might* benefit from potential inferior turbinate augmentation procedures.[32]

3. CT imaging is helpful although not diagnostic for ENS.

4. Computational fluid dynamics (CFD) studies nasal airflow by means of nasal modeling. There is significant airflow disorganization after "*surgical (or virtual) reduction of the inferior turbinate.*"[33] This newly disorganized airflow favors the middle turbinate region instead of the normal inferior turbinate region.

5. Intranasal trigeminal functional testing: It is now well known and acknowledged that it is the nasal mucosal cooling by the nasal airflow that initiates signaling through the trigeminal nerve by way of the special receptor, transient receptor potential melastatin 8 (TRPM8) also known as the menthol receptor, that signals the presence or absence of ample airflow to the brain.[33] Konstantinidis et al. noted that ENS patients had a substantial decrease in trigeminal lateralization (menthol) compared to healthy controls.[355] In 2012, Scheibe et al. examining normal individuals showed greater trigeminal sensitization of the nose anteriorly compared to trigeminal sensitivity at the posterior part of the nose.[358] Additionally, Li et al. discovered that ENS patients had poorer methanol detection thresholds compared to those in the healthy control group.[43]

6. Damage to (or the wholesale removal of) the trigeminal thermoreceptors (sensory function) such as TRPM8 located in inferior turbinate epithelium may lead to a subjective sense of nasal airway obstruction, dyspnea, and possible suffocation.

7. Testing trigeminal function can conceivably be used in diagnosing the ENS patient. The work of Eccles and Jones illustrated that menthol inhalation enhances the perception and feeling of an increased nasal airflow by stimulating the trigeminal cold receptors in the nasal mucosa. These effects occurred without affecting nasal airway resistance or inducing any decongestant effect triggered by the menthol itself.[359,360]

In summary: the physiopathology of ENS remains poorly elucidated, but several complementary hypotheses are now found in the literature. ENS may result from loss of physiological nasal functions (humidification, warming, and cleansing of inspired air) due to reduced mucosal area[74] inducing proportional loss of the sensory, tactile, and trigeminal thermoreceptors, the temporary receptor potential melastatin 8 (TRPM8) receptors, which are indispensable for physiologically managing inhaled air and experiencing the sensation of normal breathing.[33,47,74,353]

Lately, numerous studies assessing nasal airflow using CFD found noteworthy disordered (disorganized) airflow pattern distribution in ENS patients with differences in CFD findings between patients after the inferior turbinate resection some of whom develop ENS others that do not.[335,353,361,363] It is thought, by some, that perhaps at some time in the future CFD studies could be a valuable objective tool for diagnosing ENS but not at the moment.[363]

Scheithauer[28] demonstrated that ENS was associated with decreased humidification, increased warming, and reduced nasal airflow resistance. These functional losses were estimated at around 23% following turbinectomy.[74] Several studies clearly demonstrated that significantly reduced inferior turbinate volume affects nasal cavity airflow.[19,55]

These airflow changes underlie an ***alteration*** of pulmonary function. Nasal resistance plays a major role in opening peripheral bronchioles and optimizing alveolar ventilation. This in turn improves gas exchange, increases negative thoracic pressure, and enhances cardiac and pulmonary venous return.[19] Thus, normal nasal resistance during expiration helps maintain pulmonary volume, indirectly determining arterial oxygenation.[14] These alterations induce the sensation of obstruction reported by patients, which may go as far as a feeling of suffocation. The paradox between subjective congestion and reduced nasal resistance is in all likelihood due to abnormal aerodynamics and "disturbed healing" after inferior turbinate trauma as suggested by Sozansky and Houser[353] and the work of Zhao et al.[354] The sensation of pharyngeal dryness often reported by ENS patients is due to an airflow that is insufficiently humidified obviously yielding a drying of the airway mucosa.[28]

ENS is a late complication of turbinectomy varying form months to years before the functional residual capacity of the nose (FRCn) collapses. Extensive resection (total or subtotal turbinectomy) incurs the greatest risk, but ENS has also been reported secondary to partial resection, mainly partial inferior turbinectomy involving the anterior part or head of the turbinate, which plays a major role in internal nasal valve function.[20] Conservative turbinate reduction by turbinoplasty with lateralization (out-fracture) is thus recommended after (nasal obstruction resistant to well-conducted medical treatments in patients with turbinate enlargement [hypertrophy]). The amount of mucosa resected is not necessarily implicated, and the risk of ENS cannot presently be predicted; therefore, conservativism is the name of the game.

The risk of developing ENS following turbinate treatments includes mucosal resection not only to the amount of mucosa removed but also related to an undetermined individual physiological capacity and perhaps environmental factors with estimates, in the literature, ranging from 2% to 20% to as high as 35% according to the type of turbinate surgery that was performed.[2,24]

It is conjured, no conjectured, speculated that ENS affects "only a few" of the hundreds of thousands of patients who have undergone one or more endonasal procedures with the various precipitating underlying factors are only partially understood. One point of contention concerns the frequent association with psychiatric disorder and possibly psychosomatic pathologies.[55,74] A possible role of psychological stress in certain patients, as suggested in tinnitus, has been raised.[55]

1.8 Etiology of ENS

In our view, ENS remains a secondary AR, especially secondary to a total or subtotal inferior turbinectomy.[2−4,18−28,33,73,76,214] Radical turbinate resection must be condemned in the absence of disease with malignant potential since many of these patients that we have diagnosed with ENS have had a radical total or subtotal removal of an inferior turbinate as a treatment for nasal airway obstruction.

In addition to radical total or subtotal excisional turbinectomy, ENS may also arise consequent to various other turbinate treatments including: thermal coagulation (electrocautery-mucosal or submucosal), chemo-coagulation, cryosurgery, laser surgery, radiofrequency ablation, or coblation; we label these **n**on-surgical **T**urbinate **R**eductive **A**djunctive **P**rocedure (n-s TRAP). One challenging aspect of determining an accurate etiology and incidence of ENS is the fact that it may take many months to years for ENS symptoms to manifest following the inciting traumatic event; therefore, subsequent to an initial turbinate treatment, patients require observation for months to years as they may develop ENS at some time in the future before nasal functional failure is apparent.[18]

Some rare cases of ENS presented in the literature include one case of *rhinotillexomania and a single case of osteomyelitis after therapeutic turbinate trauma secondary to radiofrequency turbinoplasty reported in the Norwegian literature.[351,352] * Rhinotillexomania is a condition that causes a person to **compulsively pick their nose till they self-harm**. Picking your nose is a habit many people are familiar with. However, when it becomes an obsessive compulsion to pick your nose, it is rhinotillexomania. Definition from Google.

1.9 Pathophysiology of ENS

The most current (September 2022) and extensive systemized review of the possible pathophysiologic mechanisms causing ENS was offered by Kanjanawasee et al.[335] They studied original laboratory data on the pathophysiology of ENS attempting to elucidate the precise pathophysiology of ENS. They screened 2476 studies, included 19 studies, 13 case controlled, with 489 adult ENS patients, met their criteria for inclusion. They defined, approved, and presented nine pathophysiological subjects related to ENS. The nine pathophysiologic themes proposed for the etiology of ENS and examined by Kanjanawasee et al.[335] are:

1. Demographics
2. Symptomatology
3. Anatomic features
4. Airflow analysis
5. Mental health
6. Cognitive function
7. Diagnostic testing
8. Olfactory function
9. Mucosal physiology/inmate immunity

Because of Kanjanawasee et al.[335] scientific rigor, quality assessment, and awareness of bias risk, each one of these nine pathophysiological themes are considered and individually summarized.

1. Demographics: Climatic region had no influence on the quality of life of ENS patients.
2. Symptomatology: ENS patients had "higher symptom severity, impaired daily activity, and worse sleep function" than controls and that the ENS symptom–based 6 question questionnaire (ENS6Q) clearly and accurately described ENS patients. Some studies found higher Sinonasal Outcome Test–22 (SNOT-22) scores in ENS versus chronic rhinosinusitis (CRS) without nasal polyps, while some other investigators found similar SNOT-22 scores between CRS patients and ENS.
3. Anatomic features: They found that the postsurgical inferior turbinate reduction size was unrelated to ENS symptoms and that the inferior turbinate volume was similar between patients regardless of ENS symptoms. They found an example of where 50% of ENS patients (after inferior turbinate reduction) had evidence of concomitant sinus disease radiologically which is what was also found in the initial paper by the Mayo team in 2001.[18]
4. Airflow analysis: They found that nasal resistance and nasal airflow were comparable in patients with or without ENS after turbinate reduction.

   As expected, the minimum cross-sectional area obtained by acoustic rhinometry in the ENS group was higher (more space) than controls. Rhinomanometry calculations (measured air pressure changes divided by airflow changes) were lower in ENS patients compared to control subjects, again as expected. Using CFD analysis, when comparing patients with or without ENS after turbinate reduction, the ENS patients had a decreased (lower) nasal airflow rate at the lower (inferior) area of the nasal cavity, and while airflow (breathing) shifted upward toward the region of the middle meatus. Similarly, the wall shear force distribution (mucosal-airflow interface) was decreased in the ENS group as compared with the inferior turbinate reduction patient group without ENS and controls.
5. Mental health: They reported mental health comorbidities in some ENS patients above 50%, anxiety (73%), depression (71%), and hyperventilation syndrome (77%). Anxiety, depression, and hyperventilation correlated with ENS symptom severity.
6. Cognitive function: Functional magnetic resonance imaging (fMRI) was qualitatively different in ENS from normal controls. During normal breathing, ENS patients showed activation in emotional processing areas of the temporal lobe compared to normal controls.
7. Diagnostic testing: The menthol detection test was impaired in ENS, and cotton placement in the airway (cotton test) improved (reduced) symptoms in the ENS population.
8. Olfactory function: Subjective impairment was reported in postturbinate reduction ENS patients, but quantitative measures were similar to non-ENS patients.

9. Mucosal physiology/innate immunity: Turbinate histopathology in ENS was different compared to normal showing a tissue-remodeling pattern. nNO levels were lower in ENS patients.

Significantly and remarkably, as noted above, Kanjanawasee et al.[335] found a substantial comorbid mental health burden in ENS patients, as we did.[18] Interestingly Kanjanawasee et al.[335] emphasized the work of Freund et al.[74] who observed that when ENS patients were examined with fMRI, there was a qualitative difference between ENS patients and normal controls. This may somehow explain the comorbid mental health burden seen with ENS patients, as there was activation in the emotional processing areas of the temporal lobe compared to controls when breathing "normally."

All in all, Kanjanawasee et al.[335] concluded that yes, there is overwhelming evidence of comorbid mental health disorders in ENS patients.

Kanjanawasee et al. trying to understand the ENS patient's frequent feeling of nasal congestion with a "wide open nose" noted that since there are no specific airflow receptors in the nose, it is now known that nasal patency is perceived by the triggering of the trigeminal cool thermoreceptors (TRPM8) in the nasal mucosa.[335,354,355]

The understanding is that normal nasal airflow evaporates H_2O from the nasal epithelial lining, cooling and activating trigeminal transient receptor potential melastatin 8 (TRPM8) receptors which induce neuron depolarization thereby stimulating the respiratory center in the brain. Apparently, menthol, within its cooling effect also activates these trigeminal cool receptors (TRPM8) and by this mechanism produces the feeling of an improved breathing without altering any nasal airflow or changing nasal resistance.[47,359] They allowed that a normal trigeminal cool thermoreceptor response (TRPM8) is present in some ENS patients, but the influence of "altered airflow and the evidence of surgery as the cause for ENS are unclear."[335]

Earlier (2015), Sozansky and Houser in their study and search for the pathophysiology explaining ENS concluded that a belief in an anatomic basis for ENS "falls short" as an adequate explanation for this disorder.[353] They recognized that the typical standard measures of nasal airway obstruction did not correlate with the feeling of nasal airway obstruction. Recognizing that rhinomanometry, acoustic rhinometry, and peak nasal inspiratory flow measurements did not "measure" the physiologic mechanism that senses nasal airway patency, they explored the literature regarding thermoreceptors and nasal airflow sensation, airflow pattern behavior alternations in normal and in ENS patients along with neurosensory system aberrations all laser focused on understanding dyspnea in ENS, in the presence of a "wide open airway." They constructed an understandable explanation of this phenomena as follows: first, pharmacologic modulation of trigeminal afferents has been shown to alter the perception of nasal airway patency. For example, a topically applied nasal anesthetic produces a sensation of nasal obstruction, while topically applied menthol produces a sensation of decongestion (increased breathing) without altering nasal structural morphology, the anatomy. Concluding that the perception of nasal airway patency has a neurosensory mechanism, not anatomic. The primary physiological mechanism causing the sensation of nasal patency is the activation of trigeminal cool thermoreceptors secondary to the cooling of the nasal mucosa. The specific trigeminal cool thermoreceptor has been identified as trigeminal thermoreceptor transient receptor potential melastatin subtype 8 (TRPM8), a receptor for menthol.[354] Zhao et al. realized that the perception of nasal airway obstruction has almost no correlation to instruments for measuring nasal airflow obstruction such as rhinomanometry, acoustic rhinometry, and peak nasal inspiratory flow. They knew of prior work suggesting that the feeling of nasal airway patency resulted from trigeminal activation by cool inspiratory airflow.[354] As a consequence, they studied nasal mucosal heat loss in 22 healthy subjects constructing "real-time" CFD nasal airway models and concluded that:

"These results reveal that our noses are sensing patency via a mechanism involving localized peak nasal mucosal cooling."[354]

Remember, one of the main respiratory functions of the nose is to charge the inspired air with warmth and moisture (humidification) so that carbon dioxide (CO_2) and oxygen (O_2) exchange can occur optimally at the alveolar level. This conditioning of the inspired air is achieved through evaporation of water from the nasal mucosal epithelial surface. During expiration, a reciprocated reversal occurs, returning warmth and moisture back to the nasal airway mucosa. In other words, the perception of nasal patency involves activating these trigeminal cold thermoreceptors in the nasal mucosa by the cooling effect of nasal inspiratory airflow.

TRPM8 is triggered when "high speed" air enters the nose causing evaporation (cooling) of nasal mucosal surface fluid (H_2O) reducing the membrane fluid level which in turn fires the TRPM8 receptors causing neuronal depolarization; subsequent stimulation of its connections to the respiratory center in the brain. When the nose is topically anesthetized, the TPMP8 receptors fail to activate; therefore, the subject feels nasal congestion. Anterior nasal septal deformities, nasal valve obstructions, and nasal packing prevent (inhibit) air cooling activation of TRPM8 receptors; hence, the subject feels congested.

Apparently, the brain perceives a lack of TPMP8 receptor stimulation as the need to signal apnea, producing an increase in the work of breathing. Anything that hinders the evaporation of nasal mucosal fluid such as thick secretions or even a nasal septal deformity induces a sense of nasal airway congestion. Another way of thinking about this is that the feeling of nasal patency, easy breathing, depends on the cooling of the nasal mucosal surface which in turn activates the trigeminal cool thermoreceptor TRPM8 receptors. Some of the variables that affect nasal airflow cooling include nasal surface area, air flow characteristics (air speed, mucosal contact, and wall shear effects), and the number of trigeminal cool thermoreceptor TRPM8 receptors available to function normally.

In ENS there is reduced turbinate tissue volume and the disturbed air flow characteristics with reduced wall shear, reduced air speed, reduced normally directed turbulent airflow, reduced mucosal wall contact, reduced activation of trigeminal cool thermoreceptor TRPM8 with reduced CNS respiratory center stimulation; therefore, respiratory distress at rest ensues the sense of air hunger, apnea, dyspnea, and suffocation.

Understanding that the trigeminal nerve, which mediates nasal airflow perception, has been shown to be appreciably be impaired in patients with ENS.[355] Abnormalities in neurosensory systems may result after a surgical insult since healing may not result in full recovery with normal physiologic function; these phenomena may play a significant role in atypical sensory feelings of ENS patients.[355]

As mentioned previously, now for emphasis, Freund and coworkers observed that when an ENS patient breathes room air, there is widespread limbic system activation seen on fMRI.[74] This limbic system activation included the cerebellum, the amygdala, the para-hippocampal gyrus, the caudate/septal nuclei, and the left-sided middle occipital gyrus.

Because of the difference in brain activation in ENS patients compared to normal controls, it is thought that this abnormal brain activity may contribute to the subjective feeling of respiratory distress in ENS patients. It has been adroitly suggested that since so many ENS patients struggle with dyspnea, air hunger is a significant physical stress that a breathing preoccupation is an understandable significant emotional stress leading to a sense of fatigue, irritability, lack of concentration (aprosexia nasalis), anxiety, and depression.[353]

Thus, in ENS patients, the inspired air entering the nose fails to stimulate the trigeminal cool thermoreceptors, TRPM8 receptors, located in the nasal mucosa; however, the inspired air still reaches the lungs which activates the slowly adapting pulmonary stretch receptors (SARs) signaling the brain that adequate respiration is occurring.[339] Nerve growth factor (NGF) is an important protein, located in both the nasal epithelium and in the submucosal glands of the turbinates. NGF is critical for the preservation (neuroprotective) and restitution (repair) of both sensory and sympathetic and sensory neurons.[339,357]

If the turbinates are grossly resected or if the pseudostratified ciliated mucosal surface is savagely injured, as seen in aggressive turbinate resection surgery, the neural connections, during the healing process, are sometimes spoiled or utterly corrupted. As a consequence, these injured corrupted neurons are unable to adequately carry their electrical messages to their "correct destination" resulting in the feeling of nasal obstruction. Perhaps it is a ruined postsurgical (post-traumatic) neural recovery that answers the question, why some patients develop ENS despite an apparently identical turbinate procedure.

Jennifer Malik and colleagues used CFD studies on five patients **with** aggressive inferior turbinate reduction but **without ENS symptoms** comparing them to 12 symptomatic ENS patients also with previous aggressive inferior turbinate reduction. Twenty individuals served as healthy controls. Surgical results were established using the 22-item Sino-Nasal Outcome Test (SNOT-22) Nasal Obstruction Symptom Evaluation (NOSE) scores Empty Nose Syndrome 6-Item Questionnaire (ENS6Q) ($\geq$11 for ENS).[361]

With the 12 symptomatic ENS patients, they found an airflow imbalance with reduced wall shear stress inferiorly only little airflow in the inferior regions. These symptomatic 12 ENS patients also had impaired nasal trigeminal function, as measured by menthol lateralization detection thresholds (LDTs). On the other hand, the five patients who had the aggressive inferior turbinate reduction patients *without ENS symptoms*, their airflow was directed to the inferior region as is seen in normal controls.[361]

They concluded that:

"While turbinate tissue loss is linked with ENS, the degree of ITR that might distinguish post-operative patient satisfaction in their nasal breathing vs. development of ENS symptoms is unclear. Our results suggest that it may be a combination of distorted nasal aerodynamics and loss of mucosal sensory function potentially lead to ENS symptomology"[361]

Note: IRT is an abbreviation for inferior turbinate reduction.

1.10 Preventing ENS

Regardless of turbinate treatment strategies advocated by some surgeons, the optimal turbinate management lies in the prevention of ENS. Preservation of nasal mucosal and submucosal (lamina propria, stroma) tissue when managing the turbinates helps elude the catastrophic calamity of ENS. Unfortunately, the precise amount of nasal mucosa and submucosa (lamina propria, stroma) with the rich vascular supply that must be preserved during intranasal turbinate reduction (modification) procedures to prevent ENS is presently unknown. We should always minimize turbinate manipulation to preserve mucosal and submucosal functional tissue. Because the nasal mucosa is the functional entity involved in air conditioning, minimally invasive surgery on the turbinate that preserves the nasal mucosa is key to achieving optimal results and reducing the risk of developing ENS.

A technique that accomplishes the main goal of widening the nasal passages (for improved breathing) while preserving the trigeminal cool thermoreceptors (TRPM8 receptors) within the mucosa (for the normal sensation of breathing) and minimizes excisional and thermal trauma to the submucosal neurovascular bundles will maximize the chance to avoid ENS.

Does such a technique exist?

As previously presented, Passali et al. in a randomized comparative "technique" study on 382 patients acquiring results after four and six years showed that the best long-term results regarding free nasal breathing, quicker recovery of mucociliary clearance, and normal local IgA secretion was when they performed submucosal, nonthermal, resection (turbinoplasty) in combination with a lateralization (outfracture) of the inferior turbinate.[211,216]

Prevention largely depends upon "rational" management of the turbinates, meaning lessening inferior and middle turbinate tissue loss by minimizing turbinate trauma and limiting tissue reduction (removal) or thermal damage during reductive procedures.

1.10.1 Middle turbinate(s)

Except for inverting papilloma, juvenile angiofibroma and malignancy where excision of the lateral wall of the nose including the middle turbinate is obligatory plan on protecting the middle meatus to avoid subsequent frontal sinusitis by saving the middle turbinate when feasible. This goal may be elusive when the middle turbinate is partially destroyed by nasal polyps in CRS.

1.10.2 Inferior turbinate(s)

The work of Larrabee and Kacker[264] supported Passali et al. as the best approach for reducing the inferior turbinate.[211,216] Conservative turbinate reduction by turbinoplasty with lateralization (out-fracture) is thus recommended after (nasal obstruction resistant to well-conducted medical treatments in patients with turbinate enlargement [hypertrophy]).[211,216]

With our physiological thinking, any practitioner pursuing inferior turbinate reduction has the duty, responsibility, and obligation to preserve the pseudostratified epithelial mucociliary transport system, minimize damage to the submucosal (lamina propria, stroma) neurovascular morphologic structures avoiding adverse physiologic consequences and the resultant sequelae all the while improving the nasal airway breathing function.

Consequently, "cold-knife" techniques appear to have the edge for now, avoiding thermal trauma as submucosal vascular choking fibrosis also deprives the overlying epithelium with the necessary nutrition to maintain a healthy mucociliary transport system and the secretory deprivation robs the requisite moisture needed to charge the inspired air with heat and moisture allowing optimal exchange of O_2 and CO_2 at the alveolar level.

Prevention of ENS entails turbinate conservation during endonasal surgery including rhinoplasty, whenever turbinate reduction is considered. Turbinate conservation is fundamental to minimizing the risk of ENS.[18] Inferior turbinectomy, in the past, has been a usual procedure for nasal obstruction in cases of turbinate enlargement resistant to medical management.[28] Nevermore, please.

1.11 Medical treatment of ENS

Regarding diagnosis, we now have two validated diagnostic instruments, the ENS6Q questionnaire[31] and the cotton test.[32] With an ENS6Q[31] result over >11 and a positive cotton test[32] along with clinical history of previous turbinate surgery and physical examination, the bed rock of medical evaluation, we are able to relatively confidently diagnose patients with ENS and initiate medical management. Although noncodified, medical treatment is obviously indispensable and is the first-line prescription in all cases.

It seems that adequate medical treatments are less effective for ENS patients than for patients with secondary AR of other etiologies.[58]

The initial medical approach is focused on controlling crusting, foul odor, pain (post-traumatic neurogenic pain), and the emotional turmoil requiring psychological support since, in countless accounts, more than 50% of patients are afflicted with anxiety and depression.[18,33,62,73,74,76,334−349]

Offering a summary of the treatment strategies for the ENS, Gill and associates[33] opined:

"Nasal humidification, patient education, and treatment of possible concomitant medical conditions (e.g., depression) constitute first lines of treatment."[33]

For the crusting and foul odor, bulb syringe ("power") lavage with **hypertonic saline** is exceptionally helpful.[63] Gentamycin 80 mg in a liter of saline (Wilson solution) may also be used as necessary for controlling bacterial overgrowth and the attendant fetid malodor. Oil of sesame for moisturizing lubrication of the nasal crusting and rose geranium for the foul odor control; both may be topically applied as desired and have been used for "nasal atrophy" for over a century at the Mayo Clinic.

Pain management (post-traumatic neurogenic "phantom limb syndrome" type of pain) is challenging and must be managed by skilled experts in pain management.

Recently, from 2019 to 2022, there has been an increased awareness that many ENS patients have serious emotional pain including depression, anxiety, and suicidal ideation.[33,76,334−349] The initial Mayo paper (2001) documented that 125 of 242 (52%) of the ENS patients were diagnosed with depression by the Minnesota Multiphasic Personality Inventory (MMPI) and/or by consultation with a clinic psychiatrist.[18] In an extensive review paper by Kanjanawasee et al.[335], more than 50% of ENS patients were diagnosed with anxiety and depression, while Gill et al.[33] reported that 66% of their patients presented with some anxiety and depression, while patients reported by Kim et al.[336] had "depression prevalence of 71%."

In (2015), a paper published in the psychiatric literature labeled and treated ENS as a psychological illness: ***"Treating empty nose syndrome as a somatic symptom disorder."[346]*** Lamb et al. in the latest (2022) paper discovered 53% of ENS patients met the diagnostic criteria for a somatic symptom disorder (SSD).[334] In another new (2022) paper by Huang et al.[340] they confirmed that many ENS patents suffer significant emotional anguish. They studied 62 ENS patients and documented that 43.5% (27 of 62) had suicidal thoughts (ideation). They concluded that:

"Recognizing individuals who may carry suicidal thoughts and provide appropriate psychological interventions is critical to prevent tragedy"[340]

Doubtless, in addition to the "standard" medical approach to ENS, the new "orthodox" medical management, separately but emphatically, includes identifying and managing the emotional angst many of these ENS patients experience which, when recognized, know that optimal care is achieved by psychiatrists or psychologists qualified and skilled in treating anxiety, depression, and expressly dealing with patients precisely overwhelmed with suicidal ideation. Consultation with these professionals is at times clearly compulsory to avoid catastrophe, particularly prior to any planned surgical intervention for ENS.

In summary, the essentials of medical treatment for ENS patients include the following:

1. *Hypertonic saline* irrigations—with a bulb syringe 3 oz (90 mL) each time of application or use a powered Waterpik using at least 3 oz (90 mL) of *hypertonic saline* two to three times a day to control the dry crusted nasal mucosa. Best in shower or over a sink. In the morning upon waking-up and before bed. If additional treatment is needed, a third irrigation can be performed sometime during the day. This can be homemade; see Table 12
Or you can buy the **Neil Med sinus rinse**: It should be administered two to three times a day as a *hypertonic saline* irrigation (two packets per each administration) as noted above. The product can be viewed at the following link: Sinus Rinse Kit with 50 Packets (neilmed.com). This should be available at most retail pharmacy locations to purchase over the counter.
2. *Wilson's solution* (80 mg Gentamycin in one liter saline)—1 oz (30 mL) is used two to three times a day to control the dry crusted nasal mucosa. Best in shower or over a sink. In the morning upon waking-up and before bed. If need additional treatment, a third irrigation may be performed sometime during the day. This is obtainable from the Mayo Clinic pharmacy, Rochester, Minnesota Mayo pharmacy, Contact number: +1 (507) 284-4041.
3. *Oil of sesame with rose geranium*
For nasal odor control.
Dispense 50cc.
Apply two sprays each nostril twice daily.
This product has a 90-day expiration.
This is a special proprietary formulation obtainable from the Mayo Clinic pharmacy, Rochester, Minnesota Mayo pharmacy. Contact number: +1 (507) 284-4041.
4. **Menthol Inhaler*
Adding menthol to local treatments may provide benefit in terms of reducing the sense of nasal obstruction.[74] The menthol product can be viewed at the following link: Non Medicated Vicks VapoInhaler - Vicks.
It should be available at most retail pharmacy locations to purchase over the counter.
*Note: "The Vicks VapoInhaler is a convenient non-medicated nasal inhaler formulated with a proprietary blend of ingredients including menthol and camphor so you can experience nonmedicated soothing vapors. It's easy to use—just inhale he soothing and refreshing nonmedicated vapors through each nostril and use as often as you need to. It's also easy to carry—take it with you in your purse or pocket so you can discretely enjoy the soothing nonmedicated vapors you need to make it through the day for adults.
Not recommended for use by children under 12. Nonmedicated.
Not intended to treat cold or flu symptoms."
5. *Induction of rhinitis medicamentosa** may be considered; with topical application of nasal decongestants to consciously produce an intended nasal mucosal rebound phenomenon.

*Ramey JT, Bailen E, Lockey RF. Rhinitis medicamentosa. J Investig Allergol Clin Immunol. 2006; 16(3):148−155. PMID: 16784007

6. ***Pain control***, for post-traumatic (amputation) neurogenic pain, refer these ENS patients to a pain management center.

7. ***Emotional support,*** for the frequent incidence of emotional comorbidities including: anxiety, depression, and suicide ideation refer these ENS patients to a competent psychiatrist or psychologist interested in caring for these patients.

Catastrophically and tragically four of our own ENS patients, not previously operated by us, but in our care, committed suicide. Consider a pledge to our patients, for a conscious awareness, in addition to managing their miserable physical symptoms, for our requisite identification of the patient's emotional state of distress so they have our full attention to deliver determined comprehensive and compassionate care; that pledge is binding. During follow-up assessments, obviously, track and chart symptomatic changes, particularly the psychological status, offering the emotional sustenance, in the ample amounts these patients' plea, which can be draining of time and emotion from the physician, probably best tailored to the psychiatrist's or psychologist's office.

Just recently, in 2021, two additional supportive medical strategies, needing investigation and research evaluation, appeared in the literature that may prove useful in the future, and a third purely investigational research approach is listed below under C.

A. "Lubricants, moisturizing, cytoprotective agents could restore the perception of physiological breathing. In this regard, a ***new*** multicomponent medical device seems to be promising, as it contains D-panthenol, hyaluronic acid (HA), vitamin E, vitamin A, and biotin (Rinocross, DMG, Italy)."
From: La Rosa R, Passali D, Passali GC, Ciprandi G. A practical classification of the Empty Nose Syndrome. J Biol Regul Homeost Agents. 2021 Jan−Feb; 35(1 Suppl. 2):51−54.

B. "D-panthenol is the alcohol analog of pantothenic acid (vitamin B5) and is a provitamin of B5. In organisms, it is quickly oxidized to pantothenic acid. It is a viscous, transparent liquid at room temperature. D-panthenol is used as a moisturizer to improve wound healing in pharmaceutical and cosmetic products. It improves hydration, reduces inflammation, and accelerates mucosal wounds' rate of healing. D-panthenol readily penetrates the mucous membranes (including the intestinal mucosa), quickly oxidized to pantothenic acid. It is also used in the biosynthesis of coenzyme A, which controls a wide range of enzymatic reactions. HA is a fundamental component of the connective tissue. HA can modulate the inflammatory response, cellular proliferation, and remodeling of the extracellular matrix."

From: Maiolino L, La Mantia I, Grillo C, Grillo CT, Ciprandi G. Functional recovery in subjects undergoing nasal surgery: a *new* therapeutic strategy. J Biol Regul Homeost Agents. 2021 Jan–Feb; 35(1):363–366. https://doi.org/10.23812/20-600-L. PMID: 33624487

C. Premarin nasal sprays (**for investigational research use only**) for mucosal thickening.
Conjugated estrogen (premarin) 25 mg/30 mL nasal spray.
Concentration: 83 mcg/0.1 mL (which is equivalent to one spray).
This product is ordered in 30 mL bottles.
Typical dosing is one to three sprays each nostril once or twice a day.
This product has a 30-day expiration.
This is obtainable from the Mayo Clinic pharmacy. Rochester, Minnesota.
Mayo pharmacy, Contact number: +1 (507) 284-4041.

1.12 Surgical treatment of ENS

Of course, prevention of ENS by evading "excessive" turbinate reduction remains fundamental to thwarting iatrogenic ENS, but even unmeasurable "minimal" turbinate therapeutic trauma coupled with the inevitable aging process may eventually affect an unhappy symptomatic person with florid ENS.

Skillful medical management embraces local topical measures (detailed above) along with patient education and appropriate referrals for pain management and evaluation for the concomitant emotional mental health comorbidity using validated screening questionnaires for anxiety, Generalized Anxiety Disorder (GAD-7), and by using the Patient Health Questionnaire-9 (PHQ-9) for depression. These screening tools are important accessories to knowledgeable and compassionate clinical management.

The true incidence of ENS after therapeutic turbinate trauma is unknown, although with our experience, it seems that it is not as "rare" as some assume, many patients with ENS are conceivably undiagnosed or misdiagnosed, and the mighty misery of those ENS stricken is both physical with frequent feelings of profound difficulty breathing with feelings of suffocation, disturbed sleep, and a distressed sense of well-being linked with the emotional misery of anxiety depression and suicidal ideation.

Leong (2015) studied surgical results in 128 ENS patients from eight studies clearly expressing that ENS is a most challenging condition to treat.[73] He noted that surgical implantation of various materials for turbinate reconstruction (creating a pseudo-turbinate) often resulted in improved (reduction) patient reported symptoms, irrespective of the graft or implant material utilized. He indicated that:

"There was insufficient evidence from this review to favor any particular implant material, although it was observed that Silastic had higher extrusion rate and that hyaluronic acid gel was resorbed within 12 months."[73]

While documenting that no one implant material was superior to any another, he exhorts that authors should follow their patients and report results longer than just 12 months as not all patients were perfectly improved:

> *"Clinical response varies between patients; up to 21% may report only marginal improvement."*[73]

Merely five years later, Gill et al.[33] keenly observed that over the past several years, there has been renewed interest in understanding and treating ENS, including surgery. This recent rekindling of interest by the ENT community in ENS is evidenced by the fact that from the inception of 2019 to the first of November 2022, the PubMed database offered 45 citations with the term Empty Nose Syndrome (ENS) in the title.

With two important papers cited by Gill et al.[33] both published in 2017, one by Velasquez et al.[31] who presented a validated empty nose syndrome 6 item questionnaire (ENS6Q) and the second paper described the office cotton test by Thamboo et al.[32] The profession now had standardized screening tools by which to define, describe, and aid in diagnosing ENS patients. Prior to these two 2017 contributions, from the Stanford group, description of ENS was inconsistent and dependent upon past history of turbinate trauma associated with various clinical patient presentations and physician impressions, the prescription for misdiagnosis, resulting in an incalculable number of undiagnosed ENS patients.

Gill et al.[33] supported the cautious use of these screening tools emphasizing that they be used as accessories, adjuncts to making medical decisions. However, they did think that using the ENS6Q with the cotton test might assist in the identification of ENS patients who could possibly benefit from turbinate surgical augmentation.[33]

With the notification by Leong[73] of possible marginal surgical results of up to 21% of patients in plain view, any surgical step must be considered cautiously since the patients' pain symptoms and feeling of nasal dryness are usually ***not*** ameliorated with any type of surgery, even "successful" surgery. Additionally, abnormalities in the mucosal neurosensory systems may appear secondary to the surgical therapeutic turbinate trauma as healing may be incomplete resulting in the atypical sensory feelings that some ENS patients experience.[355]

Critically, in addition to the screening test questionnaires for anxiety and depression, a professional psychological evaluation with a competent psychologist or psychiatrist, interested in ENS patients, is ***mandatory prior to any decision to operate***, given the fact that well over 50% of ENS patients have emotional comorbidities.[18,33,334–349] Anxiety and depression were as high as 66% in one (2020) study[33] and even higher in another (2021) study with depression in 71% of their ENS patients.[336]

This emotional suffering is often first experienced years ***after*** the initiating therapeutic turbinate trauma that precipitated the launch of ENS in the first place. Because of the irrefutable evidence of monumental mental health issues in ENS patients, especially anxiety and depression with suicidal ideation, as high as 43.5%, psychologic consultation is unequivocally advocated, required, prior to contemplating any surgical intervention given the potential devastating emotional impact of an unsuccessful surgery.[340]

Surgical intercession for these ENS patients, that initial rational is for the "building or creating" of a "neo-turbinate" or "pseudo-turbinate" structure to provide increased nasal airway resistance by narrowing the airway with a graft or implant held securely within a submucosal pocket.[58,65]

Choice of the "ideal" graft or implant material combines a reduced risk of rejection and contamination with an adequate restoration and maintenance of bulk volume to the nasal airway.

These creative turbinate tissue substitutions are with biological grafts or synthetic implants have been the principal strategy for surgical reconstruction of previously resected tissues. This stratagem is itself unproven as a "cure" for ENS; "tissue replacement" has nonetheless been used for decades, including conchal cartilage and rib cartilage grafts placed submucosally along the floor of the nose, on the septum, or on the lateral wall replacing a partially resected inferior turbinate remnant. These techniques as "simplified" when residual turbinate tissue remains. Otherwise, the problem confronting the surgeon is more complex, deciding exactly where to place the graft or implant in a landmark-less field, a creator's task.

Currently, the term endonasal microplasty is used interchangeably with inferior meatus augmentation procedure (IMAP) which is used for describing a reparative endonasal surgical procedure designed to reduce the volumetric size of the nasal cavity by submucosal implantation of some graft or implant material to restore regional inferior turbinate volume.[58] The procedure is primarily designed to increase resistance to nasal airflow, reducing airflow so as to increase warmth and humidity to the inspired air, and to diverge the inspired airflow from the initial turbinate treatment site toward a healthy or nonoperated area.[20] The principle consists in positioning an implant or graft on the septum, floor, or lateral wall.[21,58,67]

Surgical therapy for ENS seeks to reestablish turbinate tissue volume (and associated nasal aerodynamics and nasal sensation) through the placement of injectable fillers, allografts, xenografts, cartilage autografts, and/or synthetic materials. Although the exact pathoetiologic mechanisms for ENS are not well understood, symptoms of ENS may be improved through the judicious patient workup, counseling, and application of selected medical and surgical treatments.

An assembly of multifarious materials, diverse and varied, including injectable fillers such as hyaluronic acid gel, carboxymethylcellulose/glycerin gel (Prolaryn), synthetic implant materials (Plastipore, Medpor, Gore-Tex, Teflon, Silastic sheets, beta-Tricalcium phosphate, hydroxyapatite and ceramic bioactive glass (Glass-BONE), allograft materials (Alloderm and Bone Source), and autologous materials (bone, costal cartilage, platelet-rich fibrin (PRF) with diced conchal cartilage, rib cartilage, muscle, fat), cadaveric rib cartilage, and even porcine small intestine submucosa (SIS) xenograft have all been tried and used for surgical reconstruction of the missing turbinate tissues.[19,62,64,72,345,366−373]

Although almost all authors claim "good" results meaning reductions of clinical nasal airway symptoms, without complications, intraoperatively or postoperatively, along with a reduction of emotional symptoms at or at some time less than one year after surgery in small published series, but the amount of volume restored by surgery and their durability and efficacy remain to be determined for the long term, optimally years into the future.[19]

Regarding pertinent pathophysiology and its relationship to surgery, Hassan et al.[371] suggested that several theories or considerations need inquiry. When turbinate mucosa and submucosa are resected or injured first, there is the loss of sensory, tactile, and thermal receptors (TRPM8)[365] along with a sweeping reduction in the number of functional neurovascular structures. A recent work, published in Laryngoscope, by Wu et al.[365] studying the histopathology of 17 ENS patients including immunohistochemical staining of transient receptor potential melastatin 8 (TRPM8) with six normal controls. In the ENS patients, they found significant squamous metaplasia, increased submucosal fibrosis, fewer submucosal glands, and a "lower expression level of thermoreceptor-like transient receptor potential channel melastatin 8 (TRPM8)."[365]

Gill et al. (2020) were aware of these new data suggesting that there is impaired trigeminal nerve function which may also play a role in the pathophysiology of ENS.[33] As a consequence of all these changes, the reduced number or injured neurovascular structures elicited a decreased humidification, decreased warming, and a decreased number of trigeminal thermoreceptors (TRPM8), with the ensuing sense of difficulty breathing, or the inability to experience a normal unobstructed breathing sensation in these ENS patients. Hassan et al.[371] let us know that in ENS, the CNS is being studied which could clarify the patient's subjective feeling of nasal airway obstruction as a disturbance of neural mucosal afferent pathways and impaired intranasal trigeminal function.[74,355]

Additionally, a reduction (a lessening) of the nasal airway resistance almost always occurs secondary to gross tissue removal, as anticipated; expected.[47] Absent the head of the inferior turbinate, the nasal resistance is reduced which may be seen, perceived, by the CNS respiratory center as respiratory distress resulting in the hyperventilation syndrome in 77% of their studied ENS patients.[13,74,358] With resistance changes, there is an alteration of pulmonary gas exchange as the nasal resistance plays a vital role in the opening of pulmonary bronchioles and physiological alveolar oxygenation as noted by Houser in 2007.[19] The next consideration includes the physical disruption of the nasal airflow, an unbalance between air distributed (flowing) primarily to the superior nasal cavity in ENS instead of toward the inferior nasal cavity along the inferior turbinate as submitted by Malik et al.[361]

Currently, **curative** and a **definitive** surgical treatment for ENS is actually **nonexistent**.

Despite the current status of surgical results, recently, the Stanford group has vigorously focused on surgical approaches to relieve these ENS patients of their onerous symptoms. All these are examples of perturbation theory, a method for attempting to continuously improve a previously obtained approximate solution to a given problem.

Thamboo et al. published a 2017 paper establishing the Cotton test as a way of confirming ENS diagnosis utilizing their validated Empty Nose Syndrome 6-Item Questionnaire ENS6Q was entitled:

"Defining surgical criteria for empty nose syndrome: validation of the office-based cotton test and clinical interpretability of the validated empty nose syndrome 6-item questionnaire."[32]

A few years later, in June 2019 another paper, also from Stanford, by Borchard et al.[366] appeared acknowledging that while augmentation of the inferior meatus has been previously proposed for ENS patients that efficacy* information with validated survey forms (questionnaires) was minimal; therefore, they wrote:

"Surgical augmentation of the inferior meatus has been proposed to treat ENS, although efficacy data with validated, disease-specific questionnaires is limited. Instead we evaluated submucosal injection of a transient, resorbable filler into the inferior meatus to favorably alter nasal aerodynamics in ENS patients."[366]

*__*Efficacy trials__ use strict inclusion and exclusion criteria to enroll a defined, homogenous patient population.*

__Effectiveness studies__ (also known as pragmatic studies) examine interventions under circumstances that more closely approach real-world practice, with more heterogeneous patient populations, less-standardized treatment protocols, and delivery in routine clinical settings.

From: Singal AG, Higgins PD, Waljee AK. A primer on effectiveness and efficacy trials. Clin Transl Gastroenterol. 2014 Jan 2; 5(1):e45. https://doi.org/10.1038/ctg. 2013.13. PMID: 24384867.

They anticipated that the submucosal instillation (injection) of carboxymethyl-cellulose/glycerin gel (Prolaryn) into the inferior meatuses of their 14 patients would be reabsorbed in a few months. Their results were excellent after three months with improvements in all their subjective measures including: ENS6Q, 22-item Sino-Nasal Outcome Test (SNOT-22), Generalized Anxiety Disorder 7-item scale (GAD-7), and Patient Health Questionnaire-9 (PHQ-9), for depression. They concluded that:

"Transient, focal airway bulking via submucosal filler injection at sites of inferior turbinate tissue loss markedly benefits ENS patients, suggesting that aberrant nasal aerodynamics from inferior turbinate tissue loss contributes to (potentially reversible) ENS symptoms."[366]

In November 2019, Talmadge et al.[345] suggested that future office injections of submucosal absorbable fillers, for "off-label" use, requiring proper informed consent, could possibly be used as a temporary "trial." Thereby confirming the office cotton test and determining the patient's satisfaction with a transient but impermanent improvement (lessening) of their ENS symptoms as the gel filler is resorbed over a 2−12-month period.[345] This would occur prior to installation of any material, organic or inorganic, graft or implant, as a more "permanent" surgical solution for ENS sufferers.

Realize that the submucosal injection of "fillers" is not without risk as rare, but significant problems may occur including thromboembolic complications[345] with tissue necrosis or blindness[122] secondary to intravascular injection. In another 2019 offering, this time by Gill et al.[76] as an update on ENS disease mechanisms, diagnostic tools, and treatment tactics they advised:

> *"Although injectable implants to augment turbinate volume show promise as a therapeutic surgical technique, there is insufficient data to fully support their use at this time."[76]*

Apparently encouraged by the results of the submucosal filler injections with carboxymethylcellulose/glycerin gel (Prolaryn) at three months, Thamboo, Dholakia, Borchard et al. (2020)[367] launched a ***pilot study*** in a series of ***10 ENS patients*** followed for ***six months*** with the Empty Nose Syndrome 6-item Questionnaire (ENS6Q), 22-item Sino-Nasal Outcome Test (SNOT-22), Generalized Anxiety Disorder 7-item scale (GAD-7), and Patient Health Questionnaire-9 (PHQ-9), for depression.

They performed 11 procedures on 10 different ENS patients using two different materials: (1) small intestine submucosa (SIS) grafts for three operations on three patients and (2) acellular dermal matrix (Alloderm) for eight operations on seven different ENS patients. They specified that an IMAP has made a considerable difference for their patients asserting that:

> *"IMAP can dramatically improve the quality of life of ENS patients regarding both ENS specific symptoms and psychological wellbeing."[367]*

With a gathering momentum, one year later, in 2021, Jennifer Malik from Ohio State University in concert with the Stanford group published a fascinating paper using CFD with ***five ENS patients*** buttressed the idea that an IMAP with costal cartilage, for example, is able to stabilize and "normalize nasal air flow patterns" in their five ENS patients. They stated that an IMAP was able to reduce "ENS symptoms in a durable manner," but how these symptomatic improvements occurred was unknown. After six months of study, they concluded:

> *"This study supports our prior working hypothesis that disordered vectors of nasal airflow congregate in the middle meatus contribute to ENS symptoms, not nasal resistance. Moreover, these data illuminate a paradoxical, but consistent, restoration of nasal airflow to the inferior meatus following the replacement of turbinate tissue volume in the inferior meatus via IMAP, potentially due to the Coandă effect."*[368]*

*The Coandă effect is the action in fluid mechanics whereby a flow along a solid surface tends to follow the curvature of the surface rather than separating. In other words, it is the tendency of a fluid jet to stay attached to a convex surface.

They acknowledged their study's limitations of a small sample size (5 ENS patients) and its nonexistent control group; however, they intend to continue to investigate altered airflow distribution and its effect on ENS symptoms.[368]

In 2021, Sachi Dholakia and colleagues from the Stanford group published a surgical treatment paper using *cadaveric rib cartilage* performed for *17 ENS patients* followed for *12 months*.[369]

Specifically, the cadaveric rib cartilage was packaged, decellularized, and irradiated which was acquired from Musculoskeletal Tissue Foundation (MTF).[369] These patients were diagnosed as having ENS based on: (1) reported discomfort with nasal breathing and/or paradoxical nasal obstruction after inferior turbinate reduction, (2) a positive ENS6Q score of at least 11, and (3) a positive cotton test. The data were collected preoperatively and at 1, 3, 6, and 12 months postoperatively. They noted that their prior practice at Stanford included injections of carboxymethylcellulose/glycerin gel (Prolaryn)[366] and other tissues, for the IMAP.[367,368] Moreover, with those procedures, their ENS patients were significantly improved regarding their anxiety and depression symptoms.[366,367] They modified their IMAP methodology in 2017 for qualms about implant resorption requiring additional surgery with complete conversion from a small intestine submucosa (SIS) graft or acellular dermal matrix (Alloderm) to cadaveric rib graft, now their preferred treatment technique. Their assessments included: four validated questionnaires: Empty Nose Syndrome 6-Item Questionnaire (ENS6Q), 22-item Sino-Nasal Outcome Test (SNOT-22), Generalized Anxiety Disorder 7-Item Scale (GAD-7), and Patient Health Questionnaire-9 (PHQ-9), for depression. Concluding that:

> *"IMAP via implant of cadaveric rib cartilage provides significant, long-term improvements in ENS-specific and general sinonasal symptoms."*[369]

Some findings of note involved the GAD-7 and PHQ-9 questionnaires as measures of anxiety and the severity of depression, respectively. Those scores were reduced but not statistically significant because anxiety and depression were in the mild ranges for those 17 patients "leaving little room for improvement from a low starting baseline." [369] Generally, their patients were clinically improved, and those results were statistically significant.

Of course, not all symptoms are ameliorated with an IMAP especially since the TRPM8 receptors, so important for the sense and feeling of normal breathing, are functionally impaired (or totally removed, excised) in patients with ENS. The evidence for the damaged TRPM8 receptors has been provided by the menthol lateralization test and histopathologic study of the inferior turbinate.[360,365,369] Laudably, their study was the first documented report of symptomatic improvement by means of validated disease-specific questionnaires in patients suffering with ENS at one year subsequent to IMAP with cadaver rib implantation.

Understandably, surgery does not restore neurological or mucosal receptor function, but it was recently shown, (2021), by the combined efforts of the group at Ohio State University and the Stanford group, that IMAP can improve (normalize) nasal airflow patterns with CFD modeling.[368]

Two other new surgical papers (2021) are mentioned for completeness. One by C.F. Chang [370] using PRF with diced cartilage in *two patients* with a *follow-up at one year* and one by Hassan et al. [371] using Bioglass (GlassBONE), in two patients, one with AR and *one with ENS* with limited *follow-up of four months*. What was uncommon was the use of a sublabial approach for submucosal placement of the Bioglass (GlassBONE) implant.

In June 2022, with a marvelous yet brief three page "How I Do It" paper in Laryngoscope, Michael Chang and colleague[372] (from the Stanford group with other colleagues outside of Stanford) described, in detail with video, the surgical technique for the IMAP with irradiated cadaveric rib for surgically treating *two ENS patients* followed for *12 months*. They emphasized that a firm diagnosis of ENS is required with a minimal ENS6Q score of >11 and positive cotton tests (blinded), on at least two occasions, where the ENS6Q score increases (improves) by 7 points on each cotton test study.[31,32,372]

In another 2022 paper, Hosokawa et al.[373] used autologous dermal fat (ADF) following *nine ENS patients* for *three months*. Arguing that using autologous tissues like rib cartilage is an invasive technique with a chest scar; however, by exploiting ADF tissue, which is essentially limitless, a surgeon has as much ADF as desired for any IMAP chosen. They claimed that their nine ENS patients were significantly improved as measured by Empty Nose Syndrome 6-Item Questionnaire (ENS6Q); however, dryness persisted, all this without complications.

Talmadge et al.[345] in a November 2019 article in Facial Plastic Surgical Clinics of North America thought that current data for surgical reconstruction of a new turbinate (neo-turbinate or pseudo-turbinate) in ENS showed possible favorable long-term effectiveness.

Despite their optimistic cheerful view, to date, 2022, no long-term results, years into the future, have appeared in the literature for ENS resembling the published work of Passali et al. for inferior turbinate treatments for 382 patients which Passali et al. recounted after four and six years postsurgery.[211,216]

We think in this current year, 2022, although injectables and various grafts and implants to augment turbinate volume show promise as a therapeutic surgical technique, there is still insufficient or long-term data to fully support their use at this time. What is desirable and needed are well designed, well planned, RCTs, with objective measures, if possible, and subjective measures of symptomatic improvement, with sufficient numbers, followed years, not merely months, into the future. All in all, this approach is indispensable and imperative to someday answer the questions surrounding surgical treatment options and alternatives for our ENS patients. Nevertheless, a realistic but empathetic approach is required considering that the current evidence is weak for enduring successful surgical intervention. Realizing that any given individual clinical response varies between patients, according to Gill et al., about 20% of patients report only marginal improvement from surgery.[33]

While these surgical studies and explorations are interesting and encouraging, they are also difficult to fully assess and implement given their limited numbers and abbreviated follow-up (often less than a year).[19,21,62,64−72,366−373]

2. Evidence-based medicine—David Sackett, MD

The ideas behind EBM come from David Sackett, MD. EBM is primarily about discovery. Discovery of the best medical evidence, for crafting clinical choices, judgments, and rational therapeutic decisions in the best interest of the patient. The entire concept of EBM is the distinction between decisions based on hard scientific evidence from well designed and competent RCTs as opposed to decisions based on expert opinion. RCTs avoid bias and placebo effects and are almost statutory for intelligently comparing competing medical practices.

Unvalidated care must not be undertaken unless in a structured evidence-based RCT. The ideal double blind placebo-controlled trial cannot easily be applied to surgical comparisons, but the optimal design of RCTs for surgery must be attempted nonetheless.[274] It is fully understood that without evidence from RCTs, there is no choice but to rely on your clinical reasoning and experience, yet awareness of a possible flawed conclusion because of a "placebo effect" must always be kept in mind.

3. Consolidated standards of reporting trials

The CONSORT statement was developed to promote consistency, clarity, accuracy, and transparency of reporting of RCTs. In this way, all interested parties, researchers, journal editors, and physicians of the general readership know exactly how the RCT was performed, with a standardized check list for the authors of trials to adhere to and for journal editors to demand before the results of RCTs are published and disseminated.[296,297]

More recently, in 2010, the checklist and flow diagram have been updated yet again and expanded to 25 essential items by the leading authorities Douglas Altman, David Moher, Kenneth Schulz, and others[299,300] with the details located at: www.consort-statement.org.

Professor Douglas Graham Altman's quote is so germane to research's expeditionary quest:

> *"To maximize the benefit to society, you need to not just do research but do it well."*

CONSORT requirements are important for clinical investigators to have an accurate repeatable standard guideline to follow for performing valid RCTs of the highest quality so ultimately practicing physicians and surgeons have proven principles to follow for effective clinical patient care. Journal editors and peer reviewers should also demand that those investigators using RCTs follow the CONSORT requirements so that the highest quality studies are transparently performed with the most accurate data published for their readership to consider when making clinical decisions.

Even after a quarter of century of demand for following the CONSORT statement, many do not adhere to those principles in their papers published in our ENT literature.

Not so long ago, in 2018, the group from McGill University evaluating RCTs in otolaryngology and adherence to the CONSORT statement concluded that the reporting of RCTs in top nine ORL-HNS journals and in the top Canadian ORL-HNS journal is "suboptimal."[301] Recall that PSM can imitate a RCT.[303,304]

4. Replacement or reversal of a medical practice

Optimally, questionable medical practices are replaced by improvements. Sound improvements are based on strong and substantial comparative trials (RCTs) where advancements overtake dubious previous practices.

Prasad et al. reviewed 2044 original articles and found that 146 (40.2%) of once verified and validated medical practices were reversed (discontinued), when at first those practices seemed "rational" when in fact they were ultimately substantiated to be flawed[271]

> *"Reversals included medications, procedures, diagnostic tests, screening tests, and even monitoring and treatment guiding devices. We were unable to identify any class of medical practice that did not have some reversal of standard of care."[271]*

When medical therapies decline in approval and are no longer practiced, it's because they are either replaced or reversed (discontinued).

1. *Replacement* (superseded) occurs when a practice is exceeded by one that's superior (better) in result.
2. *Reversal* (discontinued) occurs when a practice is stopped because it's either *unsuccessful* or *harmful.*

The solution to a treatment that was reversed (discontinued) is discovering an "improvement" by randomized controlled trials (RCTs). Proof requirements remain compulsory; therefore, the charge of our rhinologic community is to ferret out useless or harmful practices, by well-designed RCTs, the soul of EBM, principled "care research."

Admonishing the profession, with his dazzlingly provocative paper, John Ioannidis[320], from the Departments of Medicine, Health Research and Policy, and Statistics, and Meta-Research Innovation Center at Stanford (METRICS), Stanford University, asserted that most clinical research is not useful, arguing that clinical research to be useful **must** have unbiased pragmatic utility for a patient's well-being. After listing a number of "utility features" that must be met for clinical research to be useful, he concluded that:

> *"Overall, not only are most research findings false, but, furthermore, most of the true findings are not useful. Medical interventions should and can result in huge human benefit. It makes no sense to perform clinical research without ensuring clinical utility. Reform and improvement are overdue."*[320]

Accordingly, Ioannidis listed some of the features to consider and questions that need answering for clinical "care research" to be useful that included the following:[320]

Problem base: Is there a health problem that is important enough to fix?
Context: Has prior evidence been systematically assessed to inform the need for new studies?
Information gain: Is the proposed study large and long enough to be sufficiently informative?
Pragmatism: Does the research reflect real-life? If it deviates, does it matter?
Patient centeredness: Does the research reflect top patient priorities?
Value: Is the research worth the money?
Feasibility: Can this research be done?
Transparency: Are the methods, data, and analyses verifiable and unbiased?

5. Managing middle turbinate enlargement

For the current moment, in the absence of certainty from RCTs, we champion saving the middle turbinate for both its physiological function and as a critical anatomical landmark that is especially helpful for revision surgery in patients with CRS with polyps. Preservation of the middle turbinate is preferred unless there is a particular clinical scenario in which it is "sensible" to remove portions of it ("insubstantial-flimsy" structure, or obstruction to sinus outflow, involved with polys or tumors).

In managing a concha bullosa, we favor instrument collapse minimizing airway obstruction while maintaining both the medial and lateral mucosal surfaces of the middle turbinate structure since mucocele is rare. Future well-planned RCTs are required for answering these questions.

Houser (2006) described a case of ENS after left middle turbinate resection as part of functional endoscopic sinus surgery (CT scan in evidence) with the right middle turbinate untouched with both inferior turbinates in situ.[20] Houser's report and our experiences are identical as we have seen patients with ENS secondary to middle turbinate resection with both inferior turbinates in situ.[18]

6. Managing inferior turbinate enlargement ("hypertrophy")

6.1 Evidence-basedproposals

In the realm of medical management of inferior turbinate enlargement ("hypertrophy"), various treatments recommended and applied included: steroids (systemic and topical), decongestants, (systemic and topical), antihistamines, and immunotherapy. Patients who "failed" the obligatory three-month trial of medical management are candidates for surgical intervention. Principally, there are two types of "surgical" procedures for inferior turbinate reduction:

> Type 1: Transmucosal (transepithelial) approach with *epithelial* mucosal *destruction.*
> Type 2: Submucosal (turbinoplasty, turbinate reduction) approach with *epithelial* mucosal *preservation.*

The nasal mucosa (epithelium and submucosa) is composed of two distinctive strata: Fig. 5.2.

1. Epithelium is actually the outer epithelial layer and is composed of pseudostratified ciliated columnar epithelium.
2. Submucosa is called the lamina propria or deeper stromal layer located beneath the epithelial layer.

An esteemed judgment regarding inferior turbinate surgery was offered by Hol and Huizing, with the aim of reducing inferior turbinate enlargement ("hypertrophy") reducing nasal airway obstruction, thereby improving nasal breathing.[25]

> *"In our opinion, the purpose of surgically reducing the inferior turbinates should be to diminish complaints of airway obstruction, to improve breathing, all the while preserving function."*[25]

They concluded the obvious, that turbinectomy (total and subtotal), electrocautery, chemocautery, cryosurgery, and laser (surface) surgery are all transmucosal (epithelial) approaches and *should not* be used, since they are too destructive.[25] Therefore, they favored intraturbinal turbinate reduction (turbinoplasty) as the method of choice.

Specifically, as previously written, surgery is: the medical practice of managing diseases, deformities, and injuries by actually "cutting" into a part of the body, while, on the other hand, electrocautery, chemocautery, lasers, radiofrequency, coblation, or ultrasound are not surgery in the traditional sense of cold-knife "cutting" but nonetheless they are currently considered "surgery" by some authors, but we choose to call these practices the n-s TRAPs.

With evidenced-based treatment proposals in mind, Larrabee and Kacker[264] reviewed five studies that they rated as level 1 evidence (prospective and randomized trials). These include the following notable evidence-based treatment contributions.[26,27,211,230,235]

1. Passàli et al. wrote "Treatment of inferior turbinate hypertrophy: a randomized clinical trial" in 2003.[211]
2. Nease et al. wrote "Radiofrequency treatment of turbinate hypertrophy: a randomized, blinded, placebo-controlled clinical trial" in 2004.[26]
3. Liu et al. wrote "Microdebrider-assisted versus radiofrequency-assisted inferior turbinoplasy" in 2009.[235]
4. Cingi et al. wrote "Microdebrider-assisted versus radiofrequency-assisted inferior turbinoplasty: A prospective study with objective and subjective outcome measures" in 2010[230]
5. Gindros et al. wrote "Comparison of ultrasound turbinate reduction, radiofrequency tissue ablation and submucosal cauterization in inferior turbinate hypertrophy" in 2010.[27]

Therefore, to date (2022), the evidence-based treatment proposals for "surgical" management of the inferior turbinate(s) are based on five RCTs,[26,27,211,230,235] but the one favored by Larrabee and Kacker[264] was the admirable approach presented by Passali et al.[211,218] Passali and colleagues (1999, 2003) reported on the randomized outcomes for all their adult patients (n = 382) having nasal airway obstruction, secondary to inferior turbinate enlargement ("hypertrophy") who were refractory ("failed") to medical management. These patients were treated with various "surgical" procedures with the number of patients for each different procedure placed in parentheses as follows: electrocautery,[62] cryotherapy,[58] laser cautery,[54] submucosal resection without lateral displacement-out-fracture,[69] submucosal resection with lateral displacement,[94] and turbinectomy.[45] They performed objective testing including rhinomanometry and acoustic rhinometry plus measuring the mucociliary transport times and measured levels of secretory immunoglobulin A.[211,218]

And in their words:

"These data indicate that submucosal resection with lateral displacement of the inferior turbinate results in the greatest increases in airflow and nasal respiratory function with the lowest risk of long-term complications."[211] *(Bold italics added)*

They also said:

"After 6 years, only submucosal resection resulted in optimal long-term normalization of nasal patency and in restoration of mucociliary clearance and local secretory IgA production to a physiological level with few postoperative complications (p < .001)"[211]

After studying and following their 382 patients for four and six years, Passali and associates recommended, as the first-choice technique for treating nasal obstruction due to inferior turbinate hypertrophy, inferior turbinate submucosal resection (turbinoplasty) combined with out-fracture (lateral displacement).[211,216]

The older "orthodox" techniques include: turbinectomy or subtotal (partial) turbinectomy, electrocautery, laser cautery, cryotherapy, submucosal resection, and submucosal resection with lateral displacement. The newer "modern" procedures included radiofrequency-assisted turbinoplasty, coblation-assisted turbinoplasty, microdebrider-assisted turbinoplasty, and ultrasound turbinate reduction. Individually both microdebrider-assisted and ultrasound turbinate reduction (turbinoplasty) are especially effective in reducing inferior turbinate size; however, to date, 2022, a prospective RCT comparing the microdebrider-assisted turbinoplasty with ultrasound turbinoplasty has yet to be performed; accordingly, for now, the microdebrider-assisted turbinoplasty (turbinate submucosal reduction) technique is the technique of choice since the microdebrider has well-known fluency (turbinate reduction).

Surgeons should make every effort to preserve the pseudostratified epithelial mucociliary transport system, minimize damage to the submucosal (lamina propria, stroma) neurovascular morphologic structures, thereby avoiding the adverse physiologic consequences and the resultant sequelae all the while improving the nasal airway breathing (respiratory) function.

Based on physiological thinking, surgeons operating to reduce the inferior turbinate have the responsibility to preserve the pseudostratified epithelial mucociliary transport system, minimize damage to the submucosal (lamina propria, stroma) neurovascular morphologic structures avoiding adverse physiologic consequences and the resultant sequelae all the while improving the nasal airway breathing function. Therefore, as suggested by Neri et al.[256] Gindros et al.,[257] and Berger et al[258,259] with their histologic studies that "cold-knife" techniques appear to have the edge for now, by avoiding thermal trauma as submucosal vascular choking fibrosis also deprives the overlying epithelium with the necessary nutrition to maintain a healthy mucociliary transport system and the secretory deprivation robs the requisite moisture needed to charge the inspired air with heat and moisture allowing optimal exchange of O_2 and CO_2 at the alveolar level[256–259] With that said, Gindros et al.[257] noted after ultrasound treatment some patients had normally organized ciliated columnar cells in the epithelium suggesting that anatomical and functional restoration of the nasal physiology is possible.

For the future, well-planned evidence-based RCTs are indispensable and imperative to answer "all" pressing questions. We believe that in well-designed and well-performed RCTs, blinding is possible for surgical and procedural studies when the operator remains "silent" as to his/her specific involvement with subjective and objective outcome studies performed by blinded (coded study) evaluators. But until then, we think that it is the randomized controlled report of Passali et al., followed for six years, that is the first-choice technique for treating nasal obstruction due to inferior turbinate enlargement ("hypertrophy") which is inferior turbinate submucosal resection, turbinoplasty, either with a "cold knife" or with a microdebrider-assisted turbinoplasty combined with out-fracture (lateral displacement), the microdebrider-assisted turbinoplasty that is the technique of choice since the microdebrider has well-known fluency.

7. Regarding children

Regarding children, we believe that surgeons operating on the turbinates of children have an explicit moral and ethical obligation to follow, report, and publish on the trajectory of these children as they passage into adulthood. After serious study and rightful reflection regarding turbinate surgery in children, Leong, Kubba, and White[322] concluded:

> *"There is currently little evidence to support turbinate reduction surgery in children. The role of surgery, if any, has not been properly examined. Furthermore, the long-term effects on nasal airflow dynamics, nasal physiology and long-term complications remain to be studied."[322]* (Bold italics added)

Until well-executed pediatric RCTs are available, Leong et at.[322] cautioned the profession with instructions:

> *"Do not remove turbinates in children, since there is little evidence to support turbinate reduction surgery in childhood."[322]* (Bold italics added)

Nine years later in 2019, a group from Boston, Massachusetts, compared different pediatric surgical methods (turbinectomy, electrocautery, lasers, submucous microdebridement, and radiofrequency) for managing pediatric inferior turbinate hypertrophy in 1012 children.[323] After a comprehensive literature review, these authors acknowledged that surgery in children is an "escalation" in the management of inferior turbinate "hypertrophy." On the other hand, being ethically honest, these authors also acknowledged that:

> *"Still, no guidelines currently exist to help guide the escalation of management in children."[323]* (Bold italics added)

Total inferior turbinectomy for inferior turbinate enlargement ("hypertrophy") has been condemned by a number of surgeons and baptized a nasal crime by two European academic authors, Huizing and de Groot, from the Netherlands, with whom we are totally in agreement.[3,4]

We state unequivocally that total inferior turbinectomy for inferior turbinate enlargement ("hypertrophy") is a nasal crime, especially in children without the benefit of a well-designed RCT or without future follow-up into adult years.

Consider, that the primary purpose for inferior turbinate surgery is to reduce nasal airway obstruction (improve breathing), while preserving nasal function. Because guidelines from quality RCTs are presently nonexistent (for children), submucosal resection (microdebrider-submucosal) inferior turbinoplasty (without bony resection unless conchal enlargement) with out-fracture (lateralization) makes the most rational current conservative surgical alternative, after failed medical therapy; suggested by Argenbright et al.[328] for children; reinforced by Passali et al.[211] prospective randomized trial in adults with six-year follow-up with objective and subjective evaluations. Performing an adequate inferior turbinate out-fracture (lateralization), the nasal airway can be effectively enlarged and maintained (durable) for a "prolonged" period (time).[211,244−248,250,252]

Once yet again, we emphasize that ideally, all our clinical decisions should be based on EBM and the RCT. What's a surgeon to do, when trial data of an RCT is just not available or limited, incomplete, inconclusive, conflicting, or starkly nonexistent? We think there is no choice but to rely on your clinical reasoning, the rationalism of "clinical judgment," yet always aware of a possible flawed conclusion because of "placebo effects."[180]

And to reiterate, to establish concrete pediatric guidelines for inferior turbinate reduction, the profession needs principled "care research" meaning: well-designed RCTs; with sufficient numbers, objective and subjective outcome measures, followed into adulthood. Someday.

---

8. Summary, future directions, and closing thoughts

8.1 Summary

8.1.1 Definition

Defined, empty nose syndrome (ENS) is a clinical entity without a mutually agreed upon definition; however, most consider ENS as a complication of *radical inferior turbinectomy* or may also result from "lesser" inferior turbinate procedures although it has also been seen after *middle turbinectomy* alone.[18,20] The exact incidence is unknown; yet, Chhabra and Houser estimated a rate of 20% following inferior turbinate resection, which produces an "ordinary" dry nose in many patients.[19,21] Moore et al.[2] from the University of Nebraska Medical Center reported an incidence of "… at least 35% of the original 40 patients who underwent total inferior turbinectomy would be suffering unacceptable nasal symptoms at this time." The symptomatic manifestations of ENS occurred between three and five years after the turbinate excision surgery in their study.[2] It is to be distinguished from primary AR (ozena) displaying similar symptomatology. With our experience of personally caring for more than 300 *ENS* patients, we emphasize the need for *conservative* surgical intervention when treating inferior turbinate enlargement ("hypertrophy") thus avoiding, preventing, the suffering of ENS by our patients. Preventing ENS is the most important strategy when managing the turbinates.[21] Surely include middle turbinate preservation whenever possible and favor the most conservative techniques for reducing the inferior turbinates to improve breathing as suggested by Passali et al.[211]

8.1.2 Symptoms

The most common and characteristic-presenting subjective symptom is a sensation of nasal airway obstruction difficulty breathing, often associated with dyspnea (breathlessness), the so-called paradoxical nasal obstruction with a sense of suffocation despite a "wide open" nasal airway.[18,19−21,55,347]

Associated symptoms include a feeling of an empty nose or lack of nasal airflow sensation, nasal and pharyngeal dryness, crusting, epistaxis, difficulty falling asleep, disturbed ability to concentrate (aprosexia nasalis), hypersensitivity to cold air, hyperventilation, nasal pain, headaches, hyposmia, generalized fatigue, restlessness, irritability, and sweeping sense of a disturbed well-being.[21,55,58,64] Symptom intensity varies but may restrict everyday activity.[21] Do not discount the emotional toll and related symptoms experienced by our ENS patients as the incidence of this affliction is astonishingly high, over 50% in most studies, with anxiety, depression, and suicidal ideation (about 40% in one study) are the usual; a surprising comorbidity.[18,20,33,62,73,74,76,334−350]

8.1.3 Diagnosis and diagnostics
Today, ENS is more easily diagnosed when a high index of suspicion is coupled with a history of previous inferior turbinate surgery sometimes months to years after that nasal surgery, although middle turbinate trauma may also be associated with ENS.[18,20] The diagnosis is primarily clinical; based on the patient's reported subjective symptoms with a nasal cavity that is usually enlarged, meaning that normal intranasal structures are absent, or reduced, truncated in most instances.

8.1.4 Physical examination
Examination with or without endoscopy often finds the intranasal cavities enlarged secondary to the previous surgery, with turbinate structures missing or greatly reduced in volume (size). The nasal mucosa is generally pale, dry (often crusted), and is easily confirmed on examination.[55]

8.1.5 Validated diagnostic instruments
Two validated diagnostic instruments are available, one a questionnaire for ENS, the Empty Nose Syndrome 6-Item Questionnaire (ENS6Q)[31] and the cotton test.[19,21,32] With a positive cotton test and an ENS 6Q result over >11, the diagnosis of ENS is sturdily supported.[32] With the cotton test, a piece (plug) of moist cotton is placed intranasally at the estimated site of the head of inferior turbinate before it was removed. After an interval of 20−30 min, symptom reduction confirmed by repeat ENS6Q "confirms" diagnosis and suggests that surgical repair may be beneficial.

8.1.6 Imaging
Imaging, while the diagnosis is fundamentally clinical, but suggestive signs may be found on imaging. The direct coronal CT findings are variable and can range from an absence of intranasal structures, the nose is empty, devoid of intranasal structures, to sinus mucosal thickening and maxillary sinus opacity in about 50% of cases[18,24,58] (Fig. 1.2).

8.1.7 Mental health
Evidence of comorbid mental health symptoms are seen on the self-rated questionnaires: Beck anxiety inventory (BAI), Beck depression inventory, updated version,

(BDI-II) with Generalized anxiety disorder (GAD-7), and the Patient health questionnaire (PHQ-9) of depression which can be helpful diagnostically. Neuropsychological involvement is suggested by fMRI studies that demonstrated specific activation patterns in temporal and cerebellar regions and in the amygdala of ENS patients.[74]

8.1.8 Other tests

Gill et al. (2020) concluded that CT scans, CFD, and intranasal trigeminal nerve function testing currently have insufficient evidence to support routine use in the workup of ENS.[33] Rhinomanometry and acoustic rhinometry are definitely not diagnostic but generally confirms a wider nose with a reduced nasal airway resistance.[19,335,345,353] We use a modified Sumner olfactory test which is suggestive but not diagnostic for ENS.[147] The menthol detection test lower (reduced) in patients with ENS.[43,335,358,359] Low nNO levels are usually seen in ENS.[344]

8.1.9 Pathophysiology

Understanding the underlying pathophysiology is elusive, but probably involves a combination of distorted nasal aerodynamics, determined by CFD and disturbed (distorted) nasal mucosal sensory function with altered (reduced) trigeminal cool thermoreceptors, TRPM8 receptor, activation which depends on turbulent airflow with adequate mucosal cooling that does not materialize in ENS, that failure potentially leads to the complex respiratory symptoms of ENS namely dyspnea and conceivably suffocation.[354,365]

8.1.10 Management

Managing the suffering ENS patient is challenging diagnostically, additionally requiring compassionate empathetic emotional wariness. The first and primary track of treatment is medical, which involves topical lavage alongside psychological support, often requiring referral to a psychiatrist or psychologist because of the high incidence of over 50% (in many studies), of anxiety, depression, and suicidal ideation.[18,21,33,62,334–349]

8.2 Medical management

After diagnosis, first implement the full gamut of medical stratagems including: nasal hygiene by lavage with *hypertonic saline* and Wilson's solution (80 mg Gentamycin), for humidification, crust, and odor control with oil of sesame and rose geranium. Trials menthol inhalers for symptomatic relief can be effective. The induction of rhinitis medicamentosa may be considered, with the topical application of nasal decongestants. Referrals for pain control overseen by competent specialists in pain management and professional emotional support by a competent psychiatrist or psychologist is critical given the enormous incidence (over 50%) of anxiety and depression, some with suicide ideation.

8.3 Surgical management

Surgery is reserved for the most severe cases; whatever the technique, surgery aims at partial filling of the nasal airway, IMAPs also called an endonasal microplasty. Understandably, surgery does not restore neurological or mucosal receptor function or offer pain relief, but surgery may possibly improve (normalize) nasal airflow patterns as shown with CFD modeling.[368]

Additionally, as reported above, but repeated for emphasis, a pilot study (2020), with *10 patients followed six months*, ENS patients were surgically treated with an IMAP using SIS grafts in three patients and acellular dermal matrix (Alloderm) in seven patients. The authors published in the March edition of Otolaryngology Head Neck Surgery indicating that:

> *"IMAP can dramatically improve the quality of life of ENS patients regarding both ENS specific symptoms and psychological wellbeing."*[367]

While published surgical studies can be interesting and inspiring, they are difficult to fully assess and implement given their limited numbers and abbreviated follow-up (often less than a year).[19,21,62,64−72,366−373] Unfortunately, without compelling extensive data from any controlled trials, currently there are no definitive curative or restorative surgical therapies for ENS; today, there are only promises, possibilities for the future.

8.4 Future directions

8.4.1 Surgical trials for ENS

For a respectful historical perspective, homage to those before us, let's remember that Professor Maurice H. Cottle, MD (1898−1982) of Chicago used the idea of a "nasal cavity narrowing," a "nose reducing," or "smalling" operation for treating nasal atrophy, in the mid-20th century.[374] Today these "narrowing operations" are regularly termed an endonasal microplasty or an IMAP.

Cottle credited Lautenschläger's paper (1917) which recognized the benefits of narrowing the nose in patients with atrophy.*

*Lautenschläger, A.: Ueber die Technik der operativen Ozaenabenhandlung, Berlin klin. Wchnschr. 54:687, 1917.

After Lautenschläger, there were numerous modifications published by numerous surgeons using numerous materials placed primarily in submucosal pockets on the nasal floor, lateral wall, and nasal septum. Our ancestral surgeons, went, as they say, "polynomial in materials" ranging from: paraffin, starting the era of implants, celluloid, gutta percha (coagulated latex obtain from trees resembling rubber), fat, rib, cartilage, fascia, bone, ivory, acrylic resins, placenta, polyethylene and vinyl alcohol sponge, macerated spongy beef and bovine cartilage, as preambles.

When Dr. Cottle was confronted with a patient with an extremely pale (compromised blood supply) atrophic mucosal nasal floor, he suggested a *staged* elevation with immediate replacement of the mucosal flap without grafting or implanting of any materials at all. This first stage surgical elevation would theoretically increase the blood supply, thickening the mucosa, allowing for a second stage submucosal grafting at some later date, ideally avoiding extrusion due to a healthier "thicker" more vascularized mucosal covering.[374]

For him, initial treatment was always medical including lavage, corticosteroids, dietary control, vitamins, vasodilators, and antibiotics. Cottle used lobular, upper lateral cartilage, and lateral osteotomies as narrowing procedures along with the submucosal implantation of various materials including polyethylene pellets, polyvinyl plastic sponge (which ultimately extruded), cancellous bone (which absorbed), bovine cartilage, and preserved rib cartilage often using an alar facial incision to access the lateral nasal wall for the submucosal implantation.

He suggested that these procedures could be repeated as many times as necessary as long as they were safe and effective (useful), with patient determined tangible benefits, and he clearly recognized and cited the emotional benefits from these procedures. Usually the "redo" operation can be performed within a time frame interval ranging from 10 to 20 months for five to ten years. Affirming that:

> *"Clinical, social, and emotional rehabilitation can be accomplished and it is most gratefully received."*[374]

Back to the future, in 2022, we presently reason, although injectables and various grafts and implants to augment turbinate volume show promise as a therapeutic surgical technique, there are still insufficient data to fully support their use at this time. Nonetheless, as Talmadge et al.[345] previously suggested, that future office injections of submucosal absorbable fillers, "off-label" use requiring proper informed consent, could possibly be used as a temporary "trial."

That said, it may be reasonable to practice repeated injections of submucosal absorbable fillers for "off-label" use as long as they are in a "care research" protocol and is eventually proven to be both *safe* and *effective* in ameliorating the symptoms of ENS. At that future moment, it may become a "standard of care" treatment for ENS, namely "repeated intermittent injections" of submucosal absorbable fillers until the arrival of stem cell research. The reprogramming of adult somatic cells to become inducible pluripotent stem cells (iPS cells), has and continues to create the ability to produce boundless amounts of any type of human tissue cells that generate complete organs, such as an entirely normal turbinate. This may occur by seeding the area of absent or damaged turbinate tissue with iPS cells to enhance and promote the development of an organoid (the process whereby stem cells can recapitulate a human organ, such as a turbinate). Presto cure, shazam!

What to do?

Our ethical responsibility, when considering "new" innovative procedures or "reevaluations" of current procedures is to institute authorized "care research" trials. The purpose is to potentiate possible benefits while curbing adverse effects by following all the criteria, for bias elimination (placebo control), after the CONSORT statement for reporting RCTs, to avoid publishing flawed studies with conclusions that need future reversal.[4,44] The ethics of using placebos must be considered along with the distinction and differentiation between *research* and *care* as in surgical *research trials* and surgical *clinical care.* The updated (2010) CONSORT checklist is located at: www.consort-statement.org.

For surgery, Agha et al.[45] stated that CONSORT requirements are necessary when reporting RCTs:

"There is a clear need to ensure that medical research, especially relating to clinical interventions, is carried out and reported to the highest possible standards."[45]

Should we practice unproven, unvalidated procedures on unwary patients presented as appropriate certified clinical care? ***Never!!!***

Future well-planned RCTs are indispensable and imperative to answer the questions surrounding surgical treatment options and alternatives for our ENS patients. Nevertheless, a realistic but empathetic approach is required considering that the current evidence is weak for enduring successful surgical intervention for our ENS patients. Realizing that a given clinical response varies between patients and about 20% of patients report only marginal improvement from surgery.[33]

Darsaut and Raymond (2021) emphasized that our ethical medical care credo is based on reliable, repeatable interventions with proven outcomes, essentially EBM.[38] With uncertainty, Darsaut and Raymond argue that medical ethics demand that a clear distinction be made between "research" and "care." That a "separation" between the two is intended to protect patients from "research" studies designed primarily for some distant patient in some distant future. Practicing moral medicine within the context of uncertainty was their main concern; therefore, a distinction was made between *validated care* and *promising unvalidated care* offered within a clearly announced pragmatic "care research" design anticipated to: "act in the best medical interest of the patient."[38]

To establish concrete guidelines for restorative surgery for our ENS patients, we argue that the profession needs principled "care research."

What does principled "care research" mean?

We think for ENS that means patients be informed that this is "care research." Research in a well-conceived, well-designed, institutionally (preferably) approved RCT, with sufficient numbers, which may be difficult given the "rarity" of ENS, ideally with objective diagnostic and outcome measures, if ever possible, as there are currently no available agreed upon objective diagnostic methods for ENS, and subjective outcome measures, which are available with the Empty Nose Syndrome 6 question questionnaire (ENS6Q), Sino-Nasal Outcome Test-20 for the assessment of Empty Nose Syndrome (SNOT-20), the Generalized Anxiety Disorder questionnaire-7 (GAD-7), and the Patient Health Questionnaire-9 (PHQ-9) for depression. It is also required that these operated ENS patients be followed and reported to the community in the literature years into the future.

The doctor's dilemma develops when data from RCTs are unavailable since "the crucial study" was never performed. Ideally, all clinical decisions should be built on EBM with RCTs, but when RCT data are incomplete or nonexistent, there is no choice but to rely on "clinical judgment"; ever mindful that erroneous conclusions may ensue.[180] The argument of *empiricism* (evidence first) versus *rationalism* (clinical judgment) takes center stage especially when data from a "definitive" RCT are "limited, incomplete, inconclusive, conflicting, or starkly nonexistent" as it is for surgical treatment for ENS. When empirical data are unavailable, then experience and clinical judgment take over as the indispensable alternative.

Remember that Prasad et al. found that 146 (40.2%) of once verified and "validated" medical practices were reversed, when at first those practices seemed "rational" and "logical" when in fact they were ultimately proven to be flawed, useless, or harmful.[271]

All in all, proof requirements remain compulsory, to ferret out useless or harmful practices, by well-designed RCTs, the soul of EBM.

Altogether, studies need the great equalizer, the final arbitrator, "Father Time," to "weigh in" before making a "final" adjudication regarding our interventions. Duration after treatment matters before a "final" therapeutic result can be determined and "final" proclamation for therapeutic recommendation. Early favorable results may be short-lived, short-term, transitory with a number of representative examples known in our field flashing caution.

For instance, contemplate, as presented by Passali et al., that while coblation and radiofrequency improved nasal breathing in patients with enlarged ("hypertrophic") inferior turbinates "briefly," the effectiveness decreased at three years.[240] In 1985, years prior to labeling ENS, Moore et al.[2] found an overwhelming majority of patients, 35% of 40 patients, at three to five years following bilateral total inferior turbinectomy had symptoms consistent with ENS. In the exact same cohort of 40 patients, seen at the first two years following initial surgery, very few patients had symptoms suggestive of ENS only to become florid with the passage of time.[2] As previously indicated, these findings led their team to denounce total inferior turbinectomy, warning the profession that symptoms may not become obvious pending the passage of years following the initial bilateral total inferior turbinectomy.[2] Historically, with our ENS patients, there are past accounts of graft resorption, infections with necrosis, implant rejection, extrusion, some small sample-sized studies, some lacking a control group, the full tour of less than optimal reports drawn from the literature.

With time interval, length of follow up interval in mind, the 2016 work of Pelen and associates while praiseworthy comparing the "cold-knife" microdebrider reduction with radiofrequency ablation concluded that both techniques were minimally invasive and could reliably provide an improved nasal airway subjectively and objectively assessed as statistically significant without any disruption of nasal physiology.[260] The only issue of concern and disquiet was one of duration. Their post-treatment follow-up was, in their own words:

> "Nasal obstruction, the grade of turbinate hypertrophy and other symptoms were evaluated with subjective nasal obstruction scale and anterior rhinoscopy before the operation, and three days, seven days, four weeks, and eight weeks after the surgical intervention."[260] (Bold italics added)

Certainly, projecting the "long-term" effects of a given procedure based on results after eight weeks of treatment results is a startling speculative leap of faith, for "who knows" where that leap will land you?

Passali et al. set the standard by reporting outcomes at four and six years of their 382 randomized patients after treating their inferior turbinate enlargement ("hypertrophy") with various therapeutic methodologies.[211,216]

Pilot studies may be laudable with a brief follow-up of less than a year but for convincing "long-term" results we need examination and analysis somewhere between four to six years al la Passali et al.[211,216] Perhaps three to five years also seems a rational and commonsensical duration of time interval between the surgical intervention and the long-term follow-up period, all though this is perhaps open for future debate.

Before whole heartily accepting the "new" we need to heed, respect the passage of time and only then, after a respected reasonable interval, and a positive principled "care research" result we can enthusiastically and confidently accept the "new" best "approximate temporary truth." For the record, in 1799, the "approximate temporary truth" was bloodletting, blistering, and enemas.*

*On December 14, 1799, 3 prominent physicians-Craik, Brown, and Dick-gathered to examine America's first president, George Washington. He was complaining of severe throat symptoms and was being treated with bloodletting, blistering, and enemas. Dick advised performing an immediate tracheotomy to secure the airway. Both Craik and Brown were not keen on trying tracheotomy and overruled that proposal. Washington was not involved in making that decision. He most likely had acute epiglottitis that proved to be fatal at the end. If Dick had prevailed, a tracheotomy could have saved Washington's life. Human factors analysis of these events shows that his physicians were totally fixated on repeating futile treatments and could not comprehend the need for a radical alternative, like tracheotomy. That was aggravated by an impaired situational awareness and significant resistance to change. Leadership model was also based on hierarchy instead of competency, which might have also contributed to Washington's death. From: Abou-Foul AK. A Lesson on Human Factors in Airway Management Learnt From the Death of George Washington. Otolaryngol Head Neck Surg. 2020 Nov; 163(5):1000−1002. https://doi.org/10.1177/0194599820932127. Epub 2020 Jun 9. PMID: 32513057.

8.4.2 Stem cell–based technology for ENS*

Other than preventing ENS by intelligent management of symptomatic inferior turbinate enlargement ("hypertrophy"), a ***definitive curative treatment*** for ENS does not exist; surgical or otherwise. These facts require the moral and ethical search for data-driven studies that will guide rhinologists to provide successful care for our ENS patients.

A potential possibility is stem cell–based technology that will become more available and optimistically more useful at "some approaching" time in the future. Using adipocyte-derived stem cells (ADSCs) has provided ENS patients with renewed hope for the future. Xu et al. (2015) showed that these ADSCs produce cytokines that support tissue growth while diminishing mucosal injury and increasing nasal mucociliary activity in their 28 ENS study patients.[72] ADSCs have been used as an implant material as have methylcellulose hydrogels, but these materials are frequently resorbed after injection some months later requiring reinjection.[375]

To date, different types of stem cells have been employed for managing aging, wound healing, autoimmune diseases along with neurodegenerative, metabolic, and musculoskeletal disorders. Adult stem cells, derivatives of embryonic and induced pluripotent stem cells (iPS cells), have all been used clinically and are currently involved in areas of active research.

For a variety of reasons, multipotent mesenchymal stem cells (MSCs) are the primary focus of cell-based therapies today and could conceivably be expanded for ENS patients. Sources for these cell-based therapies include: bone marrow, adipose tissue, umbilical cord, and placental tissue. Stem cells have a high proliferation potential, in that they can differentiate into multiple cell types and replace damaged cells, secrete growth factors maintaining local tissue regeneration, and are able to migrate to damaged tissue sites after systemic injection. Additionally, they are able to modulate the immune system, reducing inflammation of an affected area. Neural crest-derived stem cells (NCSCs) have been suggested for therapeutic ENS tissue engineering strategies, and research is currently underway in that area too.[382]

In 2012, Shinya Yamanaka was awarded the Nobel Prize in Physiology or Medicine jointly with Sir John B. Gurdon for finding a way to "reprogram" adult cells to become stem cells; iPS cells, capable of becoming any tissue in the body, except placenta. For instance, iPS cells derived from skin or blood cells have been reprogrammed into an embryonic-like pluripotent state capable of empowering the growth of boundless amounts of any type of human tissue cell desired or required for replacing any tissue in the body. How about creating a new turbinate please? (Fig. 11.1).

8.5 Closing thoughts

We close with the humble phrase, "and the beat goes on," a modest metaphor for the rhythm of life itself, as a sustaining self-assured onward action into an unknown future, no matter whatever passing medical fads, fashions, and whims come and go, curiosity matters, integrity matters, knowledge matters based on solid scientific study (RCTs) with impeccable statistical data.

This book is more than an exploration and conversation concerning the *"empty nose syndrome"* with its diagnosis and treatment options. EBM is offered in a historical and pragmatic context with its origins, applications, and limitations especially as it relates to the direction of future rhinologic investigation and current clinical practice.

ENS is not to be ignored and discounted, especially as it can severely adversely affect a person's physical and emotional lives whose only first presenting complaint may be difficulty breathing with a sense of suffocation. ENS might be suspected

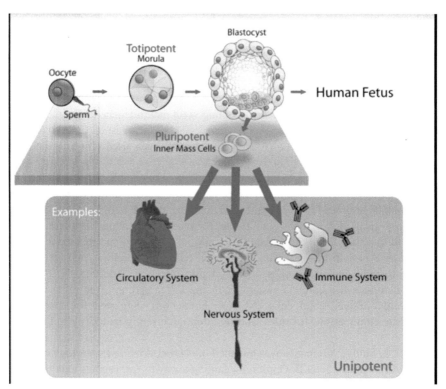

FIGURE 11.1

In 2012, Shinya Yamanaka was awarded the Nobel Prize in Physiology or Medicine jointly with Sir John B. Gurdon for finding a way to reprogram adult cells to become stem cells; induced pluripotent stem cells (iPS cells). Pluripotent, embryonic stem cells originate as inner mass cells within a blastocyst. These stem cells can become any tissue in the body, excluding a placenta. Only the morula's cells are totipotent, able to become all tissues including a placenta Mike Jones-From English Wikipedia, Original description page/is here. Comment: The source of pluripotent stem cells from developing embryos. Original works by Mike Jones for Wikipedia. CC BY-SA 2.5 hide terms File Stem cells diagram.png Created: May 3, 2006.

From English Wikipedia.

when the difficult breathing and the emotional impact seem disproportionate, exaggerated, compared to the clinical observations, yet these symptoms almost always follow some type of previous turbinate surgery, the historical clue.

8.5.1 Inferior turbinate management

Turbinoplasty, a mucosal-sparing technique, combined with out-fracture (lateralization)

In conclusion, for now, maximizing preservation of an intact turbinate mucosa is our standard advice as it is the relatively steadiest surest way to *prevent* ENS. Following the lead of Passali et al. for managing inferior turbinate enlargement ("hypertrophy") which respects the results in 382 patients, after six years, of Passali et al. with inferior turbinate submucosal resection (turbinoplasty) combined with out-fracture (lateral displacement).[211,216]

In January of this year, 2023, several authors, from academic institutions, inimitably and uniquely drew attention to the amount of "airborne particle" aerosol production ("surgery smoke plume") generated by each of the many methods of inferior turbinate reduction. Their stated goals were to determine the "ideal" method for reducing an inferior turbinate by evaluating both **outcomes and aerosol production** in the current age of:[376]

"…widespread communicable diseases, including but not limited to COVID-19, HIV, and hepatitis, additional attention is necessary to **balance outcomes** *with a degree of generation of* **airborne particles** *when selecting a technique." (Bold italics added)*

*"***Surgical management of the inferior turbinates*** includes radiofrequency ablation (RFA), microdebrider-assisted turbinoplasty (MAIT), electrocautery, laser, and ultrasound. Piezo-assisted turbinoplasty and a turbinate-specific coblation wand are new additions to the literature." (Bold italics added)*

"MAIT and RFA are comparable, although MAIT demonstrated better long-term outcomes in some studies and appears to generate fewer **airborne particles**.*" (Bold italics added)*

"Studies evaluating the production of **aerosols** *due to RFA are lacking. Ultrasound outcomes are also excellent and generate no aerosols, but the technique has not been compared against the microdebrider." (Bold italics added)*

"Electrocautery can result in increased pain and crusting for patients and causes the **highest amount of aerosols**.*" (Bold italics added)*

"Deficiencies of current studies, including a **lack of comparison of aerosol generation**, *duration of follow-up, omission of outfracture, and inadequate randomized controlled trials among existing and new techniques, have limited the identification of the best inferior turbinate reduction method." (Bold italics added)*

*"***Given the durability of MAIT* and its minimal aerosol production, it can be reinforced as the most sensible technique until further evidence is available***.*"[376] (Bold italics and asterisk added) * microdebrider-assisted turbinoplasty (MAIT)*

Unfortunately, for any patient, once turbinate tissue is resected beyond some "critical" point, the exact amount of tissue that must be preserved to conserve "optimal" function is currently unknown.

An injured or resected "organ of the nose," the mucosa, with its supporting submucosa (lamina propria, stroma) may generate persistent pain (neurogenic posttraumatic), persistent dryness, trigeminal thermoreceptor insufficiency, altered or absent TRPM8 function, with a persistent sense of dyspnea and suffocation.

Consider that, submucosal healing scar tissue secondary to thermal trauma, or tissue excision, may also lead to vascular submucosal damage, minimizing, better, compromising the post-procedure epithelium of a robust blood supply. The adverse obstructive effects of intervening scar tissue formation. Furthermore, how many of these patients will require persistent psychological maintenance?

8.5.2 Surgical treatment of ENS

Surgical treatment for ENS is still problematic since many of the various surgical interventions ***did not*** restore or return all mucosal functional integrity to normal resulting in "long-term" patient benefit. Many of the surgical interventions, although "promising," have inadequate numbers and have not been conducted as "care research" as an RCT and to date, 2022, ***have not*** been followed for a long enough duration (most often in months less than a year) to add the term, "long term" in years to the result.[19,21,62,64–72,366–373]

8.5.3 Medical management

As a consequence, the first action is to initiate medical management, recommended and detailed above, for your ENS patients along with referral for competent professional psychological support if anxiety and depression are evident and supported by the Generalized Anxiety Disorder questionnaire 7 (GAD-7) and the Patient Health Questionnaire-9 (PHQ-9) for depression as you have likely already obtained the Empty Nose Syndrome 6 question questionnaire (ENS6Q), Sino-Nasal Outcome Test-20 for the assessment of possible Empty Nose Syndrome (SNOT-20). Suicidal ideation may be lurking, perhaps prowling, just beneath a seemingly normal personality.

8.5.4 Well-planned randomized controlled trials, "care research"

Well-planned RCTs, "care research," are *indispensable* and *imperative* to answer the questions surrounding surgical treatment alternatives for our ENS patients. Short-term benefits may be reasonably tolerated if the initial surgical repair and "redo" procedures are reasonably safe and significantly helpful in inducing, enjoining, symptomatic relief. Doubtless, these decisions are for patient and surgeon to discuss and resolve. In that spirit, hopefully, future positive results from successful "care research" will provide a firm footed ethically directed successful scientific approach with either a new "long-term" (measured in years) surgical solution or the "short-term" application of repeated intermittent injections of a suitable submucosal absorbable filler or effectively using stem cell–based technology for creating a functioning "neoturbinate" to benefit our stressed and suffering ENS patients.

8.5.5 Finally

Eternally and evermore, be the questioning inquisitive skeptic, as science marches on, two steps forward one step back, buttress your thinking on the vertebral column of the next best "approximate temporary truth" from the next best RCT and apply those trial truths to that one specific, unique, and particular patient in your compassionate care.

Grapple with ethical issues related to advances in medicine especially concerning introducing "new" and "novel" surgical procedures. Our ethical responsibility, when considering "new" innovative procedures or "reevaluations" of current procedures is to institute authorized "care research" trials to potentiate possible benefits while curbing adverse effects by following all the criteria, for bias elimination (placebo control), after the CONSORT statement for reporting RCTs, to avoid publishing flawed studies with conclusions that demand future reversal.[213,266,299]

Agha et al.[269] stated that CONSORT requirements are necessary when reporting RCTs in surgery:

"There is a clear need to ensure that medical research, especially relating to clinical interventions, is carried out and reported to the highest possible standards."[266](Bold italics added)

The diagnosis of ENS is in the process of being codified, fully solidified, while surgical treatment of ENS remains "a work in progress." When dealing with turbinate surgery, prefer the least invasive turbinate procedure possible to deal with a nasal obstruction, ENS prevention.

Prasad's work[271] clarifies the fact that medicine aspires to apply the finest, most accurate, information obtainable at the time, which allows for "knowledgeable guesses," which of course, is subject to change.

"We physicians and surgeons should tolerate 'uncertainty' acknowledging the reality that medical theories and practices are subject to dislocation, disruption, continuous change and improvements since that's the nature of medical progress."[271] (Bold italics added)

Realize that there is a ***temporal quality to truth*** as described by Sir Karl R. Popper, who introduced the concept of an ***"approximate temporary truth."***

Always buttress your thinking on the vertebral column of the best "approximate temporary truth" from the best RCT, applying those truths to your patients.

Holmes (1900) writing in *The New York Medical Journal* recognized the nose as a significant organ system and that minimal resection of the inferior turbinate was superior to "extensive destruction."[80]

In closing his September 1914 paper entitled, "A plea for the conservation of the inferior turbinate," published in the *Atlanta Journal-record of Medicine*, Dr. Albert Mason beseeching readers wrote:

"In conclusion, I plead with you, both rhinologist and general practitioner, to respect the function of the inferior turbinate and to save it when possible to do so."[82] (Bold italics added)

After more than 100 years, this erudite opinion is still one with which many of us adamantly agree and unwaveringly practice. Lastly, ever since Hippocrates, the gravitational principled core of medicine has been and still is the dominating moral authority of: the interest of the patient is the only interest of concern.

Appendix

This appendix contains seven items:

1. A brief history of Professor Maurice H. Cottle, MD
2. The Empty Nose Syndrome 6-Item Questionnaire (ENS6Q)
3. The Sino-Nasal Outcome Test 20–25 (SNOT20-25) for ENS (questionnaire)
4. Nasal Obstruction Symptom Evaluation (NOSE) Instrument (questionnaire)
5. The cotton test, and how to perform it
6. The questionnaire for Generalized Anxiety Disorder (GAD-7)
7. The Patient Health Questionnaire-9 (PHQ-9) for depression

1. A brief history of Professor Maurice H. Cottle, MD (1898–1981), and his "smalling" operations for nasal atrophy from his 1958 paper[374]

Professor Maurice H. Cottle, MD, of Chicago used the idea of a "nasal cavity narrowing," a "nose reducing" or "smalling" operation for treating nasal atrophy, in the mid-20th century.[374] Today, these "narrowing operations" are regularly termed an endonasal microplasty or an inferior meatus augmentation procedure (IMAP).

Dr. Cottle, born in London England, the eldest of seven children, was the founder and first president of the American Rhinologic Society (1954) and cofounder of the International Rhinologic Society with Professor HAE van Dishoeck (1963) of the Netherlands. Cottle was an untiring educator, organizing and teaching nasal surgical dissection courses worldwide ("The Cottle Courses"),[a] incorporating live surgical demonstrations. He held the mantle as a major contributor to rhinologic thinking in the mid-20th century, urging and practicing nasal functional testing, rhinomanometry, commitment to conservative septo-rhinoplastic surgery, with the "push-down" of the nasal dorsum in rhinoplasty, now called "dorsal preservation" and turbinate conservation, whenever possible. Furthermore, as a physician and surgeon, the consummate, and most eminent rhinologist of his time, he was also a medical author, investigator as nasal physiologist, amateur musician as violinist playing in string quartets, hosting at his home musical luminaries of the day including Sergei Rachmaninov, Sergei Prokofiev, Vladimir Horowitz, Nathan Milstein, and singer Marian

---

[a] One of us (EBK) first attended the Chicago "Cottle Course" in 1967 as a student and later as a teacher for a number of years (18) until the founder's death in Chicago in May 1981.

Anderson among other personalities. He married the acclaimed Steinway artist Gitta Gradova, a Chicago born pianist, who made her debut at the age of 19 in a recital at Town Hall in New York City playing the "Dante" sonata of Liszt, Handel, Brahms, Scriabin, and Chopin Waltz (Sostenuto) in E-flat major. Together they raised two children, a son Tom, a practicing psychologist, and a daughter Judy, a noted cabaret artist. He was major collector of both Chinese ceramics, Eskenazi Ltd. (book), and Japanese woodblock prints, exhibited at several museums, among other artistic pursuits. Truly, a man for all seasons.

2. The Empty Nose Syndrome 6-Item Questionnaire strongly suggests (confirms) ENS if the score is greater than >11

The Empty Nose Syndrome 6-Item Questionnaire (ENS6Q) was validated using the Sino-Nasal Outcome test (SNOT-22), but in addition, the ENS6Q presents 6 simple questions (with a score of 1—5 points each) that can be a helpful in screening/confirming the diagnosis of ENS. A score 11 (but especially >15) out of a maximum score of 30 strongly suggests the presence of ENS in the appropriate clinical scenario.[31]

Symptom	No problem/ not applicable	Very mild	Mild	Moderate	Severe	Extremely severe
Dryness	0	1	2	3	4	5
Sense of diminished nasal airflow (cannot feel air flowing through your nose)	0	1	2	3	4	5
Suffocation	0	1	2	3	4	5
Nose feels too open	0	1	2	3	4	5
Nasal crusting	0	1	2	3	4	5
Nasal burning	0	1	2	3	4	5

ENS6Q, *Empty Nose Syndrome 6-Item Questionnaire.*

3. Sino-Nasal Outcome Test 20—25 (SNOT20-25) for ENS

This outcome test is from (Table 1):

Huang CC, Wu PW, Lee CC, Huang CC, Fu CH, Chang PH, Lee TJ. Comparison of SNOT-25 and ENS6Q in evaluating patients with empty nose syndrome.

Table 1 The Sino-Nasal Outcome Test-25 for the assessment of empty nose syndrome.[343,348]

1	Need to blow nose
2	Sneezing
3	Runny nose
4	Cough
5	Postnasal discharge
6	Thick nasal discharge
7	Ear fullness
8	Dizziness
9	Ear pain
10	Facial pain/pressure
11	Difficulty falling asleep
12	Waking up at night
13	Lack of good night's sleep
14	Waking up tired
15	Fatigue
16	Reduced productivity
17	Reduced concentration
18	Frustration/restlessness/irritability
19	Sadness
20	Embarrassment

ENS-specific symptoms

21	Dryness
22	Difficulty with nasal breathing
23	Suffocation
24	Nose is too open
25	Nasal crusting

Each question is evaluated on a Likert scale of 0–5, with 5 being most severe. ENS, empty nose syndrome.

Laryngoscope Investig Otolaryngol. February 28, 2022;7(2):342–348. https://doi.org/10.1002/lio2.767. PMID: 35434317; PMCID: PMC9008176.

4. Nasal Obstruction Symptom Evaluation Instrument
Details are found in the original source

Stewart MG, Witsell DL, Smith TL, Weaver EM, Yueh B, Hannley MT. Development and validation of the Nasal Obstruction Symptom Evaluation (NOSE) scale. *Otolaryngol Head Neck Surg.* 2004;130:157–163.

"**Conclusions and relevance:** The NOSE scale is an important tool for gauging symptoms in patients with nasal obstruction." From Lipan, MJ, Most, SP. Development of a severity classification system for subjective nasal obstruction. *Facial Plast Surg.* 2013;15(5). 358–361. https://doi.org/10.1001/jamafacial.2013.344.

The **Nasal Obstruction Symptom Evaluation (NOSE) Instrument** is a patient questionnaire that asks five questions.

1. Nasal congestion or stuffiness
2. Nasal blockage or obstruction
3. Trouble breathing through my nose
4. Trouble sleeping
5. Unable to get enough air through my nose is during exercise or insertion

The patient is asked to **grade the condition** as it affected them over the past month.

The responses may range from not a problem, scored zero (0), very mild problem, scored 1, moderate problem, scored 2, fairly bad problem, scored 3, severe problem, scored 4.

The nose score scale is calculated by the sum of the score multiplied by 5 with a possible score of 100 for an estimate of nasal obstruction as follows: Mild (range 5–25), Moderate (range 30–50), Severe (range 55–75), Extreme (range 80–100).

---

5. The cotton test, and how to perform it

Thamboo et al.[32] used the ENS6Q to validate an office-based physical examination maneuver, referred to as the cotton test, as another provocative adjunct valuable in confirming the diagnosis of ENS. For the cotton test, patients are to complete ENS6Q testing in three conditions:

1. *Precotton* placement, ENS6Q testing
2. With cotton *in place* (in situ) after 20–30 min, ENS6Q testing
3. *Postcotton* (after cotton removal), ENS6Q testing

The cotton test:

First complete the ENS6Q test prior to starting the cotton test. In an unmedicated nose, i.e., in the absence of any topical intranasal sprays, place a dry cotton (plug), usually in the region of previously resected head(s) of the inferior turbinate(s) in the patent inferior meatal space, unilaterally or bilaterally, that was partially or completely devoid of inferior turbinate tissue. The cotton remains in place for 20–30 min and with the cotton in place repeat ENS6Q testing. The cotton test is "positive" if the patient reports a reduction of their nasal symptom severity score on ENS6Q testing with the cotton in place compared to pretest the ENS6Q score.[32]

Subsequently, if patients have improvement in symptoms with the cotton test, they *might* benefit from potential inferior turbinate augmentation procedures (IMAPs).

6. Generalized Anxiety Disorder (GAD-7) test

Details are found in the original source

"**Results:** A 7-item anxiety scale (GAD-7) had good reliability, as well as criterion, construct, factorial, and procedural validity." **From the original source: Spitzer RL, Kroenke K, Williams JB, Löwe B. A brief measure for assessing generalized anxiety disorder: the GAD-7.** *Arch Intern Med.* **May 22, 2006; 166(10):1092−1097.**

The result provided by the GAD-7 is aimed at revealing whether an anxiety disorder is present and to what degree.

The original study involved a cohort of 2740 adult patients belonging to 15 primary care clinics in the United States. Following the application of the questionnaire (within a week), 965 of these patients have been referred for an interview (telephone) with a mental health professional.

Recommended usage

The GAD-7 should be used in association with other anxiety scales, such as the Hamilton scale, especially when there are concerns about the mental health status of the patient. The application of the questionnaire should be followed by other questions, related to other experiences and symptoms of the patient.

7. Patient Health Questionnaire-9 test for depression

Details are found in the original source

"**Conclusion:** In addition to making criteria-based diagnoses of depressive disorders, the PHQ-9 is also a reliable and valid measure of depression severity. These characteristics plus its brevity make the PHQ-9 a useful clinical and research tool." **From the original source: Kroenke K, Spitzer RL, Williams JB. The PHQ-9: validity of a brief depression severity measure.** *J Gen Intern Med.* **2001;16: 606−613.**

"The PHQ-9 is the 9-item depression module from the full PHQ. Major depression is diagnosed if five or more of the nine depressive symptom criteria have been present at least "more than half the days" in the past 2 weeks, and 1 of the symptoms is depressed mood or anhedonia."

"One of the nine symptom criteria ("thoughts that you would be better off dead or of hurting yourself in some way") counts if present at all, regardless of duration.

As with the original PRIME-MD, before making a final diagnosis, the clinician is expected to rule out physical causes of depression, normal bereavement, and history of a manic episode."

"For most analyses, the interpretation of the PHQ-9 score was divided into the following categories of increasing severity: 0–4, 5–9, 10–14, 15–19, and 20 or greater."

"As a severity measure, the PHQ-9 score can range from 0 to 27, since each of the 9 items can be scored from 0 (not at all) to 3 (nearly every day). An item was also added to the end of the diagnostic portion of the PHQ-9 asking patients who checked off any problems on the questionnaire: "How *difficult* have these problems made it for you to do your work, take care of things at home, or get along with other people?"

Above quotations from the original source: Kroenke K, Spitzer RL, Williams JB. The PHQ-9: validity of a brief depression severity measure. *J Gen Intern Med.* **2001;16:606–613.**

References

1. Gentles SJ, Charles C, Nicholas DB, Ploeg J, McKibbon KA. Reviewing the research methods literature: principles and strategies illustrated by a systematic overview of sampling in qualitative research. *Syst Rev*. October 11, 2016;5(1):172. https://doi.org/10.1186/s13643-016-0343-0. PMID: 27729071; PMCID: PMC5059917.

2. Moore GF, Freeman TJ, Ogren FP, Yonkers AJ. Extended follow-up of total inferior turbinate resection for relief of chronic nasal obstruction. *Laryngoscope*. September 1985;95(9 Pt 1):1095−1099.

3. Huizing EH, de Groot JAM. *Functional Reconstructive Nasal Surgery*. Thieme Stuttgart and New York Publishers; 2003.

4. Huizing EH, de Groot JAM. *Functional Reconstructive Nasal Surgery*. 2nd edition. Thieme Stuttgart, New York, Delhi: Rio de Janeiro Publishers; 2015.

5. Haight JSJ, Cole P. The site and function of the nasal valve. *Laryngoscope*. 1983;93:49−55.

6. Kasperbauer JL, Kern EB. Nasal valve physiology: implications in nasal surgery. *Otolaryngol Clin*. 1987;20:699−719.

7. Mink PJ. De neus als luchtweg. *Geneeskd Bl*. 1902;9:75−115 (Dutch translation as: The nose as airway).

8. Mink PJ. Le nez comme voie respiratoire. *Presse Otolary Belg*. 1903;21:481−496 (French translation as: The nose as respiratory tract).

9. Sulsenti G, Palma P. Tailored nasal surgery for normalization of nasal resistance. *Facial Plast Surg*. October 1996;12(4):333−345. https://doi.org/10.1055/s-2008-1064504.

10. Balakin BV, Farbu E, Kosinski P. Aerodynamic evaluation of the empty nose syndrome by means of computational fluid dynamics. *Comput Methods Biomech Biomed Eng*. 2017;20(14):1554−1561. https://doi.org/10.1080/10255842.2017.1385779.

11. Ramadan MF, Campbell IT, Linge K. The effect of nose breathing and mouth breathing on pulmonary ventilation. *Clin Otolaryngol*. 1984;9:136.

12. Flanagan P, Eccles R. Spontaneous changes of unilateral nasal airflow in man: a re-examination of the 'nasal cycle'. *Arch Otolaryngol*. 1997;117:590−595.

13. Mangin D, Coste A, Zerah-Lancner F, Bequignon E, Papon J, Devans du Mayne M. Etude de la prevalence du syndrome d'hyperventilation chez les patients atteints d'nez vide. *Annales francaises d'Oto-rhino-larygologie et de PathologieCervico-faciale*. 2014;131: A97 (French translation as: Study of the prevalence of hyperventilation syndrome in patients with empty nose.).

14. Swift AC, Campbell IT, McKown TM. Oronasal obstruction, lung volumes, and arterial oxygenation. *Lancet*. January 16, 1988;1(8577):73−75. https://doi.org/10.1016/s0140-6736(88)90282-6.

15. Cole AM, Dewan P, Ganz T. Innate antimicrobial activity of nasal secretions. *Infect Immun*. July 1999;67(7):3267−3275. https://doi.org/10.1128/IAI.67.7.3267-3275.1999. PMID: 10377100; PMCID: PMC116505.

16. Woods CM, Hooper DN, Ooi EH, Tan LW, Carney AS. Human lysozyme has fungicidal activity against nasal fungi. *Am J Rhinol Allergy*. July−August 2011;25(4):236−240. https://doi.org/10.2500/ajra.2011.25.3631. Epub June 3, 2011. PMID: 21639997.

17. Lee SH, Kim JE, Lım HH, Lee HM, Choi JO. Antimicrobial defensin peptides of the human nasal mucosa. *Ann Otol Rhinol Laryngol.* February 2002;111(2):135—141. https://doi.org/10.1177/000348940211100205. PMID: 11860065.

18. Moore EJ, Kern EB. Atrophic rhinitis: a review of 242 cases. *Am J Rhinol.* 2001;15(6): 355—361.

19. Houser SM. Surgical treatment for empty nose syndrome. *Arch Otolaryngol Head Neck Surg.* 2007;133(9):858—863.

20. Houser SM. Empty nose syndrome associated with middle turbinate resection. *Otolaryngol Head Neck Surg.* 2006;135(6):972—973.

21. Chhabra N, Houser SM. The diagnosis and management of empty nose syndrome. *Otolaryngol Clin.* 2009;42(2):311—330. ix.

22. Wang Y, Liu T, Qu Y, Dong Z, Yang Z. Empty nose syndrome. *Zhonghua Er Bi Yan Hou Ke Za Zhi.* 2001;36(3):203—205.

23. Yelenich-Huss MJ, Boyer H, Alpern JD, Stauffer WM, Schmidt D. Ozena in immigrants of differing backgrounds. *Am J Trop Med Hyg.* July 6, 2016;95(1):35—37. https://doi.org/10.4269/ajtmh.15-0885. Epub April 25, 2016. PMID: 27114295; PMCID: PMC4944704.

24. Hildenbrand T, Weber RK, Brehmer D. Rhinitis sicca, dry nose and atrophic rhinitis: a review of the literature. *Eur Arch Otorhinolaryngol.* 2011;268:17—26.

25. Hol MK, Huizing EH. Treatment of inferior turbinate pathology: a review and critical evaluation of the different techniques. *Rhinology.* 2000;38:157—166.

26. Nease C, Krempl G. Radiofrequency treatment of turbinate hypertrophy: a randomized, blinded, placebo-controlled clinical trial. *Otolaryngol Head Neck Surg.* 2004;130: 291—299.

27. Gindros G, Kantas I, Balatsouras D, Kaidoglou A, Kandiloros D. Comparison of ultrasound turbinate reduction, radiofrequency tissue ablation and submucosal cauterization in inferior turbinate hypertrophy. *Eur Arch Otorhinolaryngol.* 2010;267:1727—1733.

28. Scheithauer MO. Surgery of the turbinates and "empty nose" syndrome. *Laryngo-Rhino-Otol.* 2010;89(Suppl 1):S79—S102. https://doi.org/10.3205/cto000067. Epub April 27, 2011.

29. Chhabra N, Houser SM. The surgical management of allergic rhinitis. *Otolaryngol Clin.* 2011;44(3):779—795.

30. Hong HR, Jang YJ. Correlation between remnant inferior turbinate volume and symptom severity of empty nose syndrome. *Laryngoscope.* June 2016;126(6):1290—1295. https://doi.org/10.1002/lary.25830. Epub December 21, 2015.

31. Velasquez N, Thamboo A, Habib AR, Huang Z, Nayak JV. The Empty Nose Syndrome 6-Item Questionnaire (ENS6Q): a validated 6-item questionnaire as a diagnostic aid for empty nose syndrome. patients. *Int Forum Allergy Rhinol.* 2017;7(01):64—71.

32. Thamboo A, Velasquez N, Habib AR, Zarabanda D, Paknezhad H, Nayak JV. Defining surgical criteria for empty nose syndrome: validation of the office-based cotton test and clinical interpretability of the validated Empty Nose Syndrome 6-Item Questionnaire. *Laryngoscope.* 2017;127(08):1746—1752.

33. Gill AS, Said M, Tollefson TT, Strong EB, Nayak JV, Steele TO. Patient-reported outcome measures and provocative testing in the workup of empty nose syndrome-advances in diagnosis: a systematic review. *Am J Rhinol Allergy.* January 2020;34(1): 134—140. https://doi.org/10.1177/1945892419880642. First published Epub October 8, 2019.

34. Benignus VA, Prah JD. Olfaction: anatomy, physiology and behavior. *Environ Health Perspect.* April 1982;44:15−21. https://doi.org/10.1289/ehp.824415. PMID: 7084147; PMCID: PMC1568955.

35. Sarafoleanu C, Mella C, Georgescu M, Perederco C. The importance of the olfactory sense in the human behavior and evolution. *J Med Life.* April-June 2009;2(2): 196−198. PMID: 20108540; PMCID: PMC3018978.

36. Rhee JS, Arganbright JM, McMullin BT, Hannley M. Evidence supporting functional rhinoplasty or nasal valve repair: a 25 year systematic review. *Otolaryngol Head Neck Surg.* July 2008;139(1):10−20. https://doi.org/10.1016/j.otohns.2008.02.007.

37. Mertz JS, McCaffrey TV, Kern EB. Objective evaluation of anterior septal surgical reconstruction. *Otolaryngol Head Neck Surg.* 1984;92:308−311.

38. Huart C, Eloy P, Collet S, Rombaux P. Chemosensory function assessed with psychophysical testing and event-related potentials in patients with atrophic rhinitis. *Eur Arch Oto-Rhino-Laryngol Off J Eur Federation Oto-Rhino-Laryngol Societies (EUFOS): Affiliated with the German Society for Oto-Rhino-Laryngology - Head and Neck Surgery.* 2011.

39. Wu X, Myers AC, Goldstone AC, Togias A, Sanico AM. Localization of nerve growth factor and its receptors in the human nasal mucosa. *J Allergy Clin Immunol.* 2006; 118(2):428−433.

40. Clarke RW, Jones AS. Nasal airflow sensation. *Clin Otolaryngol Allied Sci.* 1995;20(2): 97−99.

41. Woolf CJ, Shortland P, Coggeshall RE. Peripheral nerve injury triggers central sprouting of myelinated afferents. *Nature.* January 2, 1992;355(6355):75−78.

42. Wrobel BB, Leopold DA. Olfactory and sensory attributes of the nose. *Chronic Rhinosinusitis.* 2005;38(6):1163−1170.

43. Li C, Farag AA, Maza G, et al. Investigation of the abnormal nasal aerodynamics and trigeminal functions among empty nose syndrome patients. *Int Forum Allergy Rhinol.* March 2018;8(3):444−452. https://doi.org/10.1002/alr.22045.

44. Elad D, Naftali S, Rosenfeld M, Wolf M. Physical stresses at the air-wall interface of the human nasal cavity during breathing. *J Appl Physiol.* 2006;100(3):1003−1010.

45. Grutzenmacher S, Lang C, Mlynski G. The combination of acoustic rhinometry, rhinoresistometry and flow simulation in noses before and after turbinate surgery: a model study. *ORL J Oto-Rhino-Laryngol Relat Specialties.* 2003;65(6):341−347.

46. Chen XB, Leong SC, Lee HP, Chong VF, Wang DY. Aerodynamic effects of inferior turbinate surgery on nasal airflow−a computational fluid dynamics model. *Rhinology.* 2010;48(4):394−400.

47. Naftali S, Rosenfeld M, Wolf M, Elad D. The air-conditioning capacity of the human nose. *Ann Biomed Eng.* 2005;33(4):545−553.

48. Chen XB, Lee HP, Chong VF, Wang de Y. Numerical simulation of the effects of inferior turbinate surgery on nasal airway heating capacity. *Am J Rhinol Allergy.* 2010;24(5): e118−e122.

49. Lindemann J, Keck T, Wiesmiller KM, Rettinger G, Brambs HJ, Pless D. Numerical simulation of intranasal air flow and temperature after resection of the turbinates. *Rhinology.* 2005;43(1):24−28.

50. Kastl KG, Rettinger G, Keck T. The impact of nasal surgery on air-conditioning of the nasal airways. *Rhinology.* 2009;47(3):237−241.

51. Fontanari P, Burnet H, Zattara-Hartmann MC, Jammes Y. Changes in airway resistance induced by nasal inhalation of cold dry, dry, or moist air in normal individuals. *J Appl Physiol*. 1996;81(4):1739−1743.

52. Churchill SE, Shackelford LL, Georgi JN, Black MT. Morphological variation and airflow dynamics in the human nose. *Am J Hum Biol Off J Human Biol Council*. 2004;16(6):625−638.

53. Mlynski G, Grutzenmacher S, Plontke S, Mlynski B, Lang C. Correlation of nasal morphology and respiratory function. *Rhinology*. 2001;39(4):197−201.

54. Doorly DJ, Taylor DJ, Gambaruto AM, Schroter RC, Tolley N. Nasal architecture: form and flow. *Phil Trans Math Phys Eng Sci*. 2008;366(1879):3225−3246.

55. Payne SC. Empty nose syndrome: what are we really talking about? *Otolaryngol Clin*. 2009;42(2):331−337. ix-x.

56. Di MY, Jiang Z, Gao ZQ, Li Z, An YR, Lv W. Numerical simulation of airflow fields in two typical nasal structures of empty nose syndrome: a computational fluid dynamics study. *PLoS One*. December 18, 2013;8(12):e84243. https://doi.org/10.1371/journal.pone.0084243. PMID: 24367645; PMCID: PMC3867489.

57. Naclerio RM, Pinto J, Assanasen P, Baroody FM. Observations on the ability of the nose to warm and humidify inspired air. *Rhinology*. 2007;45(2):102−111.

58. Jang YJ, Kim JH, Song HY. Empty nose syndrome: radiologic findings and treatment outcomes of endonasal microplasty using cartilage implants. *Laryngoscope*. 2011; 121(6):1308−1312.

59. Tos M, Mogensen C. Changes of the nasal mucosa in altered airflow illustrated by blind quantitative histology. *J Laryngol Otol*. 1978;92(8):667−680.

60. Jang YJ, Myong NH, Park KH, Koo TW, Kim HG. Mucociliary transport and histologic characteristics of the mucosa of deviated nasal septum. *Arch Otolaryngol Head Neck Surg*. 2002;128(4):421−424.

61. deShazo RD, Stringer SP. Atrophic rhinosinusitis: progress toward explanation of an unsolved medical mystery. *Curr Opin Allergy Clin Immunol*. 2011;11(1):1−7.

62. Manji J, Nayak JV, Thamboo A. The functional and psychological burden of empty nose syndrome. *Int Forum Allergy Rhinol*. 2018;XX:1−6.

63. Brown CL, Graham SC. Nasal irrigation: good or bad? *Curr Opin Otolaryngol Head Neck Surg*. 2004;12:9−13.

64. Modrzynski M. Hyaluronic acid gel in the treatment of empty nose syndrome. *Am J Rhinol Allergy*. 2011;25(2):103−106.

65. Jung JH, Baguindali MA, Park JT, Jang YJ. Costal cartilage is a superior implant material than conchal cartilage in the treatment of empty nose syndrome. *Otolaryngol Head Neck Surg*. September 2013;149(3):500−505.

66. Goldenberg D, Danino J, Netzer A, Joachims HZ. Plastipore implants in the surgical treatment of atrophic rhinitis: technique and results. *Otolaryngology-Head Neck Surg*. 2000;122(6):794−797.

67. Rice DH. Rebuilding the inferior turbinate with hydroxyapatite cement. *Ear Nose Throat J*. 2000;79(4):276−277.

68. Jiang C, Shi R, Sun Y. Study of inferior turbinate reconstruction with Medpor for the treatment of empty nose syndrome. *Laryngoscope*. May 2013;123(5):1106−1111.

69. Bastier PL, Bennani-Baiti AA, Stoll D, de Gabory L. beta-Tricalcium phosphate implant to repair empty nose syndrome: preliminary results. *Otolaryngology-Head and Neck Surgery*. March 2013;148(3):519−522.

70. Saafan ME. Acellular dermal (alloderm) grafts versus silastic sheets implants for management of empty nose syndrome. *Eur Arch Otorhinolaryngol*. February 2013;270(2): 527−533.

71. Kim DY, Hong HR, Choi EW, Yoon SW, Jang YJ. Efficacy and safety of autologous stromal vascular fraction in the treatment of empty nose syndrome. *Clin Exp Otorhinolaryngol*. December 2018;11(4):281−287. https://doi.org/10.21053/ceo.2017.01634. Epub May 16, 2018. PMID: 29764011.

72. Xu X, Li L, Wang C, et al. The expansion of autologous adipose-derived stem cells in vitro for the functional reconstruction of nasal mucosal tissue. *Cell Biosci*. September 17, 2015;5:54. https://doi.org/10.1186/s13578-015-0045-7.

73. Leong SC. The clinical efficacy of surgical interventions for empty nose syndrome: a systematic review. *Laryngoscope*. 2015;125:1557−1562.

74. Freund W, Wunderlich AP, Stocker T, Schmitz BL, Scheithauer MO. Empty nose syndrome: limbic system activation observed by functional magnetic resonance imaging. *Laryngoscope*. 2011;121(9):2019−2025.

75. Patel P, Most SP. . Functionally crippled nose. *Facial Plast Surg*. 2020;36(01):66−71. https://doi.org/10.1055/s-0040-1701488.

76. Gill AS, Said M, Tollefson TT, Steele TO. Update on empty nose syndrome me: disease mechanisms, diagnostic tools, and treatment strategies. *Curr Opin Otolaryngol Head Neck Surg*. August 2019;27(4):237−242.

77. Jarvis WMC. Removal of hypertrophied turbinated tissue by ecrasement with the cold wire. *Arch Laryngol*. 1882;3:I05−I111.

78. Jones TC. "Turbinotomy in cases of deafness and tinnitus aurinm": the lancet 2. *Br Med Assoc*. August 24, 1895:496.

79. Jones MN. Turbinal hypertrophy: the lancet. *Fifth Int Congress Otol*. October 5, 1895: 879.

80. Holmes CR. Hypertrophy of the turbinated bodies. *N Y Med J*. 1900;72:529.

81. Freer OT. The inferior turbinate; its longitudinal resection for chronic intumescence. *Laryngoscope*. 1911;21(12):1136−1144.

82. Mason A. A plea for the conservation of the inferior turbinate. *Atlanta J-record Med*. September 1914;61:245−249.

83. Spielberg W. The treatment of nasal obstruction by submucosal resection of the inferior turbinate. *Laryngoscope*. 1924;34:197−205.

84. House HP. Submucous resection of the inferior turbinal bone. *Laryngoscope*. July 1951; 61(7):637−648. https://doi.org/10.1288/00005537-195107000-00005. PMID: 14851737.

85. Fry HJH. Judicious turbinectomy for nasal obstruction. *Aust N Z J Surg*. February 1973; 42(3):291−294.

86. Goode RL. Surgery of the turbinates. *J Otolaryngol*. June 1978;7(3):262−268. PMID: 691091.

87. Pollock RA, Rohrich RJ. Inferior turbinate surgery: an adjunct to successful treatment of nasal obstruction in 408 patients. *Plast Reconstr Surg*. August 1984;74(2):227−236. PMID: 6463147.

88. Fanous N. Anterior turbinectomy. A new surgical approach to turbinate hypertrophy: a review of 220 cases. *Arch Otolaryngol Head Neck Surg*. August 1986;112(8): 850−852. https://doi.org/10.1001/archotol.1986.03780080050010. PMID: 3718689.

89. Mabry RL. "How I do it" – plastic surgery. Practical suggestions on facial plastic surgery. Inferior turbinoplasty. *Laryngoscope*. April 1982;92(4):459–461. https://doi.org/10.1288/00005537-198204000-00019. PMID: 7070189.

90. Mabry RL. Surgery of the inferior turbinates: how much and when? *Otolaryngol Head Neck Surg*. October 1984;92(5):571–576. https://doi.org/10.1177/019459988409200512. PMID: 6438588.

91. Mabry RL. Inferior turbinoplasty. *Arch Otolaryngol Head Neck Surg*. October 1988; 114(10):1189. https://doi.org/10.1001/archotol.1988.01860220123041. PMID: 3415833.

92. Grymer LF, Illum P, Hilberg O. Septoplasty and compensatory inferior turbinate hypertrophy: a randomized study evaluated by acoustic rhinometry. *J Laryngol Otol*. 1993; 107:413–417.

93. Illum P. Septoplasty and compensatory inferior turbinate hypertrophy: long-term results after randomized turbinoplasty. *Eur Arch Otorhinolaryngol*. 1997;254(Suppl 1): S89–S92. https://doi.org/10.1007/BF02439733. PMID: 9065637.

94. Marks S. Endoscopic inferior turbinoplasty. *Am J Rhinol*. November-December 1998; 12(6):405–407. https://doi.org/10.2500/105065898780708017. PMID: 9883296.

95. Courtiss EH, Goldwyn RM, OBrien JJ. Resection of obstructing inferior nasal turbinates. *Plast Reconstr Surg*. 1978;62-2:249–257.

96. Courtiss EH, Goldwyn RM. Resection of obstructing inferior turbinates: a 6-year follow-up. *Plast Reconstr Surg*. 1983;72:913.

97. Courtiss EH, Gargan TJ, Courtiss GB. Nasal physiology. *Ann Plast Surg*. September 1984;13(3):214–223. https://doi.org/10.1097/00000637-198409000-00008. PMID: 6497269.

98. Courtiss EH, Goldwyn RM. Resection of obstructing inferior nasal turbinates: a 10-year follow-up. *Plast Reconstr Surg*. 1990;86:152–154.

99. Dawes PJ. The early complications of inferior turbinectomy. *J Laryngol Otol*. November 1987;101(11):1136–1139. https://doi.org/10.1017/s002221510010338x. PMID: 3320236.

100. Ophir D, Shapira A, Marshak G. Total inferior turbinectomy for nasal airway obstruction. *Arch Otolaryngol*. 1985;111:93–95.

101. Ophir D. Resection of obstructing inferior turbinates following rhinoplasty. *Plast Reconstr Surg*. May 1990;85(5):724–727. https://doi.org/10.1097/00006534-199005000-00012. PMID: 2326355.

102. Ophir D, Schindel D, Halperin D, Marshak G. Long-term follow-up of the effectiveness and safety of inferior turbinectomy. *Plast Reconstr Surg*. 1992;90:980–984.

103. Martinez SA, Nissen AJ, Stock CR, et al. Nasal turbinate resection for relief of nasal obstruction. *Laryngoscope*. 1983;93:871–875.

104. Olarinde O. Total inferior turbinectomy: operative results and technique. *Ann Otol Rhinol Laryngol*. July 2001;110(7 Pt 1):700. PMID: 11465832.

105. Talmon Y, Samet A, Gilbey P. Total inferior turbinectomy: operative results and technique. *Ann Otol Rhinol Laryngol*. December 2000;109(12 Pt 1):1117–1119. https://doi.org/10.1177/000348940010901206. PMID: 11130822.

106. Eliashar R. Total inferior turbinectomy: operative results and technique. *Ann Otol Rhinol Laryngol*. July 2001;110(7 Pt 1):700. PMID: 11465833.

107. Persky MA. Possible hemorrhage after inferior turbinectomy. *Plast Reconstr Surg*. September 1993;92(4):770. https://doi.org/10.1097/00006534-199309001-00055. PMID: 8356150.

108. Yue J, Tan H, Zeng J, Huang X. Choice of the methods for inferior turbinectomy. *Lin Chuang Er Bi Yan Hou Ke Za Zhi*. February 2002;16(2):58–59. Chinese. PMID: 15510628.

109. Downs BW. The inferior turbinate in rhinoplasty. *Facial Plast Surg Clin N Am*. May 2017;25(2):171–177. https://doi.org/10.1016/j.fsc.2016.12.003. Epub February 21, 2017. PMID: 28340648.

110. Oburra HO. Complications following bilateral turbinectomy. *East Afr Med J*. February 1995;72(2):101–102. PMID: 7796746.

111. Thompson AC. Surgical reduction of the inferior turbinate in children: extended follow-up. *J Laryngol Otol*. June 1989;103(6):577–579. https://doi.org/10.1017/s0022215100109375. PMID: 2769023.

112. Wight RG, Jones AS, Beckingham E. Trimming of the inferior turbinates: a prospective long-term study. *Clin Otolaryngol Allied Sci*. August 1990;15(4):347–350. https://doi.org/10.1111/j.1365-2273.1990.tb00481.x. PMID: 2225505.

113. Segal S, Eviatar E, Berenholz L, Kessler A, Shlamkovitch N. Inferior turbinectomy in children. *Am J Rhinol*. March-April 2003;17(2):69–73. discussion 69. PMID: 12751699.

114. Salam MA, Wengraf C. Concho-antropexy or total inferior turbinectomy for hypertrophy of the inferior turbinates? A prospective randomized study. *J Laryngol Otol*. December 1993;107(12):1125–1128. https://doi.org/10.1017/s0022215100125460. PMID: 8289001.

115. Garth RJ, Cox HJ, Thomas MR. Haemorrhage as a complication of inferior turbinectomy: a comparison of anterior and radical trimming. *Clin Otolaryngol Allied Sci*. June 1995;20(3):236–238. https://doi.org/10.1111/j.1365-2273.1995.tb01856.x. PMID: 7554335.

116. Berenholz L, Kessler A, Sarfati S, Eviatar E, Segal S. Chronic sinusitis: a sequela of inferior turbinectomy. *Am J Rhinol*. July-August 1998;12(4):257–261. https://doi.org/10.2500/105065898781390046. PMID: 9740918.

117. Elwany S, Harrison R. Inferior turbinectomy: comparison of four techniques. *J Laryngol Otol*. March 1990;104(3):206–209. https://doi.org/10.1017/s0022215100112290. PMID: 2187941.

118. Carrie S, Wright RG, Jones AS, Stevens JC, Parker AJ, Yardley MP. Long-term results of trimming of the inferior turbinates. *Clin Otolaryngol Allied Sci*. April 1996;21(2):139–141. https://doi.org/10.1111/j.1365-2273.1996.tb01318.x. PMID: 8735399.

119. Jackson LE, Koch RJ. Controversies in the management of inferior turbinate hypertrophy: a comprehensive review. *Plast Reconstr Surg*. January 1999;103(1):300–312. https://doi.org/10.1097/00006534-199901000-00049. PMID: 9915195.

120. Mabry RL. Visual loss after intranasal corticosteroid injection. Incidence, causes, and prevention. *Arch Otolaryngol*. August 1981;107(8):484–486. https://doi.org/10.1001/archotol.1981.00790440024006. PMID: 7247820.

121. Byers B. Blindness secondary to steroid injections into the nasal turbinates. *Arch Ophthalmol*. January 1979;97(1):79–80. https://doi.org/10.1001/archopht.1979.01020010019004. PMID: 758896.

122. Moss WJ, Kjos KB, Karnezis TT, Lebovits MJ. Intranasal steroid injections and blindness: our personal experience and a review of the past 60 years. *Laryngoscope*. April 2015;125(4):796–800. https://doi.org/10.1002/lary.25000. Epub November 6, 2014. PMID: 25376695.

123. Sen H. Observations on the alternate erectility of the nasal mucous membrane. *Lancet.* 1901;1:564.

124. Heetderks DL. Observations on the reaction of normal nasal mucous membrane. *Am J Med Sci.* 1927;174:231−244.

125. Stoksted P. Rhinometric measurements for determination of the nasal cycle. *Acta Otolaryngol.* 1953;109(Suppl):159−175.

126. Hasegawa M, Kern EB. The human nasal cycle. *Mayo Clin Proc.* 1977;52:28−34.

127. Eccles R. The central rhythm of the nasal cycle. *Acta Otolaryngol.* 1978;86:464−468.

128. Williams MR, Eccles R. The nasal cycle and age. *Acta Otolaryngol.* August 2015; 135(8):831−834. https://doi.org/10.3109/00016489.2015.1028592. Epub March 24, 2015. PMID: 25803147.

129. Williams M, Eccles R. A model for the central control of airflow patterns within the human nasal cycle. *J Laryngol Otol.* January 2016;130(1):82−88. https://doi.org/10.1017/S0022215115002881. Epub October 20, 2015. PMID: 26482243.

130. Eccles R. A role for the nasal cycle in respiratory defence. *Eur Respir J.* February 1996; 9(2):371−376. https://doi.org/10.1183/09031936.96.09020371. PMID: 8777979.

131. Eccles R. Nasal airflow in health and disease. *Acta Otolaryngol.* 2000;120:580−595.

132. Adams DR, Ireland WP. Structure and organization of the subepithelial microvasculature in the canine nasal-mucosa. *Microvasc Res.* 1990;39:307−314.

133. Cauna N. In: Proctor DF, Andersen I, eds. *Blood and Nerve Supply of the Nasal Lining: The Nose, Upper Airways Physiology and the Atmospheric Environment.* Amsterdam: Elsevier; 1982:45−69.

134. Dahlstrom A, Fuxe K. The adrenergic innervation of the nasal mucosa of certain mammals. *Acta Otolaryngol.* 1964;59:65−72.

135. Anggard A, Edwall L. The effects of sympathetic nerve stimulation on the tracer disappearance rate and local blood content in the nasal mucosa of the cat. *Acta Otolaryngol.* 1974;77:131−139.

136. Malm L. Sympathetic influence on the nasal mucosa. *Acta Otolaryngol.* 1977;83: 20−21.

137. Lacroix JS, Stjarne P, Anggard A, Lundberg JM. Sympathetic vascular control of the pig nasal mucosa(III): co-release of noradrenaline and neuropeptide Y. *Acta Physiol Scand.* 1989;135:17−28.

138. van Dishoek HAE, Leiden MD. The part of the valve and the turbinates in total nasal resistance. *Int Rhinol.* 1965;3:19−26.

139. Bridger GP. Physiology of the nasal valve. *Arch Otolaryngol.* 1970;92:543−553.

140. Cole P. *The respiratory role of the upper airways. A Selective Clinical and Pathological Review.* St Louis, MO: Mosby Year Book; 1993:164.

141. Schulte DL, Sherris DA, Kern EB. *M-plasty correction of nasal valve obstruction. Facial Plastic Surgery Clinics of North America.* W. B. Saunders; August 1999.

142. Farmer SEJ, Eccles R. Chronic inferior turbinate enlargement and the implications for surgical intervention. *Rhinology.* December 2006;44(4):234−238.

143. Pandya VK, Tiwari RS. Nasal mucociliary clearance in health and disease. *Indian J Otolaryngol Head Neck Surg.* October 2006;58(4):332−334.

144. Duchateau GS, Graamans K, Zuidema J, Merkus FW. Correlation between nasal ciliary beat frequency and mucus transport rate in volunteers. *Laryngoscope.* July 1985;95(7 Pt 1):854−859. PMID: 401042.

145. Stupp F, Weigel A, Hoffmann TK, Sommer F, Grossi AS, Lindemann J. Schirmer test for determining the moisture status of the nasal mucosa. *HNO.* May 2019;67(5):

379−384. NOTE: This test will further investigations on the nasal patients with nasal atrophy, e. g. empty nose syndrome or Sjogren's syndrome.

146. Stevens S. Schirmer's test. *Community Eye Health*. December 2011;24(76):45. NOTE: Measurement of tears secretion has utility in patients suspected of "dry eyes".

147. Sumner D. On testing the sense of smell. *Lancet*. November 3, 1962;2(7262):895−897.

148. Doty RL. Psychophysical testing of smell and taste function. *Handb Clin Neurol*. 2019; 164:229−246.

149. Grymer LF. Clinical applications of acoustic rhinometry. *Rhinol Suppl*. December 2000;16:35−43.

150. Wong EH, Eccles R. Comparison of the classic and Broms methods of rhinomanometry using model noses. *Eur Arch Oto-Rhino-Laryngol*. January 2015;272(1):105−110.

151. Santiago-Diez de Bonilla J, McCaffrey TV, Kern EB. The nasal valve: a rhinomanometric evaluation of maximum nasal inspiratory flow and pressure curves. *Ann Otol Rhinol Laryngol*. May-June 1986;95:229−232.

152. van Spronsen E, Ebbens FA, Fokkens WJ. Normal peak nasal inspiratory flow rate values in healthy children aged 6 to 11 years in the Netherlands. *Rhinology*. March 2012;50(1):22−25.

153. Ottaviano G, Fokkens WJ. Measurements of nasal airflow and patency: a critical review with emphasis on the use of peak nasal inspiratory flow in daily practice. *Allergy*. February 2016;71(2):162−174. https://doi.org/10.1111/all.12778.

154. Radulesco T, Meister L, Bouchet G, et al. Functional relevance of computational fluid dynamics in the field of nasal obstruction: a literature review. *Clin Otolaryngol*. 2019; 44(5):801−809.

155. Kirkeby L, Rasmussen TT, Reinholdt J, Kilian M. Immunoglobulins in nasal secretions of healthy humans: structural integrity of secretory immunoglobulin A1 (IgA1) and occurrence of neutralizing antibodies to IgA1 proteases of nasal bacteria. *Clin Diagn Lab Immunol*. January 2000;7(1):31−39. Note: Levels of IgE and IgD, are present at low levels in nasal secretions of healthy people.

156. Gassner HG, Ponikau JU, Sherris DA, Kern EB. CSF rhinorrhea: 95 consecutive surgical cases with long term follow-up at the Mayo Clinic. *Am J Rhinol*. 1999;13(6): 439−447.

157. Malmberg H, Holopainen E. Nasal smear as a screening test for immediate-type nasal allergy. *Allergy*. October 1979;34(5):331−337.

158. Cole P. Rhinomanometry: practice and trends. *Laryngoscope*. 1989;99:311−315.

159. Cole P. Stability of nasal airflow resistance. *Clin Otolaryngol*. 1989;14:177−182. https://doi.org/10.1111/j.1365-2273.1989.tb00357.x.

160. Thoma A, Eaves 3rd FF. A brief history of evidence-based medicine (EBM) and the contributions of Dr. David Sackett. *Aesthetic Surg J*. November 2015;35(8): NP261−N263. https://doi.org/10.1093/asj/sjv130. Epub July 9, 2015. PMID: 26163313.

161. Sackett DL, Rosenberg WM, Gray JA, Haynes RB, Richardson WS. Evidence based medicine: what it is and what it isn't. *BMJ*. 1996;312(7023):71−72.

162. Sackett DL, Strauss SE, Richardson WS, Rosenberg W, Haynes RB. *Evidence-based Medicine: How to Practice and Teach EBM*. 2nd ed. Edinburgh, Scotland: Churchill Livingston; 2000.

163. Sackett D. How to read clinical journals: I. why to read them and how to start reading them critically. *Can Med Assoc J*. 1981;124(5):555−558.

164. Guyatt G, Rennie D, Meade MO, Cook DJ. *Users' Guides to the Medical Literature: A Manual for Evidence-Based Clinical Practice*. 2nd ed. New York: McGraw-Hill Professional; 2008.

165. The periodic health examination. Canadian Task force on the Periodic Health Examination. *Can Med Assoc J*. 1979;121:1191−1254.

166. Burns PB, Rohrich RJ, Chung KC. The levels of evidence and their role in evidence-based medicine. *Plast Reconstr Surg*. July 2011;128(1):305−310. https://doi.org/10.1097/PRS.0b013e318219c171. PMID: 21701348; PMCID: PMC3124652.

167. Sackett DL. Rules of evidence and clinical recommendations on the use of antithrombotic agents. *Chest*. 1989;95(2 Suppl):2S−4S.

168. American Society of Plastic Surgeons. Scales for rating levels of evidence. Available at: http://www.plasticsurgery.org/Medical_Professionals/Health_Policy_and_Advocacy/Health_Policy_Resources/Evidencebased_GuidelinesPractice_Parameters/Description_and_Development_of_Evidence-based_Practice_Guidelines/ASPS_Evidence_Rating_Scales.html.

169. Centre for Evidence Based Medicine (Web site). Available at: http://www.cebm.net. Oxford Centre for Evidence-based Medicine. Levels of evidence. March 2009. http://www.cebm.net/oxford-centre-evidence-based-medicine-levels-evidence-march-2009.

170. Jadad AR, Moore RA, Carroll D, et al. Assessing the quality of reports of randomized clinical trials: is blinding necessary? *Contr Clin Trials*. 1996;17:1−12.

171. Concato J, Shah N, Horwitz RI. Randomized, controlled trials, observational studies, and the hierarchy of research designs. *N Engl J Med*. 2000;342:1887−1892.

172. Ackley BJ, Swan BA, Ladwig G, Tucker S. *Evidence-based Nursing Care Guidelines: Medical-Surgical Interventions*. St. Louis, MO: Mosby Elsevier; 2008:7.

173. Straus SE, Sackett DL. Getting research findings into practice: using research findings in clinical practice. *BMJ*. 1998;317:339−342.

174. El Dib RP, Atallah AN, Andriolo RB. Mapping the Cochrane evidence for decision making in health care. *J Eval Clin Pract*. August 2007;13(4):689−692. https://doi.org/10.1111/j.1365-2753.2007.00886.x. PMID: 17683315.

175. Al Deek NF. Rethinking evidence-based medicine in plastic and reconstructive surgery. *Plast Reconstr Surg*. September 2018;142(3):429e. https://doi.org/10.1097/PRS.0000000000004643. PMID: 29965927.

176. Swanson E. In defense of evidence-based medicine in plastic surgery. *Plast Reconstr Surg*. April 2019;143(4):898e−899e. https://doi.org/10.1097/PRS.0000000000005470. PMID: 30707152.

177. Croft P, Malmivaara A, van Tulder M. The pros and cons of evidence-based medicine. *Spine*. August 1, 2011;36(17):E1121−E1125. https://doi.org/10.1097/BRS.0b013e318223ae4c. PMID: 21629165.

178. Freddi G, Romàn-Pumar JL. Evidence-based medicine: what it can and cannot do. *Ann Ist Super Sanita*. 2011;47(1):22−25. https://doi.org/10.4415/ANN_11_01_06. PMID: 21430334.

179. Sniderman AD, LaChapelle KJ, Rachon NA, Furberg CD. The necessity for clinical reasoning in the era of evidence-based medicine. *Mayo Clin Proc*. October 2013;88(10):1108−1114. https://doi.org/10.1016/j.mayocp.2013.07.012. PMID: 24079680.

180. Bakwin H. Pseudodoxia Pediatrica. *N Engl J Med*. 1945;232:691−697. https://doi.org/10.1056/NEJM194506142322401.

181. Proust M. *The Guermantes Way. Volume 1. of 7 Volumes*. New York: Boni; 1930:929.

182. Wigand ME, Steiner W, Jaumann MP. Endonasal sinus surgery with endoscopical control: from radical operation to rehabilitation of the mucosa. *Endoscopy*. 1978;10: 255–260. https://doi.org/10.1055/s0028-1098304.

183. Biedlingmeier JP. Endoscopic middle turbinate resection: results and complications. *Ear Nose Throat J*. 1993;72:351–355.

184. Marchioni D, Alicandri-Ciufelli M, Mattioli F, et al. Middle turbinate preservation versus middle turbinate resection in endoscopic surgical treatment of nasal polyposis. Acta Otolaryngol. September 2008;128(9):1019–1026. https://doi.org/10.1080/00016480701827541. PMID: 19086309.

185. Messerklinger W. Endoscopic diagnosis and surgery of recurrent sinusitis. In: Krajira Z, ed. *Advances in Nose and Sinus Surgery*. Zagreb: Zagreb University; 1985.

186. Ramadan HH, Allen GC. Complications of endoscopic sinus surgery in a residency training program. *Laryngoscope*. 1995;105:376–379. https://doi.org/10.1288/00005537-199504000-00007.

187. Stammberger H, Posawetz W. Functional endoscopic sinus surgery. Concept, indications and results of the Messerklinger technique. *Eur Arch Otorhinolaryngol*. 1990; 247(2):63–76. https://doi.org/10.1007/BF00183169. PMID: 2180446.

188. Swanson P, Lanza DC, Kennedy DW, Vining EM. The effect of middle turbinate resection upon frontal sinus disease. *Am J Rhinol*. 1995;9:191–195. https://doi.org/10.2500/105065895781873737.

189. Zhou C, Li B. The effect of partial middle turbinectomy upon the frontal sinus. *Lin Chuang Er Bi Yan Hou Ke Za Zhi*. June 1999;13(6):261–262. Chinese. PMID: 12563980.

190. Fortune DS, Duncavage JA. Incidence of frontal sinusitis following partial middle turbinectomy. *Ann Otol Rhinol Laryngol*. 1998;107:447–453.

191. Havas TE, Lowinger DS. Comparison of functional endonasal sinus surgery with and without partial middle turbinate resection. *Ann Otol Rhinol Laryngol*. 2000;109: 634–640.

192. Giacchi RJ, Lebowitz RA, Jacobs JB. Middle turbinate resection:issues and controversies. *Am J Rhinol*. 2000;14(3):193–197. https://doi.org/10.2500/105065800782102726.

193. Shih C, Chin G, Rice DH. Middle turbinate resection: impact on outcomes in endoscopic sinus surgery. *Ear Nose Throat J*. 2003;82:796–797.

194. Kennedy DW. Middle turbinate resection. Evaluating the issues – should we resect normal middle turbinates? *Arch Otolaryngol Head Neck Surg*. 1998;124:107.

195. Rice DH. Middle turbinate resection. Weighing the decision. *Arch Otolaryngol Head Neck Surg*. 1998;124:106.

196. Stewart MG. Middle turbinate resection. *Arch Otolaryngol Head Neck Surg*. 1998;124: 104–106.

197. Nurse LA, Duncavage JA. Surgery of the inferior and middle turbinates. *Otolaryngol Clin*. April 2009;42(2):295–309. https://doi.org/10.1016/j.otc.2009.01.009. PMID: 19328894.

198. Rice DH, Kern EB, Marple BF, Mabry RL, Friedman WH. The turbinates in nasal and sinus surgery: a consensus statement. *Ear Nose Throat J*. February 2003;82(2):82–84. PMID: 12619458.

199. Clement WA, White PS. Trends in turbinate surgery literature: a 35-year review. *Clin Otolaryngol*. 2001;26:124–128.

200. Hudon MA, Wright ED, Fortin-Pellerin E, Bussieres M. Resection versus preservation of the middle turbinate for chronic rhinosinusitis with nasal polyposis: a randomized controlled trial. *J Otolaryngol Head Neck Surg.* November 8, 2018;47(1):67. https://doi.org/10.1186/s40463-018-0313-8. PMID: 30409178; PMCID: PMC6225688.

201. Camacho M, Zaghi S, Certal V, et al. Inferior turbinate classification system, grades 1 to 4: development and validation study. *Laryngoscope.* February 2015;125(2):296−302. https://doi.org/10.1002/lary.24923. Epub September 12, 2014. PMID: 25215619.

202. Friedman M, Tanyeri H, Lim J, Landsberg R, Caldarelli D. A safe, alternative technique for inferior turbinate reduction. *Laryngoscope.* November 1999;109(11):1834−1837. https://doi.org/10.1097/00005537-199911000-00021. PMID: 10569417.

203. Leitzen KP, Brietzke SE, Lindsay RW. Correlation between nasal anatomy and objective obstructive sleep apnea severity. *Otolaryngol Head Neck Surg.* February 2014; 150(2):325−331. https://doi.org/10.1177/0194599813515838. Epub December 13, 2013. PMID: 24334963.

204. Uzun L, Ugur MB, Savranlar A, Mahmutyazicioglu K, Ozdemir H, Beder LB. Classification of the inferior turbinate bones: a computed tomography study. *Eur J Radiol.* September 2004;51(3):241−245. https://doi.org/10.1016/j.ejrad.2004.02.013. PMID: 15294331.

205. Yao F, Singer M, Rosenfeld RM. Randomized controlled trials in otolaryngology journals. *Otolaryngol Head Neck Surg.* October 2007;137(4):539−544. https://doi.org/10.1016/j.otohns.2007.07.018. PMID: 17903567.

206. Ah-See KW, Molony NC, Maran AG. Trends in randomized controlled trials in ENT: a 30-year review. *J Laryngol Otol.* July 1997;111(7):611−613. https://doi.org/10.1017/s0022215100138101. PMID: 9282195.

207. Banglawala SM, Lawrence LA, Franko-Tobin E, Soler ZM, Schlosser RJ, Ioannidis J. Recent randomized controlled trials in otolaryngology. *Otolaryngol Head Neck Surg.* March 2015;152(3):418−423. https://doi.org/10.1177/0194599814563518. Epub December 30, 2014. PMID: 25550226.

208. Joyce KM, Joyce CW, Kelly JC, Kelly JL, Carroll SM. Levels of evidence in the plastic surgery literature: a citation analysis of the top 50 'classic' papers. *Arch Plast Surg.* July 2015;42(4):411−418. https://doi.org/10.5999/aps.2015.42.4.411. Epub July 14, 2015. PMID: 26217560; PMCID: PMC4513048.

209. Eggerstedt M, Brown HJ, Shay AD, et al. Level of evidence in facial plastic surgery research: a procedure-level analysis. *Aesthetic Plast Surg.* 2020;44:1531−1536. https://doi.org/10.1007/s00266-020-01720-3.

210. Batra PS, Seiden AM, Smith TL. Surgical management of adult inferior turbinate hypertrophy: a systematic review of the evidence. *Laryngoscope.* September 2009;119(9):1819−1827. https://doi.org/10.1002/lary.20544. PMID: 19521999.

211. Passàli D, Passàli FM, Damiani V, Passàli GC, Bellussi L. Treatment of inferior turbinate hypertrophy: a randomized clinical trial. *Ann Otol Rhinol Laryngol.* August 2003; 112(8):683−688. https://doi.org/10.1177/000348940311200806. PMID: 12940665.

212. Cavaliere M, Mottola G, Iemma M. Monopolar and bipolar radiofrequency thermal ablation of inferior turbinates: 20-month follow-up. *Otolaryngol Head Neck Surg.* 2007;137:256−263.

213. Peters JP, Hooft L, Grolman W, Stegeman I. Assessment of the quality of reporting of randomised controlled trials in otorhinolaryngologic literature - adherence to the CONSORT statement. *PLoS One.* March 20, 2015;10(3):e0122328. https://doi.org/10.1371/journal.pone.0122328. PMID: 25793517; PMCID: PMC4368673.

214. Abdullah B, Singh S. Surgical interventions for inferior turbinate hypertrophy: a comprehensive review of current techniques and technologies. *Int J Environ Res Publ Health.* March 26, 2021;18(7):3441. https://doi.org/10.3390/ijerph18073441. PMID: 33810309; PMCID: PMC8038107.

215. Silkoff PE, Chakravorty S, Chapnik J, Cole P, Zamel N. Reproducibility of acoustic rhinometry and rhinomanometry in normal subjects. *Am J Rhinol.* March-April 1999; 13(2):131−135. https://doi.org/10.2500/105065899782106689. PMID: 10219442.

216. Passàli D, Lauriello M, Anselmi M, Bellussi L. Treatment of hypertrophy of the inferior turbinate: long-term results in 382 patients randomly assigned to therapy. *Ann Otol Rhinol Laryngol.* June 1999;108(6):569−575. https://doi.org/10.1177/000348949910800608. PMID: 10378525.

217. Janda P, Sroka R, Baumgartner R, Grevers G, Leunig A. Laser treatment of hyperplastic inferior nasal turbinates: a review. *Laser Surg Med.* 2001;28(5):404−413. https://doi.org/10.1002/lsm.1068. PMID: 11413552.

218. Sroka R, Janda P, Killian T, Vaz F, Betz CS, Leunig A. Comparison of long term results after Ho:YAG and diode laser treatment of hyperplastic inferior nasal turbinates. *Laser Surg Med.* April 2007;39(4):324−331. https://doi.org/10.1002/lsm.20479. PMID: 17304563.

219. Kisser U, Stelter K, Gürkov R, et al. Diode laser versus radiofrequency treatment of the inferior turbinate - a randomized clinical trial. *Rhinology.* December 2014;52(4): 424−430. https://doi.org/10.4193/Rhin14.001. PMID: 25479227.

220. Prokopakis EP, Koudounarakis EI, Velegrakis GA. Efficacy of inferior turbinoplasty with the use of CO(2) laser, radiofrequency, and electrocautery. *Am J Rhinol Allergy.* May-June 2014;28(3):269−272. https://doi.org/10.2500/ajra.2014.28.4044. PMID: 24980241.

221. Puterman MM, Segal N, Joshua BZ. Endoscopic, assisted, modified turbinoplasty with mucosal flap. *J Laryngol Otol.* 2012;126:525−528. https://doi.org/10.1017/S0022215112000163.

222. Barham HP, Knisely A, Harvey RJ, Sacks R. How I do it: medial flap inferior turbinoplasty. *Am J Rhinol Allergy.* 2015;29:314−315. https://doi.org/10.2500/ajra.2015.29.4168.

223. Hamerschmidt R, Hamerschmidt R, Moreira AT, Tenorio SB, Timi JR. Comparison of turbinoplasty surgery efficacy in patients with and without allergic rhinitis. *Braz J Otorhinolaryngol.* 2016;82:131−139. https://doi.org/10.1016/j.bjorl.2015.10.010.

224. Sindwani R, Manz R. Technological innovations in tissue removal during rhinologic surgery. *Am J Rhinol Allergy.* 2012;26:65−69. https://doi.org/10.2500/ajra.2012.26.3722.

225. Joniau S, Wong I, Rajapaksa S, Carney SA, Wormald PJ. Long-term comparison between submucosal cauterization and powered reduction of the inferior turbinates. *Laryngoscope.* 2006;116:1612−1616. https://doi.org/10.1097/01.mlg.0000227999.76713.d3.

226. Huang TW, Cheng PW. Changes in nasal resistance and quality of life after endoscopic microdebrider-assisted inferior turbinoplasty in patients with perennial allergic rhinitis. *Arch Otolaryngol Head Neck Surg.* 2006;132:990−993. https://doi.org/10.1001/archotol.132.9.990.

227. Lee CF, Chen TA. Power microdebrider-assisted modification of endoscopic inferior turbinoplasty: a preliminary report. *Chang Gung Med J.* 2004;27:359−365.

228. El Henawi Del D, Ahmed MR, Madian YT. Comparison between power-assisted turbinoplasty and submucosal resection in the treatment of inferior turbinate hypertrophy. *Orl J Otorhinolaryngol Relat Spec.* 2011;73:151−155. https://doi.org/10.1159/000327607.

229. Woloszko J, Gilbride C. Coblation technology: plasma-mediated ablation for otolaryngology applications. In: Anderson RR, Bartels KE, Bass LS, eds. *Proceedings of the SPIE: Lasers in Surgery: Advanced Characterization, Therapeutics, and Systems X.* Vol 3907. Bellingham, WA, USA: SPIE−The International Society for Optical Engineering; 2000:306−316.

230. Cingi C, Ure B, Cakli H, Ozudogru E. Microdebrider-assisted versus radiofrequency-assisted inferior turbinoplasty: a prospective study with objective and subjective outcome measures. *Acta Otorhinolaryngol Ital.* 2010;30:138−143.

231. Utley DS, Goode RL, Hakim I. Radiofrequency energy tissue ablation for the treatment of nasal obstruction secondary to turbinate hypertrophy. *Laryngoscope.* 1999;109:683−686. https://doi.org/10.1097/00005537-199905000-00001.

232. Li KK, Powell NB, Riley RW, Troell RJ, Guilleminault C. Radiofrequency volumetric tissue reduction for treatment of turbinate hypertrophy: a pilot study. *Otolaryngol Head Neck Surg.* 1998;119:569−573. https://doi.org/10.1016/S0194-5998(98)70013-0.

233. Bakshi SS, Shankar Manoharan K, Gopalakrishnan S. Comparison of the long-term efficacy of radiofrequency ablation and surgical turbinoplasty in inferior turbinate hypertrophy: a randomized clinical study. *Acta Otolaryngol.* 2017;137:856−861. https://doi.org/10.1080/00016489.2017.1294764.

234. Vijay Kumar K, Kumar S, Garg S. A comparative study of radiofrequency assisted versus microdebrider assisted turbinoplasty in cases of inferior turbinate hypertrophy. *Indian J Otolaryngol Head Neck Surg.* 2014;66:35−39. https://doi.org/10.1007/s12070-013-0657-3.

235. Liu CM, Tan CD, Lee FP, Lin KN, Huang HM. Microdebrider-assisted versus radiofrequency assisted-inferior turbinoplasty. *Laryngoscope.* 2009;119:414−418. https://doi.org/10.1002/lary.20088.

236. Means C, Camacho M, Capasso R. Long-term outcomes of radiofrequency ablation of the inferior turbinates. *Indian J Otolaryngol Head Neck Surg.* 2016;68:424−428. https://doi.org/10.1007/s12070-015-0912-x.

237. Acevedo JL, Camacho M, Brietzke SE. Radiofrequency ablation turbinoplasty versus microdebrider-assisted turbinoplasty: a systematic review and meta-analysis. *Otolaryngol Head Neck Surg.* 2015;153:951−956. https://doi.org/10.1177/0194599815607211.

238. Garzaro M, Landolfo V, Pezzoli M, et al. Radiofrequency volume turbinate reduction versus partial turbinectomy: clinical and histological features. *Am J Rhinol Allergy.* 2012;26:321−325. https://doi.org/10.2500/ajra.2012.26.3788.

239. Harrill WC, Pillsbury 3rd HC, McGuirt WF, Stewart MG. Radiofrequency turbinate reduction: a NOSE evaluation. *Laryngoscope.* 2007;117:1912−1919. https://doi.org/10.1097/MLG.0b013e3181271414.

240. Passali D, Loglisci M, Politi L, Passali GC, Kern E. Managing turbinate hypertrophy: coblation vs. radiofrequency treatment. *Eur Arch Otorhinolaryngol.* 2016;273:1449−1453. https://doi.org/10.1007/s00405-015-3759-6.

241. Farmer SE, Quine SM, Eccles R. Efficacy of inferior turbinate coblation for treatment of nasal obstruction. *J Laryngol Otol.* 2009;123:309−314. https://doi.org/10.1017/S0022215108002818.

242. Leong SC, Farmer SE, Eccles R. Coblation inferior turbinate reduction: a long-term follow-up with subjective and objective assessment. *Rhinology.* 2010;48:108−112.

243. Singh S, Ramli RR, Wan Mohammad Z, Abdullah B. Coblation versus microdebrider-assisted turbinoplasty for endoscopic inferior turbinates reduction. *Auris Nasus Larynx.* August 2020;47(4):593−601. https://doi.org/10.1016/j.anl.2020.02.003. Epub February 19, 2020. PMID: 32085929.

244. Moss WJ, Lemieux AJ, Alexander TH. Is inferior turbinate lateralization effective? *Plast Reconstr Surg.* November 2015;136(5):710e−711e. https://doi.org/10.1097/PRS.0000000000001687. PMID: 26182178.

245. Aksoy F, Yıldırım YS, Veyseller B, Ozturan O, Demirhan H. Midterm outcomes of out-fracture of the inferior turbinate. *Otolaryngol Head Neck Surg.* October 2010;143(4):579−584. https://doi.org/10.1016/j.otohns.2010.06.915. PMID: 20869571.

246. Marquez F, Cenjor C, Gutierrez R, Sanabria J. Multiple submucosal out-fracture of the inferior turbinates: evaluation of the results by acoustic rhinometry. *Am J Rhinol.* 1996;10:387−391.

247. Buyuklu F, Cakmak O, Hizal E, Donmez FY. Outfracture of the inferior turbinate: a computed tomography study. *Plast Reconstr Surg.* June 2009;123(6):1704−1709. https://doi.org/10.1097/PRS.0b013e31819b69b1. Epub March 23, 2009.

248. O'Flynn PE, Milford CA, Mackay IS. Multiple submucosal out-fractures of interior turbinates. *J Laryngol Otol.* March 1990;104(3):239−240. https://doi.org/10.1017/s002221510011237x. PMID: 2341781.

249. Thomas PL, John DG, Carlin WV. The effect of inferior turbinate outfracture on nasal resistance to airflow in vasomotor rhinitis assessed by rhinomanometry. *J Laryngol Otol.* February 1988;102(2):144−145. https://doi.org/10.1017/s0022215100104359. PMID: 3346593.

250. Zhang QX, Zhou WG, Zhang HD, Ke YF, Wang QP. Relationship between inferior turbinate outfracture and the improvement of nasal ventilatory function. *Zhonghua Er Bi Yan Hou Tou Jing Wai Ke Za Zhi.* May 2013;48(5):422−425. Chinese. PMID: 24016569.

251. Sinno S, Mehta K, Lee ZH, Kidwai S, Saadeh PB, Lee MR. Inferior turbinate hypertrophy in rhinoplasty: systematic review of surgical techniques. *Plast Reconstr Surg.* September 2016;138(3):419e−429e. https://doi.org/10.1097/PRS.0000000000002433. PMID: 27556616.

252. Lee DC, Jin SG, Kim BY, et al. Does the effect of inferior turbinate outfracture persist? *Plast Reconstr Surg.* February 2017;139(2):386e−391e. https://doi.org/10.1097/PRS.0000000000002934. PMID: 28121862.

253. Lee KC, Lee SS, Lee JK, Lee SH. Medial fracturing of the inferior turbinate: effect on the osteomeatal unit and uncinate process. *Eur Arch Otorhinolaryngol.* 2009;266:857−861.

254. Jung D, Gray ST. Silent sinus syndrome after lateral fracture of the inferior turbinate. *Otolaryngol Head Neck Surg.* May 2012;146(5):863−864. https://doi.org/10.1177/0194599811424041. Epub September 27, 2011. PMID: 21952356.

255. Kökoğlu K, Vural A. Evaluation of the effect of inferior turbinate outfracture on nasolacrimal transit time by saccharin test. *Eur Arch Otorhinolaryngol.* June 2019;276(6):1671−1675. https://doi.org/10.1007/s00405-019-05382-z. Epub March 15, 2019. PMID: 30877421.

256. Neri G, Cazzato F, Mastronardi V, et al. Ultrastructural regenerating features of nasal mucosa following microdebrider-assisted turbinoplasty are related to clinical recovery. *J Transl Med.* 2016;14:164. https://doi.org/10.1186/s12967-016-0931-8.

257. Gindros G, Kantas I, Balatsouras DG, Kandiloros D, Manthos AK, Kaidoglou A. Mucosal changes in chronic hypertrophic rhinitis after surgical turbinate reduction. *Eur Arch Otorhinolaryngol.* September 2009;266(9):1409−1416. https://doi.org/10.1007/s00405-009-0916-9. Epub January 30, 2009. PMID: 19184076.

258. Berger G, Gass S, Ophir D. The histopathology of the hypertrophic inferior turbinate. *Arch Otolaryngol Head Neck Surg.* 2006;132:588−594. https://doi.org/10.1001/archotol.132.6.588.

259. Berger G, Ophir D, Pitaro K, Landsberg R. Histopathological changes after coblation inferior turbinate reduction. *Arch Otolaryngol Head Neck Surg.* August 2008;134(8):819−823. https://doi.org/10.1001/archotol.134.8.819. PMID: 18711054.

260. Pelen A, Tekin M, Özbilen Acar G, Özdamar Oİ. Comparison of the effects of radio-frequency ablation and microdebrider reduction on nasal physiology in lower turbinate surgery. *Kulak Burun Bogaz Ihtis Derg.* November-December 2016;26(6):325−332. https://doi.org/10.5606/kbbihtisas.2016.26964. PMID: 27983900.

261. Smith GCS, Pell JP. Parachute use to prevent death and major trauma related to gravitational challenge: systematic review of randomized controlled trials. *BMJ.* 2003;327:20−72.

262. Leong SC, Eccles R. Inferior turbinate surgery and nasal airflow: evidence-based management. *Curr Opin Otolaryngol Head Neck Surg.* February 2010;18(1):54−59. https://doi.org/10.1097/MOO.0b013e328334db14. PMID: 19915466.

263. Wasserman JM, Wynn R, Bash TS, Rosenfeld RM. Levels of evidence in otolaryngology journals. *Otolaryngol Head Neck Surg.* May 2006;134(5):717−723. https://doi.org/10.1016/j.otohns.2005.11.049. PMID: 16647522.

264. Larrabee YC, Kacker A. Which inferior turbinate reduction technique best decreases nasal obstruction? *Laryngoscope.* April 2014;124(4):814−815. https://doi.org/10.1002/lary.24182. Epub September 19, 2013. PMID: 24105730.

265. Jose J, Coatesworth AP. Inferior turbinate surgery for nasal obstruction in allergic rhinitis after failed medical treatment. *Cochrane Database Syst Rev.* December 8, 2010;(12):CD005235. https://doi.org/10.1002/14651858.CD005235.pub2. PMID: 21154359.

266. Agha R, Cooper D, Muir G. The reporting quality of randomised controlled trials in surgery: a systematic review. *Int J Surg.* December 2007;5(6):413−422. https://doi.org/10.1016/j.ijsu.2007.06.002. Epub October 29, 2007. PMID: 18029237.

267. Glasziou P, Chalmers I, Rawlins M, McCulloch P. When are randomised trials unnecessary? Picking signal from noise. *BMJ.* February 17, 2007;334(7589):349−351. https://doi.org/10.1136/bmj.39070.527986.68. PMID: 17303884; PMCID: PMC1800999.

268. Kenny SE, Shankar KR, Rintala R, Lamont GL, Lloyd DA. Evidence-based surgery: interventions in a regional paediatric surgical unit. *Arch Dis Child.* January 1997;76(1):50−53. https://doi.org/10.1136/adc.76.1.50. PMID: 9059162; PMCID: PMC1717052.

269. Lanier WL, Rajkumar SV. Empiricism and rationalism in medicine: can 2 competing philosophies coexist to improve the quality of medical care? *Mayo Clin Proc.* October 2013;88(10):1042−1045. https://doi.org/10.1016/j.mayocp.2013.08.005. PMID: 24079675.

270. Farley R. A is for aphorism–'good judgment comes from experience; experience comes from bad judgment'. *Aust Fam Physician*. August 2013;42(8):587−588. PMID: 23971071.

271. Prasad V, Vandross A, Toomey C, et al. A decade of reversal: an analysis of 146 contradicted medical practices. *Mayo Clin Proc*. 2013;88(8):790−798.

272. Prasad V. Regarding empiricism and rationalism in medicine and 2 medical worldviews. *Mayo Clin Proc*. January 2014;89(1):137. https://doi.org/10.1016/j.mayocp.2013.10.019. PMID: 24388033.

273. Ross DG. Two medical worldviews. *Mayo Clin Proc*. January 2014;89(1):137−138. https://doi.org/10.1016/j.mayocp.2013.11.004. PMID: 24388032.

274. Stirrat GM, Farrow SC, Farndon J, Dwyer N. The challenge of evaluating surgical procedures. *Ann R Coll Surg Engl*. March 1992;74(2):80−84. PMID: 1567147; PMCID: PMC2497523.

275. Stirrat GM. Ethics and evidence based surgery. *J Med Ethics*. April 2004;30(2): 160−165. https://doi.org/10.1136/jme.2003.007054. PMID: 15082810; PMCID: PMC1733841.

276. Black N. Evidence-based surgery: a passing fad? *World J Surg*. August 1999;23(8): 789−793. https://doi.org/10.1007/s002689900581. PMID: 10415204.

277. Darsaut TE, Raymond J. Ethical care requires pragmatic care research to guide medical practice under uncertainty. *Trials*. February 15, 2021;22(1):143. https://doi.org/10.1186/s13063-021-05084-0. PMID: 33588946; PMCID: PMC7885344.

278. Finniss DG, Kaptchuk TJ, Miller F, Benedetti F. Biological, clinical, and ethical advances of placebo effects. *Lancet*. February 20, 2010;375(9715):686−695. https://doi.org/10.1016/S0140-6736(09)61706-2. PMID: 20171404; PMCID: PMC2832199.

279. Beecher HK. The powerful placebo. *J Am Med Assoc*. December 24, 1955;159(17): 1602−1606. https://doi.org/10.1001/jama.1955.02960340022006. PMID: 13271123.

280. Blease C, Colloca L, Kaptchuk TJ. Are open-label placebos ethical? Informed consent and ethical equivocations. *Bioethics*. July 2016;30(6):407−414. https://doi.org/10.1111/bioe.12245. Epub February 3, 2016. PMID: 26840547; PMCID: PMC4893896.

281. Savulescu J, Wartolowska K, Carr A. Randomised placebo-controlled trials of surgery: ethical analysis and guidelines. *J Med Ethics*. December 2016;42(12):776−783. https://doi.org/10.1136/medethics-2015-103333. Epub October 24, 2016. PMID: 27777269; PMCID: PMC5256399.

282. Probst P, Grummich K, Harnoss JC, et al. Placebo-controlled trials in surgery: a systematic review and meta-analysis. *Medicine (Baltim)*. April 2016;95(17):e3516. https://doi.org/10.1097/MD.0000000000003516. PMID: 27124060; PMCID: PMC4998723.

283. Nelson E, Shadbolt C, Bunzli S, Cochrane A, Choong P, Dowsey M. The effect of animated consent material on participants' willingness to enroll in a placebo-controlled surgical trial: a protocol for a randomised feasibility study. *Pilot Feasibility Stud*. February 8, 2021;7(1):46. https://doi.org/10.1186/s40814-021-00782-7. PMID: 33557951; PMCID: PMC7869245.

284. Miller FG. Sham surgery: an ethical analysis. *Am J Bioeth*. 2003;3(4):41−48. https://doi.org/10.1162/152651603322614580. PMID: 14744332.

285. Cotton P, Pauls Q, Wood A, Durkalski-Mauldin V. Maintaining the blind in sham controlled interventional trials: lessons from the EPISOD study. *Endosc Int Open*. November 2019;7(11):E1322−E1326. https://doi.org/10.1055/a-0900-3789. Epub October 22, 2019. PMID: 31673601; PMCID: PMC6805196.

286. Tenery R, Rakatansky H, Riddick Jr FA, et al. Surgical "placebo" controls. *Ann Surg*. February 2002;235(2):303—307. https://doi.org/10.1097/00000658-200202000-00021. PMID: 11807373; PMCID: PMC1422430.

287. Demange MK, Fregni F. Limits to clinical trials in surgical areas. *Clinics*. 2011;66(1): 159—161. https://doi.org/10.1590/s1807-59322011000100027. PMID: 21437453; PMCID: PMC3044561.

288. Rothwell PM. External validity of randomized controlled trials: "to whom do the results of this trial apply?". *Lancet*. January 1—7, 2005;365(9453):82—93. https://doi.org/10.1016/S0140-6736(04)17670-8. PMID: 15639683.

289. Cochrane AL. Archie cochrane in his own words. Selections arranged from his 1972 introduction to "effectiveness and efficiency: random reflections on the health services" 1972. *Contr Clin Trials*. December 1989;10(4):428—433. https://doi.org/10.1016/0197-2456(89)90008-1. PMID: 2691208.

290. Horton R. Common sense and figures: the rhetoric of validity in medicine (Bradford Hill Memorial Lecture 1999). *Stat Med*. December 15, 2000;19(23):3149—3164. https://doi.org/10.1002/1097-0258(20001215)19:23<3149::aid-sim617>3.0.co;2-e. PMID: 11113950.

291. Ashton CM, Wray NP, Jarman AF, Kolman JM, Wenner DM, Brody BA. Ethics and methods in surgical trials. *J Med Ethics*. September 2009;35(9):579—583. https://doi.org/10.1136/jme.2008.028175. PMID: 19717699; PMCID: PMC2736392.

292. Wenner DM, Brody BA, Jarman AF, Kolman JM, Wray NP, Ashton CM. Do surgical trials meet the scientific standards for clinical trials? *J Am Coll Surg*. November 2012;215(5):722—730. https://doi.org/10.1016/j.jamcollsurg.2012.06.018. Epub July 21, 2012. PMID: 22819638; PMCID: PMC3478478.

293. Barkun JS, Aronson JK, Feldman LS, et al. Evaluation and stages of surgical innovations. *Lancet*. September 26, 2009;374(9695):1089—1096. https://doi.org/10.1016/S0140-6736(09)61083-7. PMID: 19782874.

294. Ergina PL, Cook JA, Blazeby JM, et al. Challenges in evaluating surgical innovation. *Lancet*. September 26, 2009;374(9695):1097—1104. https://doi.org/10.1016/S0140-6736(09)61086-2. PMID: 19782875; PMCID: PMC2855679.

295. McCulloch P, Altman DG, Campbell WB, et al. No surgical innovation without evaluation: the IDEAL recommendations. *Lancet*. September 26, 2009;374(9695): 1105—1112. https://doi.org/10.1016/S0140-6736(09)61116-8. PMID: 19782876.

296. Altman DG. Better reporting of randomised controlled trials: the CONSORT statement. *BMJ*. September 7, 1996;313(7057):570—571. https://doi.org/10.1136/bmj.313.7057.570. PMID: 8806240; PMCID: PMC2352018.

297. Begg C, Cho M, Eastwood S, et al. Improving the quality of reporting of randomized controlled trials. The CONSORT statement. *JAMA*. August 28, 1996;276(8): 637—639. https://doi.org/10.1001/jama.276.8.637. PMID: 8773637.

298. Moher D, Schulz KF, Altman DG. The CONSORT statement: revised recommendations for improving the quality of reports of parallel-group randomised trials. *Lancet*. April 14, 2001;357(9263):1191—1194. PMID: 11323066.

299. Schulz KF, Altman DG, Moher D, for the CONSORT group. CONSORT 2010 statement: updated guidelines for reporting parallel group randomised trials. *BMJ*. 2010; 340:c332. https://doi.org/10.1136/bmj.c332.

300. Moher D, Hopewell S, Schulz KF, for the CONSORT group, et al. CONSORT 2010 explanation and elaboration: updated guidelines for reporting parallel groups randomized trials. *BMJ*. 2010;340:c869. https://doi.org/10.1136/bmj.c869.

301. Huang YQ, Traore K, Ibrahim B, Sewitch MJ, Nguyen LHP. Reporting quality of randomized controlled trials in otolaryngology: review of adherence to the CONSORT statement. *J Otolaryngol Head Neck Surg*. May 15, 2018;47(1):34. https://doi.org/10.1186/s40463-018-0277-8. PMID: 29764496; PMCID: PMC5952888.

302. Prasad A, Shin M, Carey RM, et al. Propensity score matching in otolaryngologic literature: a systematic review and critical appraisal. *PLoS One*. 2020;15(12):e0244423. https://doi.org/10.1371/journal.pone.0244423.

303. Lonjon G, Boutron I, Trinquart L, et al. Comparison of treatment effect estimates from prospective nonrandomized studies with propensity score analysis and randomized controlled trials of surgical procedures. *Ann Surg*. January 2014;259(1):18−25. https://doi.org/10.1097/SLA.0000000000000256. PMID: 24096758.

304. Austin PC. An introduction to propensity score methods for reducing the effects of confounding in observational studies. *Multivariate Behav Res*. May 2011;46(3):399−424. https://doi.org/10.1080/00273171.2011.568786. Epub June 8, 2011. PMID: 21818162; PMCID: PMC3144483.

305. Loss J, Nagel E. Bedeutet Evidenz-basierte Chirurgie eine Abkehr von der ärztlichen Therapiefreiheit? [Does evidence-based surgery harm autonomy in clinical decision making?]. *Zentralbl Chir*. February 2005;130(1):1−6. https://doi.org/10.1055/s-2004-836267. German. PMID: 15717232.

306. Barrett B. Evidence, values, guidelines and rational decision-making. *J Gen Intern Med*. February 2012;27(2):238−240. https://doi.org/10.1007/s11606-011-1903-6. Epub October 5, 2011. PMID: 21971602; PMCID: PMC3270230.

307. Woolf SH, Grol R, Hutchinson A, Eccles M, Grimshaw J. Clinical guidelines: potential benefits, limitations, and harms of clinical guidelines. *BMJ*. February 20, 1999;318(7182):527−530. https://doi.org/10.1136/bmj.318.7182.527. PMID: 10024268; PMCID: PMC1114973.

308. Jevsevar DS, Bozic KJ. Orthopaedic healthcare worldwide: using clinical practice guidelines in clinical decision making. *Clin Orthop Relat Res*. September 2015;473(9):2762−2764. https://doi.org/10.1007/s11999-015-4336-4. Epub May 16, 2015. PMID: 25981712; PMCID: PMC4523514.

309. Timmermans S. From autonomy to accountability: the role of clinical practice guidelines in professional power. *Perspect Biol Med*. 2005;48(4):490−501. https://doi.org/10.1353/pbm.2005.0096. PMID: 16227662.

310. Sun GH. Conflict of interest reporting in otolaryngology clinical practice guidelines. *Otolaryngol Head Neck Surg*. August 2013;149(2):187−191. https://doi.org/10.1177/0194599813490894. Epub May 23, 2013. PMID: 23702973.

311. Horn J, Checketts JX, Jawhar O, Vassar M. Evaluation of industry relationships among authors of otolaryngology clinical practice guidelines. *JAMA Otolaryngol Head Neck Surg*. 2018;144(3):194−201. https://doi.org/10.1001/jamaoto.2017.2741.

312. Tunkel DE. Payments, conflict of interest, and trustworthy otolaryngology clinical practice guidelines. *JAMA Otolaryngol Head Neck Surg*. March 1, 2018;144(3):201−202. https://doi.org/10.1001/jamaoto.2017.2740. PMID: 29270627.

313. Pathak N, Fujiwara RJT, Mehra S. Assessment of nonresearch industry payments to otolaryngologists in 2014 and 2015. *Otolaryngol Head Neck Surg*. June 2018;158(6):1028−1034. https://doi.org/10.1177/0194599818758661. Epub February 13, 2018. PMID: 29437524.

314. Morse E, Berson E, Mehra S. Industry involvement in otolaryngology: updates from the 2017 open payments database. *Otolaryngol Head Neck Surg*. August 2019;161(2):

265–270. https://doi.org/10.1177/0194599819838268. Epub March 26, 2019. PMID: 30909808.

315. Brems JH, Davis AE, Clayton EW. Analysis of conflict of interest policies among organizations producing clinical practice guidelines. *PLoS One.* April 30, 2021;16(4): e0249267. https://doi.org/10.1371/journal.pone.0249267. PMID: 33930893; PMCID: PMC8087455.

316. Denneny 3rd JC, Brereton J, Satterfield L. American academy of otolaryngology-head and neck surgery foundation clinical practice guideline development process. *Otolaryngol Head Neck Surg.* May 2018;158(5):781–782. https://doi.org/10.1177/0194599818765914. Epub March 20, 2018. PMID: 29558242.

317. Taylor C. The use of clinical practice guidelines in determining standard of care. *J Leg Med.* 2014;35(2):273–290. https://doi.org/10.1080/01947648.2014.913460. PMID: 24896315.

318. Prasad V, Cifu A. Medical reversal: why we must raise the bar before adopting new technologies. *Yale J Biol Med.* December 2011;84(4):471–478. PMID: 22180684; PMCID: PMC3238324.

319. Prasad V, Cifu A, Ioannidis JP. Reversals of established medical practices: evidence to abandon ship. *JAMA.* January 4, 2012;307(1):37–38. https://doi.org/10.1001/jama.2011.1960. PMID: 22215160.

320. Ioannidis JP. Why most clinical research is not useful. *PLoS Med.* June 21, 2016;13(6): e1002049. https://doi.org/10.1371/journal.pmed.1002049. PMID: 27328301; PMCID: PMC4915619.

321. Coccheri S. Error, contradiction and reversal in science and medicine. *Eur J Intern Med.* June 2017;41:28–29. https://doi.org/10.1016/j.ejim.2017.03.026. Epub April 11, 2017. PMID: 28408071.

322. Leong SC, Kubba H, White PS. A review of outcomes following inferior turbinate reduction surgery in children for chronic nasal obstruction. *Int J Pediatr Otorhinolaryngol.* January 2010;74(1):1–6. https://doi.org/10.1016/j.ijporl.2009.09.002. Epub October 8, 2009. PMID: 19818515.

323. Komshian SR, Cohen MB, Brook C, Levi JR. Inferior turbinate hypertrophy: a review of the evolution of management in children. *Am J Rhinol Allergy.* March 2019;33(2): 212–219. https://doi.org/10.1177/1945892418815351. Epub December 17, 2018. PMID: 30554518.

324. Bhattacharyya N, Kepnes LJ. Clinical effectiveness of coblation inferior turbinate reduction. *Otolaryngol Head Neck Surg.* October 2003;129(4):365–371. https://doi.org/10.1016/s0194-5998(03)00634-x. PMID: 14574290.

325. Bitar MA, Kanaan AA, Sinno S. Efficacy and safety of inferior turbinates coblation in children. *J Laryngol Otol.* July 2014;128(Suppl 2):S48–S371. https://doi.org/10.1017/S0022215114000206. Epub February 26, 2014. PMID: 24572324.

326. Yuen SN, Leung PP, Funamura J, Kawai K, Roberson DW, Adil EA. Complications of turbinate reduction surgery in combination with tonsillectomy in pediatric patients. *Laryngoscope.* 2017;127:1920–1923. https://doi.org/10.1002/lary.26421.

327. Manzi B, Sykes KJ, Wei JL. Sinonasal quality of life in children after outfracture of inferior turbinates and submucous inferior turbinoplasty for chronic nasal congestion. *JAMA Otolaryngol Head Neck Surg.* May 1, 2017;143(5):452–457. https://doi.org/10.1001/jamaoto.2016.3889. PMID: 28152126; PMCID: PMC5824307.

328. Arganbright JM, Jensen EL, Mattingly J, Gao D, Chan KH. Utility of inferior turbinoplasty for the treatment of nasal obstruction in children: a 10-year review. *JAMA*

Otolaryngol Head Neck Surg. October 2015;141(10):901–904. https://doi.org/10.1001/jamaoto.2015.1560. PMID: 26334516.

329. Ioannidis JP. Why most published research findings are false. *PLoS Med.* August 2005; 2(8):e124. https://doi.org/10.1371/journal.pmed.0020124. Epub August 30, 2005. PMID: 16060722; PMCID: PMC1182327.

330. Ioannidis JP. How to make more published research true. *PLoS Med.* 2014;11(10): e1001747. https://doi.org/10.1371/journal.pmed.1001747.

331. Superchi C, González JA, Solà I, Cobo E, Hren D, Boutron I. Tools used to assess the quality of peer review reports: a methodological systematic review. *BMC Med Res Methodol.* March 6, 2019;19(1):48. https://doi.org/10.1186/s12874-019-0688-x. PMID: 30841850; PMCID: PMC6402095.

332. Rennie D. Let's make peer review scientific. *Nature.* July 7, 2016;535(7610):31–33. https://doi.org/10.1038/535031a. PMID: 27383970.

333. Buckwalter JA, Tolo VT, O'Keefe RJ. How do you know it is true? Integrity in research and publications: AOA critical issues. *J Bone Joint Surg Am.* January 7, 2015;97(1):e2. https://doi.org/10.2106/JBJS.N.00245. PMID: 25568400; PMCID: PMC4279030.

334. Lamb M, Bacon DR, Zeatoun A, et al. Mental health burden of empty nose syndrome compared to chronic rhinosinusitis and chronic rhinitis. *Int Forum Allergy Rhinol.* March 25, 2022. https://doi.org/10.1002/alr.22997. Epub ahead of print. PMID: 35333009.

335. Kanjanawasee D, Campbell RG, Rimmer J, et al. Empty nose syndrome pathophysiology: a systematic review. *Otolaryngol Head Neck Surg.* September 2022;167(3): 434–451. https://doi.org/10.1177/01945998211052919. Epub October 19, 2021. PMID: 34665687.

336. Kim CH, Kim J, Song JA, Choi GS, Kwon JH. The degree of stress in patients with empty nose syndrome, compared with chronic rhinosinusitis and allergic rhinitis. *Ear Nose Throat J.* February 2021;100(2):NP87–NP92. https://doi.org/10.1177/0145561319858912. Epub July 4, 2019. PMID: 31272211.

337. Fu CH, Chen HC, Huang CC, Chang PH, Lee TJ. Serum high-sensitivity C-reactive protein is associated with postoperative psychiatric status in patients with empty nose syndrome. *Diagnostics.* December 18, 2021;11(12):2388. https://doi.org/10.3390/diagnostics11122388. PMID: 34943627; PMCID: PMC8700485.

338. Tian P, Hu J, Ma Y, et al. The clinical effect of psychosomatic interventions on empty nose syndrome secondary to turbinate-sparing techniques: a prospective self-controlled study. *Int Forum Allergy Rhinol.* June 2021;11(6):984–992. https://doi.org/10.1002/alr.22726. Epub November 5, 2020. PMID: 33151634.

339. Maul X, Thamboo A. The clinical effect of psychosomatic interventions on empty nose syndrome secondary to turbinate-sparing techniques: a prospective self-controlled study. *Int Forum Allergy Rhinol.* May 2021;11(5):955–956. https://doi.org/10.1002/alr.22724. Epub November 5, 2020. PMID: 33151623.

340. Huang CC, Wu PW, Lee CC, Chang PH, Huang CC, Lee TJ. Suicidal thoughts in patients with empty nose syndrome. *Laryngoscope Investig Otolaryngol.* January 19, 2022;7(1):22–28. https://doi.org/10.1002/lio2.730. PMID: 35155779; PMCID: PMC8823180.

341. Huang CC, Wu PW, Lee YS, et al. Impact of sleep dysfunction on psychological burden in patients with empty nose syndrome. *Int Forum Allergy Rhinol.* June 5, 2022. https://doi.org/10.1002/alr.23040. Epub ahead of print. PMID: 35665478.

342. Huang CC, Wu PW, Fu CH, Huang CC, Chang PH, Lee TJ. Impact of psychologic burden on surgical outcome in empty nose syndrome. *Laryngoscope*. 2021;131(3): E694—E701.

343. Huang CC, Wu PW, Fu CH, et al. What drives depression in empty nose syndrome? A sinonasal outcome test-25 subdomain analysis. *Rhinology*. December 1, 2019;57(6): 469—476. https://doi.org/10.4193/Rhin19.085. PMID: 31502597.

344. Fu CH, Wu CL, Huang CC, Chang PH, Chen YW, Lee TJ. Nasal nitric oxide in relation to psychiatric status of patients with empty nose syndrome. *Nitric Oxide*. November 1, 2019;92:55—59. https://doi.org/10.1016/j.niox.2019.07.005. Epub 10. PMID: 31408674.

345. Talmadge J, Nayak JV, Yao W, Citardi MJ. Management of postsurgical empty nose syndrome. *Facial Plast Surg Clin N Am*. November 2019;27(4):465—475. https:// doi.org/10.1016/j.fsc.2019.07.005. PMID: 31587766.

346. Lemogne C, Consoli SM, Limosin F, Bonfils P. Treating empty nose syndrome as a somatic symptom disorder. *Gen Hosp Psychiatr*. 2015;37, 273.e9—273.e10.

347. Manji J, Nayak JV, Thamboo A. The functional and psychological burden of empty nose syndrome. *Int Forum Allergy Rhinol*. 2018;8:707—712.

348. Lee TJ, Fu CH, Wu CL, et al. Evaluation of depression and anxiety in empty nose syndrome after surgical treatment. *Laryngoscope*. 2016;126:1284—1289.

349. Mangin D, Bequignon E, Zerah-Lancner F, et al. Investigating hyperventilation syndrome in patients suffering from empty nose syndrome. *Laryngoscope*. 2017;127: 1983—1988. https://doi.org/10.1002/lary.26599. Epub April 13, 2017. PMID: 28407251.

350. Hopkins C, Gillett S, Slack R, Lund VJ, Browne JP. Psychometric validity of the 22-item sinonasal outcome test. *Clin Otolaryngol*. October 2009;34(5):447—454. https:// doi.org/10.1111/j.1749-4486.2009.01995.x. PMID: 19793277.

351. Tranchito E, Chhabra N. Rhinotillexomania manifesting as empty nose syndrome. *Ann Otol Rhinol Laryngol*. January 2020;129(1):87—90. https://doi.org/10.1177/ 0003489419870832. Epub August 16, 2019. PMID: 31416334.

352. Alnæs M, Andreassen BS.. Osteomyelitis after radiofrequency turbinoplasty. *Tidsskr Nor Laegeforen*. May 16, 2019;139(9). https://doi.org/10.4045/tidsskr.18.0843. Norwegian, English. PMID: 31140260. Note: One patient developed "empty nose syndrome".

353. Sozansky J, Houser SM. Pathophysiology of empty nose syndrome. *Laryngoscope*. January 2015;135825(1):70—74. https://doi.org/10.1002/lary.24813. Epub June 30, 2014. PMID: 24978195.

354. Zhao K, Jiang J, Blacker K, Lyman B, Dalton P. Regional peak mucosal cooling predicts the perception of nasal patency. *Laryngoscope*. 2014;124:589—595. https:// doi.org/10.1002/lary.24265. Epub June 28, 2013. PMID:23775640; PMCID: PMC3841240.

355. Konstantinidis I, Tsakiropoulou E, Chatziavramidis A, Ikonomidis C, Markou K. Intranasal trigeminal function in patients with empty nose syndrome. *Laryngoscope*. 2017; 127:1263—1267.

356. Schelegl ES, Green JF. An overview of the anatomy and physiology of slow adapting pulmonary stretch receptors. *Respir Physiol*. 2001;125:17—31.

357. Sofroniew MV, Howe CL, Mobley WC. Nerve growth factor signaling, neuroprotection, and neural repair. *Annu Rev Neurosci*. 2001;24:1217—1281.

358. Scheibe M, Schmidt A, Hummel T. Investigation of the topographical differences in somatosensory sensitivity of the human nasal mucosa. *Rhinology*. 2012;50:290—293.

359. Eccles R, Jones AS. The effect of menthol on nasal resistance to air flow. *J Laryngol Otol*. August 1983;97(8):705−709. https://doi.org/10.1017/s002221510009486x. PMID: 6886530.

360. Baraniuk JN, Merck SJ. New concepts of neural regulation in human nasal mucosa. *Acta Clin Croat*. 2009;48:65−73.

361. Malik J, Li C, Maza G, et al. Computational fluid dynamic analysis of aggressive turbinate reductions: is it a culprit of empty nose syndrome? *Int Forum Allergy Rhinol*. 2019;9:891−899.

362. Li C, Farag AA, Leach J, et al. Computational fluid dynamics and trigeminal sensory examinations of empty nose syndrome patients. *Laryngoscope*. 2017;127:E176−E184.

363. Maza G, Li C, Krebs JP, et al. Computational fluid dynamics after endoscopic endonasal skull base surgery—possible empty nose syndrome in the context of middle turbinate resection. *Int Forum Allergy Rhinol*. 2019;9:204−211.

364. Leong SC, Chen XB, Lee HP, Wang DY. A review of the implications of computational fluid dynamic studies on nasal airflow and physiology. *Rhinology*. June 2010;48(2):139−145. https://doi.org/10.4193/Rhin09.133. PMID: 20502749.

365. Wu CL, Fu CH, Lee TJ. Distinct histopathology characteristics in empty nose syndrome. *Laryngoscope*. January 2021;131(1):E14−E18. https://doi.org/10.1002/lary.28586. Epub March 3, 2020. PMID: 32125703.

366. Borchard NA, Dholakia SS, Yan CH, Zarabanda D, Thamboo A, Nayak JV. Use of intranasal submucosal fillers as a transient implant to alter upper airway aerodynamics: implications for the assessment of empty nose syndrome. *Int Forum Allergy Rhinol*. June 2019;9(6):681−687. https://doi.org/10.1002/alr.22299. Epub February 4, 2019. PMID: 30715801.

367. Thamboo A, Dholakia SS, Borchard NA, et al. Inferior meatus augmentation procedure (IMAP) to treat empty nose syndrome: a pilot study. *Otolaryngol Head Neck Surg*. March 2020;162(3):382−385. https://doi.org/10.1177/0194599819900263. Epub January 14, 2020. PMID: 31935161.

368. Malik J, Dholakia S, Spector BM, et al. Inferior meatus augmentation procedure (IMAP) normalizes nasal airflow patterns in empty nose syndrome patients via computational fluid dynamics (CFD) modeling. *Int Forum Allergy Rhinol*. May 2021;11(5):902−909. https://doi.org/10.1002/alr.22720. Epub November 29, 2020. PMID: 33249769; PMCID: PMC8062271.

369. Dholakia SS, Yang A, Kim D, et al. Long-term outcomes of inferior meatus augmentation procedure to treat empty nose syndrome. *Laryngoscope*. November 2021;131(11):E2736−E2741. https://doi.org/10.1002/lary.295.

370. Chang CF. Using platelet-rich fibrin scaffolds with diced cartilage graft in the treatment of empty nose syndrome. *Ear Nose Throat J*. September 25, 2021:1455613211045567. doi: 10.1177/01455613211045567. Epub ahead of print. PMID: 34569297.

371. Hassan CH, Malheiro E, Béquignon E, Coste A, Bartier S. Sublabial bioactive glass implantation for the management of primary atrophic rhinitis and empty nose syndrome: operative technique. *Laryngoscope Investig Otolaryngol*. December 8, 2021;7(1):6−11. https://doi.org/10.1002/lio2.713. PMID: 35155777; PMCID: PMC8823167.

372. Chang MT, Bartho M, Kim D, et al. Inferior meatus augmentation procedure (IMAP) for treatment of empty nose syndrome. *Laryngoscope*. June 2022;132(6):1285−1288. https://doi.org/10.1002/lary.30001. Epub January 24, 2022. PMID: 35072280.

373. Hosokawa Y, Miyawaki T, Omura K, et al:Surgical treatment for empty nose syndrome using autologous dermal fat: evaluation of symptomatic improvement. *Throat J*.

September 29, 2022:1455613221130885. https://doi.org/10.1177/01455613221130885. Online ahead of print. PMID: 36174975.

374. Cottle MH. Nasal atrophy, atrophic rhinitis, ozena: medical and surgical treatment: repair of septal perforations. *J Int Coll Surg*. April 1958;29(4):472−484. PMID: 13539430.

375. Gordiienko IM, Gubar OS, Sulik R, Kunakh T, Zlatskiy I, Zlatska A. Empty nose syndrome pathogenesis and cell-based biotechnology products as a new option for treatment. *World J Stem Cell*. September 26, 2021;13(9):1293−1306. https://doi.org/10.4252/wjsc.v13.i9.1293. PMID: 34630863; PMCID: PMC8474723.

376. Smith DH, Daines BS, Cazzaniga J, Bhandarkar ND. Surgical management of inferior turbinate hypertrophy in the era of widespread communicable disease. *Cureus*. January 27, 2023;15(1):e34280. https://doi.org/10.7759/cureus.34280. PMID: 36855496. PMCID: PMC9968500.

Index

Note: Page numbers followed by "f" indicate figures and "t" indicate tables.

A

Adenoidectomy, 169
Adenotonsillectomy, 169
Adipocyte-derived stem cells (ADSCs), 66, 226–227
Aggravated anxiety, 67
Aggressive surgery, 3
Aging, 53
Airflow analysis, 195
Allografts, 66
Alveolar ventilation, 25
American Academy of Pediatrics, 180
American Journal of Rhinology, 173
American Medical Association (AMA), 147
American Rhinologic Society, 1, 20, 185
Antimicrobial proteins, 25–28, 186
Approximate temporary truth, 2, 7, 116, 167
Atrophic rhinitis, 40–54, 71, 181
    primary, 47–49
    secondary, 49
Autism, 180
Autoimmune diseases, 50–51
Autologous dermal fat (ADF), 211
Autologous stromal vascular fraction (SVF), 65
Autonomic nervous system, 28

B

Beck Anxiety Inventory (BAI), 187, 190
Beck Depression Inventory, updated version, (BDI-II), 187
Belmont report, 138–139
Beta-tricalcium phosphate, 66
Bextra, 179
Bias, 4, 177
Bilateral concha bullosa, 113, 113f
Biopsy, 80t, 95–96
B lymphocytes, 28
Breathing (respiration), 185
    tests, 189
Breathlessness, 33
British Medical Association, 69–70
British Medical Journal, 97, 155
Bronchospasm, 59

C

The Canadian Medical Association Journal, 97–98
Canadian Task Force on the Periodic Health Examination, 98, 98t
Carbon dioxide exchange, 25
Celebrex, 179
Centers for Disease Control and Prevention, 180
CFD. *See* Computational fluid dynamics (CFD)
Chronic rhinosinusitis (CRS), 112, 195
Churg-Strauss syndrome, 50–51
Clinical judgment, 144
Clinical practice guidelines (CPGs), 4, 158–165, 183
    abstract, 161–165
    defined, 160
    key points, 161
    nonobedience, 160
Clinical reasoning, 104
Clinical surgical care, 147
Clustered regularly interspaced short palindromic repeats (CRISPR), 7
Coblation-assisted turbinoplasty (CAT), 125–126
Cochrane Methodology Register, 176–177
Cognitive function, 195
Cold-knife techniques, 200
Computational fluid dynamics (CFD), 25, 190, 192
Computational models, 59
Computerized tomography (CT), 8, 8f, 10f, 188–189, 192
    cavernous expansion, of intranasal airway, 33, 34f
    inferior turbinates, 33, 34f–35f, 40f–41f
        reduction of, 38f
    maxillary sinus, 33, 39f
    middle turbinates, 33, 35f–38f, 40f–41f, 107–108, 108f–109f
        after septectomy and subtotal resection, 110f
        atrophic change of, 38f
        bilateral concha bullosa, 113, 113f, 116f
        frontal sinusitis, 111f
    nasal septal deformity, 33, 37f
    rhinoplasty, 33, 42f–44f
    turbinate tissue, 58
Concha bullosa, 87
Conflict of interest (COI), 4, 162, 183
Confounding variable, 158

Conservative turbinoplasty, 6
Consolidated Standards of Reporting Trials
(CONSORT) statement, 4, 6, 155–157,
183, 212–213, 223
Copernicus, 179
Cotton test, 55, 189, 236–237
CPGs. *See* Clinical practice guidelines (CPGs)
Crime and Punishment, 7
Cryosurgery, 86
Cryotherapy, 123
Cyclooxygenase-2 (COX-2), 179
Cytokines, 28, 66, 186

D

David Kennedy, MD, 173
David Sackett, M.D ("father" of evidence-based
medicine, EBM), 3, 97–106, 212
Declaration of Helsinki, 138, 147–148
Defensins, 25–28, 185
Depression, 237–238
Desiderio Passali, MD, 6, 121–122, 128–129,
131, 135, 137, 140, 183, 199–200, 203,
211, 216–219, 225–226, 228–229
Diffusor function, 76, 185
Disease tolerance, 61
Dorsal preservation, 233–234
D-panthenol, 203–204
Duncavage technique, 112
Dyspnea (breathlessness), 181

E

EBM. *See* Evidence-based medicine (EBM)
Editors, 175
Efficacy trials, 208
Egbert Huizing, MD, 7, 29, 49, 75–77, 118, 128,
130, 138, 215, 218
Electrocautery, 86, 122, 127
Empiricism, 140–142, 224–225
Empty nose syndrome (ENS), 8f, 40–54, 181,
227–231
computerized tomography (CT), 8, 8f
definition of, 33, 219
diagnosis/diagnostics of, 39, 54–56,
220
emotional torment, 181
etiology of, 193–194
exists, 185
features of, 1
free online encyclopedia, 9, 9f
iatrogenic condition, 33
imaging, 189, 220

incidence of, 1
management, 221
medical treatments, 63–65, 200–204, 221, 230
D-panthenol, 203–204
emotional support, 203
hypertonic saline, 201–202
nasal irrigations, 64
nasal mucosal moistening agents, 64, 64t
pain management, 201
premarin nasal sprays, 204
rhinitis medicamentosa, 202–203
saline irrigations, 64
Wilson's solution, 202
mental health, 220–221
mucopurulent postnasal discharge, 39, 47f
nasal endoscopy, 189
pathophysiology of, 57–58, 194–199, 221
airflow analysis, 195
anatomic features, 195
cognitive function, 195
computational models, 59
computerized tomography (CT), 58
demographics, 195
diagnostic testing, 195
mental health, 195
mucociliary apparatus, 61
mucosal physiology/innate immunity,
196
nerve growth factor (NGF), 198
olfactory function, 195
phantom limb pain, 58
physiologic and pathologic conditions,
59
suffocation, 59
symptomatology, 195
wide open airway, 196–197
pertinent nasal physiology, 185–186
phantom limb pain, 58
physical examination, 220
physiopathology of, 192
preliminary treatment, 182
prevention, 3, 67–68, 199–200
inferior turbinate(s), 200
middle turbinate(s), 200
PubMed database, 9, 11t–19t
regarding children, 218–219
replacement, of medical practice, 213–214
reversal, of medical practice, 213–214
Sino-Nasal Outcome Test 20-25 (SNOT20-25)
for, 234–235, 235t
stem cell-based technology, 226–227

surgical treatment, 65–67, 204–211, 222, 230
surgical trials for, 222–226
symptoms of, 39, 45t, 55, 186–188, 219–220
  diagnostic investigations for, 187
  history and, 188
  indicators, 186
  suicidal ideation (thoughts), 187
testing in, 189–193
  breathing tests, 189
  computational fluid dynamics (CFD), 190
  cotton test, 189
  menthol test, 189
  nasal nitric oxide test levels, 189
  olfactory test, 189
  psychological testing, 190
  tissue biopsy, 190–193
validated diagnostic instruments, 220
Empty Nose Syndrome 6 Questionnaire (ENS6Q)
    questionnaire, 55, 188, 191, 200
ENS. *See* Empty nose syndrome (ENS)
ENS web sites (multiple languages), 1, 20
Environmental irritants, 93
Eosinophilic granulomatosis with polyangiitis
    (formerly Churg- Strauss syndrome),
    50–51, 52t
Epithelial mucosal destruction, 118
  cryotherapy, 123
  electrocautery, 122
  lasers, 122
  treatment groups, 121
Epithelial mucosal preservation, 118, 123–127
  coblation, 125–126
  conchal bone reduction only, 124
  electrocautery, 127
  microdebrider, 124–125
  radiofrequency turbinoplasty, 125
  soft tissue and conchal bone reduction, 124
  submucosal soft tissue reduction only, 123–124
  ultrasound, 126–127
Ethmoid sinus, 33, 37f
Evidence-based medicine (EBM), 97, 117–118,
    135–136, 182–183, 212
  clinical reasoning, 104
  Cochrane Collaboration, 103
  criticism, 104
  defined, 97
  empiricism, 141
  expert opinion, 97
  grading system, 100, 101t
  levels of evidence (LOEs), 98, 98t–99t
    for prognostic studies, 99t
    for therapeutic studies, 100t

randomized controlled trials (RCTs), 98
  rationalism, 141
  scientific evidence, 97
External validity, 152

F
Facebook, 9
Ferris Smith forceps, 113, 115f
Food and Drug Administration (FDA), 153
Functional magnetic resonance imaging (fMRI),
    195
Functional residual capacity of the nose (FRCn),
    85–86, 193

G
Generalized Anxiety Disorder (GAD 7), 187, 190,
    204
Genetic engineering, 7
Gentamycin, 201
Geriatric rhinitis, 53
Granulomatosis with polyangiitis (formerly
    Wegener's granulomatosis), 50–51, 52t
Granulomatous disorders, 49–50
Guideline development groups (GDGs), 160–161

H
Hamilton Anxiety Scale, 190
Hamilton Depression Scale, 190
Heinz Stammberger, MD, 107
High sensitivity C-reactive protein (hsCRP),
    11t–19t
Human beta-defensin 1 (hBD-1), 186
Hyaluronic acid (HA), 65
Hydroxyapatite, 66
Hyperplasia (increase in cell number), 94–95
Hypertonic saline irrigations (home recipes), 64,
    201–202, 221
Hypertrophy (increase in cell size), 3, 49, 69–70,
    94–95, 117, 138–139

I
Iatrogenic wonderland, 56
Idiopathic midline granuloma, 49–50
Immunoglobulins (IgA), 186
Immunoglobulins (IgG), 186
Induced pluripotent stem cells (iPS cells), 227,
    228f
Inferior meatus augmentation procedure (IMAP),
    206
Inferior turbinates, 33, 34f–35f, 40f–41f, 200
  anatomy of, 88–92
    anterior mask rhinomanometry, 93f–94f

Inferior turbinates (*Continued*)
  in females, 88
  intranasal mucosal biopsy, 88, 88f
  in males, 88
  nasal cycle, 89, 91f–92f
  nasal mucus membrane, 89f
  nasal respiratory cilia, 90f
  nasal venous sinuses, 91
  subepithelial layer, 89
  venous capacitance vessels, 90
enlargement, 117, 215–217
  clinical practice guidelines (CPGs), 158–165
  CONSORT requirements, 155–157
  empiricism *vs.* rationalism, 140–142
  evidence-based proposals, 215–217
  obligations and accountability, 154
  placebo effects, 145–146
  practice replacement, 165–168
  propensity score matching (PSM), 157–158
  randomized controlled trials (RCTs), 136–137
  reversal, 165–168
  "sham" surgery, 149–151
  surgical innovations, 154
epithelial mucosal destruction, 118
  cryotherapy, 123
  electrocautery, 122
  lasers, 122
  treatment groups, 121
epithelial mucosal preservation, 118, 123–127
  coblation, 125–126
  conchal bone reduction only, 124
  electrocautery, 127
  microdebrider, 124–125
  radiofrequency turbinoplasty, 125
  soft tissue and conchal bone reduction, 124
  submucosal soft tissue reduction only, 123–124
  ultrasound, 126–127
epithelium, 119
external surgical resection, 120
histopathology, 131–134
management, 228–230
out-fracture (lateralization) techniques, 127–131
reduction, 38f, 117–134, 119t, 169
  adults, 169
  children, 169
  conservative inferior turbinoplasty approach, 170–172
  outcomes for, 172t
  radiofrequency volumetric tissue reduction (RVTR), 170
  study characteristics, 171t
  symptom grading tools, 170–172

submucosa, 119
surgical and nonsurgical procedures, 117–134, 119t
treatment, 118
turbinoplasty, 120
Inflammatory response, 25–28
Institute of Medicine (IOM), 160
Interleukins (Ils), 28
Internally validity, 152
Internal nasal valve, 21–29, 22f, 24f
International Journal of Pediatric Otorhinolaryngology, 169
International Peer Review Congress, 5–6
Intranasal atrophy, 39, 45f, 48f
  diagnostic workup for, 51
Intranasal biopsy, 60
Intranasal crusting, 39, 46f
Intranasal trigeminal functional testing, 192
Intraturbinal turbinoplasty, 76

J

The Journal of General Internal Medicine, 159
Journal of Medical Ethics, 143–144
Journals, 175. *See also* Medical journals

K

Klebsiella pneumoniae ozaenae, 25–28, 43, 47–49, 181
Klebsiella pneumoniae rhinoscleromatis, 43

L

Lactoferrin (Lf), 186
The Lancet, 25, 69–70
The Laryngoscope, 7
Laser surgery, 86
Legal Aid Board, 180
Leprosy, 49–50
Lethal midline granuloma, 49–50
Levels of evidence (LOEs), 98, 98t–99t
  clinical question, 102–103
  for prognostic studies, 99t
  for therapeutic studies, 100t
The Logic of Scientific Discovery, 2, 167
Lung hyperventilation, 25
Lymphoma, 49–50
Lysozyme (Ly), 186

M

Malodor control agents, 63
Maurice Cottle, MD ("father" of modern rhinology), 85, 187, 222–223

Maxillary sinus, 33, 37f, 39f
Mayo Clinic, 1, 8f, 10f, 21—24, 33, 34f—41f,
      44f—46f, 48f, 53—54, 108f—111f, 110,
      128, 201—202
Measles, mumps, and rubella (MMR) vaccine, 180
Medical journals, 5
   editors, 175
   funding mechanisms, 175
   peer review, 176—177
   piercing perspicacious questions, 176
   problems in, 177
   responsibilities, 176
   tools, 177
Medical treatments, 63—65
   nasal irrigations, 64
   nasal mucosal moistening agents, 64, 64t
   saline irrigations, 64
Medpor, 66
Mental health, 195, 220—221
Menthol test, 189
Mesenchymal stem cells (MSCs), 227
Metaplasia, 94—95
Microdebrider-assisted turbinoplasty (MAT),
      124—125
Middle turbinates, 33, 35f—38f, 40f—41f, 200
   anatomy of, 87—88
      classification, 88
      concha bullosa, 87
      osseous skeleton, 87
   atrophic change of, 38f
   enlargement, 214
   management of, 107—116, 114f
      airway obstruction, 113
      bone scissor cut, 114f
      chronic rhinosinusitis (CRS), 112
      collapse of, 115f
      computerized tomography (CT), 107—108,
         108f—109f
      Duncavage technique, 112
      Ferris Smith forceps, 113, 115f
      inflammatory process, 112
      olfactory cribriform region, 107
      outcomes, 110
      preservation, 107
      retrospective analysis, 112
      secondary frontal sinusitis, 110, 111f
Minnesota Multiphasic Personality Inventory
      (MMPI), 53—54, 190, 201
Moisturizing agents, 63
Monika Stenkvist, MD, 33
Mucociliary apparatus, 61
Mucopurulent postnasal discharge, 39, 47f

Mucosal physiology/innate immunity, 196
Mycobacterial tuberculosis, 49—50

N
Nasal aerodynamics, 59
Nasal airway obstruction, 39
Nasal airway resistance, 25
Nasal anatomy, 185
Nasal atrophy, differential diagnosis of, 49—54, 52t
Nasal breathing, 2—3, 24
Nasal crime, 3, 7, 29, 218
Nasal cripple, 1, 20
Nasal cycle, 89, 91f—92f, 93
Nasal dryness, 53, 53t
   symptoms of, 58
Nasal endoscopy, 189
Nasal epithelium, 132
Nasal irrigations, 64
Nasal mucosa, 2, 25—28, 60f, 132, 186
Nasal mucosal moistening agents, 64, 64t
Nasal nitric oxide test levels, 189
Nasal obstruction, 66
Nasal Obstruction Symptom Evaluation (NOSE),
      235—236
Nasal physiology, 21—29
Nasal resistance, 25, 193
Nasal respiratory cilia, 90f
Nasal septal deformity, 33, 37f
Nasopulmonary reflex, 59
National Institute of Health (NIH), 183—184
Nebulizer (spray) method, 64
Neglect external validity, 152
Neil Med sinus rinse, 202
Nerve growth factor (NGF), 58—59, 198
Neural-crest derived stem cells (NCSCs), 227
Non-surgical turbinate reduction adjunctive pro-
      cedures (n-sTRAPs), 2, 33, 40—43,
      53—54, 189, 194

O
Olfaction, 21—29, 185
   function, 195
   test, 189
Open Payments Database (OPD), 164
Osseous skeleton, 87
Out-fracture (lateralization) techniques, 127—131
   combined with other procedures, 128—131
   solitary-isolated and sole intervention, 128
Oxford Centre for Evidence-Based Medicine, 103
Oxygen exchange, 25
Ozena, 47—49, 81. *See also* Primary atrophic
      rhinitis

P

Pain management, 179
Paradoxical nasal obstruction, 25, 181, 219
Paradoxical obstruction, 33
Partial turbinectomy, 86–87
Patient Health Questionnaire (PHQ-9), 187, 190, 204
   depression, 237–238
Pediatric surgery, 6
Peer Review Congress, 5–6, 177
Peer reviewers, 5, 175–176
   comprehension, 177
   tools, 176–177
Peptides, 25–28
Pertinent nasal physiology, 185–186
Phantom limb pain, 58
Physiologic disease entity, 55
Placebo effects
   ethics of using
      medicine, 147
      surgery, 147–148
   in research and practice outcomes, 145–146
Plagiarism, 6, 175–180
Plastipore, 66
Polymorphic reticulosis, 49–50
Postnasal surgery dysfunction community, 1
Primary atrophic rhinitis, 43, 47–49, 81
   incidence, 47–49
   symptoms, 47–49
Propensity score matching (PSM), 4, 157–158, 183
Pseudodoxia Epidemica, 104–105
PSM. *See* Propensity score matching (PSM)
Psychological testing, 190
Psychosocial distress, 61
Ptolemy's work, 179
PubMed database, 1, 11t–19t, 185, 205
Pulmonary function, 193

R

Radical inferior turbinectomy, 219
Radical turbinate resection, 193–194
Radiofrequency turbinoplasty, 125
Radiofrequency volumetric tissue reduction (RVTR), 170
Randomized controlled trials (RCTs), 2, 4, 136–137, 182–184, 213, 230
   absolute criteria, 143
   bias elimination, 6

"care research" trial, 145
   clinical judgment, 144
   CONSORT, 156
   empiricism, 141
   evidence-based medicine (EBM), 98
   evidence first, 144–145
   levels of evidence (LOEs), 100
   limitations, 151–153
      external validity, 152
      generalizability, 152
      internally validity, 152
      neglect external validity, 152
   not needed, 139–140
   peer review process, 177
   placebo control, 6
   propensity score matching (PSM), 158
   randomization in surgical practice, 142
   rationalism, 141
   relative criteria, 143
   reversal, 4–5
   surgical and invasive procedures, 153–154
Rationalism, 140–142, 224–225
RCTs. *See* Randomized controlled trials (RCTs)
Realistic management, 63
Replacement/reversal, of medical practice, 213–214
Research surgical trials, 147
   "sham" surgery, 149–151
Resistor function, 76, 185
Respiration, 25
Rhinitis medicamentosa, 93
Rhinoplasty, 233–234
Rhinoscleroma, 43
Rhinotillexomania, 194
Risk of Bias tool, 177

S

Saline irrigations, 64
Sarcoidosis, 49–50
Secondary atrophic rhinitis, 2, 40–43, 49, 71, 80–81
   aging, 53
   nonsurgical turbinate reduction procedures, 50t
   surgical turbinate reduction procedures, 50t
   treatment modalities, 49, 51t
Secondary frontal sinusitis, 110, 111f
Secretory IgA, 121–122, 139, 216
Secretory phospholipase A2, 25–28
Self-rated questionnaires, 190
Senile rhinitis, 53
"Sham" surgery, 149–151
   clinical research, 150

medical care, 150
proved, 149
Silent sinus syndrome, 130–131
Sino-Nasal Outcome Test-22 (SNOT-22), 195, 198
Sino-Nasal Outcome Test 20-25 (SNOT20-25), 234–235
Sir Karl Raimund Popper, 2, 7, 167, 184, 231
Sjogren's syndrome, 50–51
Somatic symptom disorder (SSD), 201
Squamous metaplasia, 47–49, 94–95
    mucociliary apparatus, 61
Statherin, 25–28
Stem cell-based technology, 226–227
Steven Houser, MD, 43, 66, 121–122, 193, 196–197, 207, 214, 219
Submucosal (lamina propria, stroma) tissue, 25–28, 33, 47–49, 54–55, 87, 88f–89f, 90, 118–120, 133, 181, 186, 199, 217, 229–230
Submucosal turbinoplasty, 189
Suffocation, 59
Suicide, 1, 187
Surgical clinical care, 183–184
Surgical research trials, 183–184
Surgical treatments, 65–67
Syphilis, 49–50

T

Therapeutic turbinate trauma (TTT), 181–182, 194, 204–206
The Three Musketeers, 178
Tissue biopsy, 190–193
T lymphocytes, 28
Tonsillectomy, 169
Total inferior turbinectomy, 3, 7, 39, 46f, 69–70, 80, 86–87
Transient receptor potentials melastatin 8 (TRPM8), 186, 191, 196–197, 207
Treponema pallidum, 49–50
Turbinates
    anatomy, 87–92
        inferior turbinate, 88–92
        middle turbinate, 87–88
    biopsy, 80t, 95–96
    diagnostic assessment tests, 80t, 95–96
    diffusor function, 76
    enlargement, 70
    inferior turbinate, 117–134
        classification, 117

reduction, 117–134
    injections, 86
    middle turbinate, 107–116, 114f
        airway obstruction, 113
        bone scissor cut, 114f
        chronic rhinosinusitis (CRS), 112
        collapse of, 115f
        computerized tomography (CT), 107–108, 108f–109f
        Duncavage technique, 112
        Ferris Smith forceps, 113, 115f
        inflammatory process, 112
        olfactory cribriform region, 107
        outcomes, 110
        preservation, 107
        retrospective analysis, 112
        secondary frontal sinusitis, 110, 111f
    out-fracture (lateralization), 86
    physical examination, 93–95
    resistor function, 76
Turbinate swelling, 93
Turbinate trauma, 20–21
Turbinectomy, 136, 193
    defined, 121
Turbinoplasty, 86–87, 120
    coblation-assisted turbinoplasty (CAT), 125–126
    microdebrider-assisted turbinoplasty (MAT), 124–125
    radiofrequency, 125
Turbulent air flow, 25

U

Ultrasound, 126–127
    turbinoplasty, 120, 216–217
Upper lateral cartilage (ULC), 24f

V

Vagus nerve, 59
Vioxx, 179
Visual analog scale (VAS), 86, 122–123, 127, 129, 139

W

Walter Messerklinger, MD, 107
Wikipedia, 9, 9f, 176
William M. Jarvis, MD, 69

Y

YouTube, 9